**WORLD HEALTH ORGANIZATION**
**INTERNATIONAL AGENCY FOR RESEARCH ON CANCER**

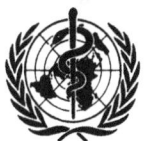

# *IARC Monographs on the Evaluation of Carcinogenic Risks to Humans*

## VOLUME 85
## Betel-quid and Areca-nut Chewing and Some Areca-nut-derived Nitrosamines

This publication represents the views and expert opinions
of an IARC Working Group on the
Evaluation of Carcinogenic Risks to Humans,
which met in Lyon,

11–18 June 2003

2004

# IARC MONOGRAPHS

In 1969, the International Agency for Research on Cancer (IARC) initiated a programme on the evaluation of the carcinogenic risk of chemicals to humans involving the production of critically evaluated monographs on individual chemicals. The programme was subsequently expanded to include evaluations of carcinogenic risks associated with exposures to complex mixtures, life-style factors and biological and physical agents, as well as those in specific occupations.

The objective of the programme is to elaborate and publish in the form of monographs critical reviews of data on carcinogenicity for agents to which humans are known to be exposed and on specific exposure situations; to evaluate these data in terms of human risk with the help of international working groups of experts in chemical carcinogenesis and related fields; and to indicate where additional research efforts are needed.

The lists of IARC evaluations are regularly updated and are available on Internet: http://monographs.iarc.fr/

This project was supported by Cooperative Agreement 5 UO1 CA33193 awarded by the United States National Cancer Institute, Department of Health and Human Services. Additional support has been provided since 1993 by the United States National Institute of Environmental Health Sciences.

©International Agency for Research on Cancer, 2004

Distributed by IARC*Press* (Fax: +33 4 72 73 83 02; E-mail: press@iarc.fr)
and by the World Health Organization Marketing and Dissemination, 1211 Geneva 27
(Fax: +41 22 791 4857; E-mail: publications@who.int)

Publications of the World Health Organization enjoy copyright protection in accordance with the provisions of Protocol 2 of the Universal Copyright Convention.

All rights reserved. Application for rights of reproduction or translation, in part or *in toto*, should be made to the International Agency for Research on Cancer.

**IARC Library Cataloguing in Publication Data**

Betel-quid and areca-nut chewing and some areca-nut-derived nitrosamines /
IARC Working Group on the Evaluation of Carcinogenic Risks to Humans
(2003 : Lyon, France)

(IARC monographs on the evaluation of carcinogenic risks to humans ; v. 85)

1. Areca – adverse effects   2. Carcinogens   3. Esophageal neoplasms   4. Mouth neoplasms   5. Neoplasms   6. Nitrosamines – toxicity   7. Pharyngeal neoplasms   8. Tobacco, smokeless   I. IARC Working Group on the Evaluation of Carcinogenic Risks to Humans   II. Series

ISBN 92 832 1285 1                                     (NLM Classification: W1)
ISSN 1017-1606

PRINTED IN FRANCE

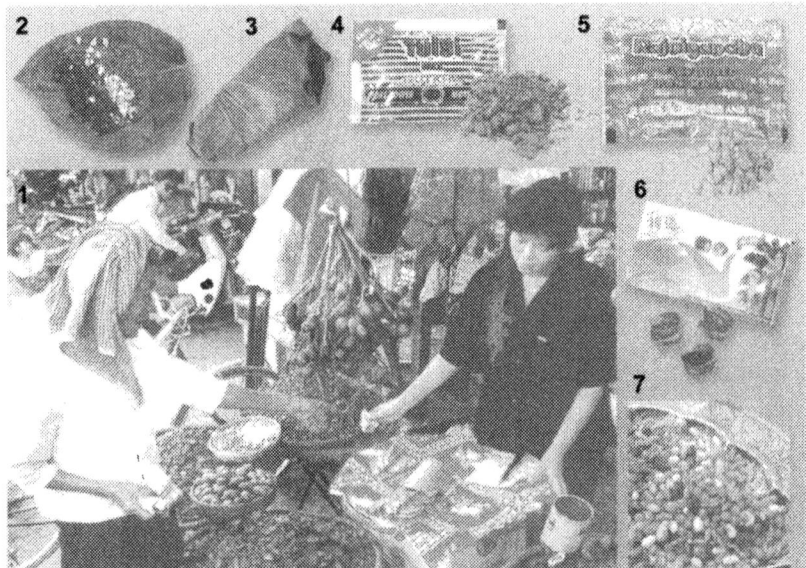

1     Betel quid stand at a Phnom Penh local market (provided by Peter Reichart)
2     Betel quid, unfolded
3     Betel quid, folded
4     *Gutka*, as commercially manufactured and sold in Southeast Asia
5     *Pan masala*, as commercially manufactured and sold in Southeast Asia
6     *Lao-hwa* areca nuts, as sold in Taiwan, China (provided by Peter Reichart)
7     *Pan masala*, as served in restaurants after the meal

Cover design by Georges Mollon, IARC

# CONTENTS

NOTE TO THE READER ................................................................................................1

LIST OF PARTICIPANTS .............................................................................................3

PREAMBLE ..................................................................................................................7
   1. Background .........................................................................................................9
   2. Objective and Scope ...........................................................................................9
   3. Selection of Topics for Monographs ................................................................10
   4. Data for Monographs ........................................................................................11
   5. The Working Group ..........................................................................................11
   6. Working Procedures .........................................................................................11
   7. Exposure Data ...................................................................................................12
   8. Studies of Cancer in Humans ...........................................................................14
   9. Studies of Cancer in Experimental Animals .....................................................17
  10. Other Data Relevant to an Evaluation of Carcinogenicity
      and its Mechanisms ..........................................................................................20
  11. Summary of Data Reported .............................................................................22
  12. Evaluation ........................................................................................................23
  13. References .......................................................................................................28

GENERAL REMARKS ...............................................................................................33

THE MONOGRAPHS .................................................................................................37
**Betel-quid and Areca-nut Chewing** .........................................................................39
   1. Exposure Data ...................................................................................................41
      1.1 Composition of betel quid ...........................................................................41
          1.1.1   Betel quid ........................................................................................41
          1.1.2   Areca nut .........................................................................................42
          1.1.3   Betel leaf ........................................................................................50
          1.1.4   Betel inflorescence ........................................................................50
          1.1.5   Slaked lime ....................................................................................50
          1.1.6   Catechu ..........................................................................................51
          1.1.7   Tobacco .........................................................................................51
          1.1.8   Miscellaneous additives and contaminants ..................................51
      1.2 Areca nut-based industrial packaged products ...........................................52
      1.3 Consumption by geographical region .........................................................52

       1.3.1   India .................................................................................................52
              (a) Adults ....................................................................................53
              (b) Children and adolescents ....................................................59
       1.3.2   Pakistan ..........................................................................................61
       1.3.3   Bangladesh .....................................................................................62
       1.3.4   Sri Lanka ........................................................................................62
       1.3.5   Maldives .........................................................................................63
       1.3.6   People's Republic of China ...........................................................63
       1.3.7   Taiwan, China ................................................................................64
       1.3.8   Myanmar .........................................................................................68
       1.3.9   Thailand ..........................................................................................68
       1.3.10 Lao People's Democratic Republic ..............................................69
       1.3.11 Cambodia .......................................................................................69
       1.3.12 Malaysia .........................................................................................69
       1.3.13 Singapore .......................................................................................70
       1.3.14 Indonesia ........................................................................................70
       1.3.15 The Philippines ..............................................................................71
       1.3.16 Papua New Guinea ........................................................................71
       1.3.17 Palau ...............................................................................................72
       1.3.18 Guam ...............................................................................................73
       1.3.19 Others ..............................................................................................73
       1.3.20 Migrant populations .......................................................................74
              (a) South Africa ...........................................................................74
              (b) United Kingdom .....................................................................75
              (c) Others ......................................................................................78
       1.3.21 Placement of the quid in the mouth ..............................................78
  1.4 Regulations and legislation ........................................................................78
      Regulation of import and sale of areca-containing products ..................79
              (a) India ........................................................................................79
              (b) North America .......................................................................79
              (c) European Union .....................................................................79
              (d) Limited bans in other countries .............................................80
2. Studies of Cancer in Humans .................................................................................80
  2.1 Oral cancer .................................................................................................80
       2.1.1   India, Pakistan and Sri Lanka .......................................................80
              (a) Descriptive studies and case series .......................................80
              (b) Cohort studies ........................................................................86
              (c) Case–control studies .............................................................87
              (d) Cross-sectional surveys .......................................................101
              (e) Synergism .............................................................................101
       2.1.2   Taiwan, China ..............................................................................104
              (a) Descriptive study .................................................................104

|  |  | (b) Case–control studies ........................................................105 |
|---|---|---|
|  | 2.1.3 | South-East Asia...........................................................108 |
|  |  | (a) Malaysia................................................................108 |
|  |  | (b) Myanmar ..............................................................110 |
|  |  | (c) Thailand................................................................110 |
|  | 2.1.4 | Papua New Guinea ......................................................111 |
|  | 2.1.5 | Migrant populations ....................................................112 |
|  |  | (a) South Africa .........................................................112 |
|  |  | (b) United Kingdom...................................................112 |
| 2.2 | Some betel quid-associated lesions, and precancerous lesions and conditions ................................................................................113 |
|  | 2.2.1 | Introduction.................................................................113 |
|  | 2.2.2 | Betel quid-associated oral lesions................................113 |
|  | 2.2.3 | Leukoplakia and erythroplakia ....................................113 |
|  |  | (a) India ......................................................................114 |
|  |  | (b) Taiwan, China ......................................................116 |
|  |  | (c) South-East Asia ....................................................123 |
|  |  | (d) Migrants ...............................................................123 |
|  | 2.2.4 | Oral submucous fibrosis ..............................................123 |
|  |  | (a) India and Pakistan ................................................123 |
|  |  | (b) People's Republic of China ..................................127 |
|  |  | (c) Taiwan, China ......................................................128 |
|  |  | (d) South-East Asia ....................................................128 |
|  |  | (e) Migrants ...............................................................128 |
|  | 2.2.5 | Oral lichen planus .......................................................129 |
|  |  | (a) India ......................................................................129 |
|  |  | (b) South-East Asia ....................................................130 |
|  | 2.2.6 | Multiple and mixed lesions..........................................130 |
|  | 2.2.7 | Malignant transformation ............................................131 |
|  |  | (a) India and Pakistan ................................................131 |
|  |  | (b) Taiwan, China ......................................................132 |
|  |  | (c) Migrants ...............................................................132 |
| 2.3 | Other upper aerodigestive cancer ............................................132 |
|  | 2.3.1 | India ............................................................................132 |
|  | 2.3.2 | Taiwan, China .............................................................137 |
| 2.4 | Other cancers...........................................................................137 |
|  | 2.4.1 | Stomach cancer............................................................137 |
|  | 2.4.2 | Lung cancer.................................................................137 |
|  | 2.4.3 | Cervical cancer............................................................139 |
|  | 2.4.4 | Liver cancer ................................................................139 |
|  |  | (a) Taiwan, China ......................................................139 |
|  |  | (b) Thailand ................................................................140 |

3. Studies of Cancer in Experimental Animals...............................................142
   3.1 Oral administration ...........................................................................142
       3.1.1 Mouse ........................................................................................142
       3.1.2 Rat..............................................................................................145
       3.1.3 Hamster .....................................................................................146
   3.2 Skin application................................................................................147
       Mouse .....................................................................................................147
   3.3 Subcutaneous administration ...........................................................147
       3.3.1 Mouse ........................................................................................147
       3.3.2 Rat..............................................................................................148
   3.4 Intraperitoneal administration .........................................................148
       Mouse .....................................................................................................148
   3.5 Administration to the oral mucosa or cheek pouch .........................149
       3.5.1 Rat..............................................................................................149
       3.5.2 Hamster......................................................................................149
       3.5.3 Baboon ......................................................................................154
   3.6 Intravaginal instillation ....................................................................154
       Mouse .....................................................................................................154
   3.7 Administration with known carcinogens or modifiers of cancer risk ..154
       3.7.1 Mouse ........................................................................................154
       3.7.2 Rat .............................................................................................156
       3.7.3 Hamster......................................................................................156
4. Other Data Relevant to an Evaluation of Carcinogenicity
   and its Mechanisms ..................................................................................160
   4.1 Absorption, distribution, metabolism and excretion........................160
       4.1.1 Humans .....................................................................................160
             (a) Constituents of betel quid ................................................160
             (b) Biomarkers of constituents of betel quid.........................162
       4.1.2 Experimental systems ..............................................................166
             (a) Areca nut/arecoline ..........................................................166
             (b) Betel leaf/hydroxychavicol/eugenol ................................168
             (c) Formation of nitrosamines ...............................................169
             (d) Formation of reactive oxygen species from betel-quid
                 ingredients ........................................................................170
             (e) Antioxidant effects...........................................................172
   4.2 Physiological and toxic effects ........................................................173
       4.2.1 Humans......................................................................................173
             (a) Psychopharmacological effects ........................................173
             (b) Effects on oral hard and soft tissues ................................173
             (c) Effects on various physiological systems ........................175
             (d) Other effects.....................................................................180

        4.2.2   Experimental systems .................................................................180
                (a) In-vivo studies ............................................................180
                (b) In-vitro studies ..........................................................186
    4.3 Reproductive and developmental effects ....................................190
        4.3.1   Humans ............................................................................190
        4.3.2   Experimental systems .................................................................191
                (a) *Pan masala*................................................................191
                (b) Areca nut ....................................................................192
                (c) Arecoline ...................................................................192
                (d) Stems of *Piper betle*................................................193
                (e) Nicotine ....................................................................193
    4.4 Genetic and related effects ....................................................194
        4.4.1   Humans ............................................................................194
                (a) Genotoxicity and mutagenicity ............................194
                (b) Genomic instability ..................................................196
                (c) Oncogenes and tumour-suppressor genes ..............196
                (d) Polymorphism in carcinogen-metabolizing enzymes ........203
        4.4.2   Experimental systems .................................................................213
                (a) Genotoxicity and mutagenicity ............................213
                (b) Oncogenes and tumour-suppressor genes ..............226
                (c) Polymorphisms in carcinogen metabolizing genes ...........227
                (d) Markers of tumour promotion ...................................227
                (e) Preventive effects...................................................227
    4.5 Mechanistic considerations ....................................................228
5.  Summary of Data Reported and Evaluation...........................................230
    5.1 Exposure data ..........................................................................230
    5.2 Human carcinogenicity data ....................................................231
    5.3 Animal carcinogenicity data ....................................................232
    5.4 Other relevant data ..................................................................235
    5.5 Evaluation ..............................................................................238
6.  References...........................................................................................239

**Some Areca-nut-derived *N*-Nitrosamines** .......................................................279
1.  Exposure Data......................................................................................281
    1.1 Chemical and physical data ....................................................281
        1.1.1   Synonyms and structural and molecular formulae..................281
        1.1.2   Chemical and physical properties..............................................282
    1.2 Production ..............................................................................282
    1.3 Occurrence ..............................................................................283
    1.4 Analysis..................................................................................284
2.  Studies of Cancer in Humans ..............................................................284

3. Studies of Cancer in Experimental Animals ..................................................284
   3.1 3-Methylnitrosaminopropionaldehyde .................................................284
   3.2 3-Methylnitrosaminopropionitrile .......................................................284
       3.2.1 Oral application ........................................................................284
       3.2.2 Subcutaneous administration ...................................................285
       3.2.3 Administration with known carcinogens or modifiers
             of cancer risk ...........................................................................285
   3.3 *N*-Nitrosoguvacoline ..........................................................................286
       3.3.1 Oral administration ..................................................................286
       3.3.2 Administration with known carcinogens or modifiers
             of cancer risk ...........................................................................286
4. Other Data Relevant to an Evaluation of Carcinogenicity
   and its Mechanisms .......................................................................................287
   4.1 Absorption, distribution, metabolism and excretion ............................287
       4.1.1 Humans .....................................................................................287
       4.1.2 Experimental systems ..............................................................287
   4.2 Toxic effects ........................................................................................287
       4.2.1 Humans .....................................................................................287
       4.2.2 Experimental systems ..............................................................287
   4.3 Reproductive and developmental effects .............................................288
   4.4 Genetic and related effects ...................................................................288
       4.4.1 Humans .....................................................................................288
       4.4.2 Experimental systems ..............................................................288
5. Summary of Data Reported and Evaluation .................................................291
   5.1 Exposure data .......................................................................................291
   5.2 Human carcinogenicity data .................................................................291
   5.3 Animal carcinogenicity data ................................................................291
   5.4 Other relevant data ..............................................................................292
   5.5 Evaluation ............................................................................................292
6. References .....................................................................................................293

GLOSSARY A ......................................................................................................295

GLOSSARY B ......................................................................................................297

CUMULATIVE INDEX TO THE *MONOGRAPHS* SERIES ...............................301

# NOTE TO THE READER

The term 'carcinogenic risk' in the *IARC Monographs* series is taken to mean the probability that exposure to an agent will lead to cancer in humans.

Inclusion of an agent in the *Monographs* does not imply that it is a carcinogen, only that the published data have been examined. Equally, the fact that an agent has not yet been evaluated in a monograph does not mean that it is not carcinogenic.

The evaluations of carcinogenic risk are made by international working groups of independent scientists and are qualitative in nature. No recommendation is given for regulation or legislation.

Anyone who is aware of published data that may alter the evaluation of the carcinogenic risk of an agent to humans is encouraged to make this information available to the Unit of Carcinogen Identification and Evaluation, International Agency for Research on Cancer, 150 cours Albert Thomas, 69372 Lyon Cedex 08, France, in order that the agent may be considered for re-evaluation by a future Working Group.

Although every effort is made to prepare the monographs as accurately as possible, mistakes may occur. Readers are requested to communicate any errors to the Unit of Carcinogen Identification and Evaluation, so that corrections can be reported in future volumes.

# IARC WORKING GROUP ON THE EVALUATION OF CARCINOGENIC RISKS TO HUMANS: BETEL-QUID AND ARECA-NUT CHEWING AND SOME ARECA-NUT-DERIVED NITROSAMINES

Lyon, 11–18 June 2003

## LIST OF PARTICIPANTS

**Members**

Rajani A. Bhisey, Cancer Research Institute, Tata Memorial Centre, Kharghar, Navi Mumbai 410210, India

Barbara J. Boucher, Department of Diabetes and Metabolic Medicine, Alexandra Wing, Royal Hospital London, Whitechapel, London E1 1BB, United Kingdom

Tony Hsiu-Hsi Chen, Institute of Preventive Medicine, College of Public Health, National Taiwan University, Room 207, 2F No. 19, Suchow Road, Taipei, Taiwan 100, Taiwan, China

Vendhan Gajalakshmi, Epidemiological Research Center, 37 Outer Circular Road, Kilpauk Garden Colony, Chennai 600 010, Tamil Nadu, India

Prakash C. Gupta, Tata Institute of Fundamental Research, Homi Bhabha Road, Bombay 400 005, India (*Subgroup Chair: Cancer in Humans*)

Stephen S. Hecht, University of Minnesota Cancer Center, Mayo Mail Code 806, 420 Delaware St, SE, Minneapolis, MN 55455, USA (*Chairman*)

Jiiang-Huei Jeng, Laboratory of Dental Pharmacology and Toxicology, Graduate Institute of Clinical Dental Science, National Taiwan University, No. 1 Chang-Te Street, Taipei, Taiwan, China

Jagadeesan Nair, Division of Toxicology and Cancer Risk Factors C01O, German Cancer Research Centre (DKFZ), Im Neuenheimer Feld 280, 69120 Heidelberg, Germany (*Subgroup Chair: Other Relevant Data*)

Urmila J. Nair, Division of Toxicology and Cancer Risk Factors C01O, German Cancer Research Centre (DKFZ), Im Neuenheimer Feld 280, 69120 Heidelberg, Germany

Ranju Ralhan, Department of Biochemistry, All India Institute of Medical Sciences, Ansari Nagar, New Delhi 110029, India

A. Ramesha Rao, Cancer and Radiation Biology Laboratory, School of Life Sciences, Jawaharlal Nehru University, New Delhi 110067, India

Peter A. Reichart, Charité, Medizinische Fakultät der Humboldt-Universität zu Berlin, Föhret Str 15, 13353 Berlin, Germany

Pieter J. Slootweg, Department of Pathology, H04.312, University Medical Center, Heidelberglaan 100, P.O. Box 85500, 3508 GA Utrecht, The Netherlands (*Subgroup Chair: Cancer in Experimental Animals*)

Ilse Stander[1], previously at Division of Biostatistics, Medical Research Council, P.O. Box 19070, Tygerberg 7505, South Africa

Saman Warnakulasuriya, Guy's, King's and St Thomas' Dental Institute, Caldecot Road, London SE5 9RW, United Kingdom (*Subgroup Chair: Exposure Data*)

Werner van Wyk[2], Centre for Stomatological Research, School of Dentistry, University of Pretoria, Dr Savage Road, P.O. Box 1288, Pretoria 0002, South Africa

Kui-Hua Zhang, Peking University School of Stomatology, Wei Gong Cun, Haidian District, 100081 Beijing, People's Republic of China

**IARC Secretariat**

Robert Baan, Unit of Carcinogen Identification and Evaluation (*Rapporteur, subgroup on other relevant data*)

Vincent Cogliano, Unit of Carcinogen Identification and Evaluation (*Head of Programme*)

Fatiha El Ghissassi, Unit of Carcinogen Identification and Evaluation (*Co-Rapporteur, subgroup on other relevant data*)

Marlin Friesen, Unit of Nutrition and Cancer

Yann Grosse, Unit of Carcinogen Identification and Evaluation (*Rapporteur, subgroup on cancer in experimental animals*)

Mia Hashibe, Unit of Environmental Cancer Epidemiology

Nikolai Napalkov[3]

Linda Northrup (*Editor*)

Hiroshi Ohshima, Unit of Endogenous Cancer Risk Factors

Rengaswamy Sankaranarayanan, Unit of Descriptive Epidemiology

Béatrice Secretan, Unit of Carcinogen Identification and Evaluation (*Rapporteur, subgroup on exposure data*)

Kurt Straif, Unit of Carcinogen Identification and Evaluation (*Responsible Officer; Rapporteur, subgroup on cancer in humans*)

Sean Tavtigian, Unit of Genetic Cancer Susceptibility

Salvatore Vaccarella, Unit of Field and Intervention Studies

*Post-meeting scientific assistance*
Catherine Cohet

---

[1] Unable to attend
[2] Deceased
[3] Present address: Director Emeritus, Petrov Institute of Oncology, Pesochny-2, 197758 St Petersburg, Russia

*Technical assistance*
Sandrine Egraz
Martine Lézère
Jane Mitchell (*Co-Editor*)
Elspeth Perez
Annick Rivoire

# PREAMBLE

# IARC MONOGRAPHS PROGRAMME ON THE EVALUATION OF CARCINOGENIC RISKS TO HUMANS

## PREAMBLE

### 1. BACKGROUND

In 1969, the International Agency for Research on Cancer (IARC) initiated a programme to evaluate the carcinogenic risk of chemicals to humans and to produce monographs on individual chemicals. The *Monographs* programme has since been expanded to include consideration of exposures to complex mixtures of chemicals (which occur, for example, in some occupations and as a result of human habits) and of exposures to other agents, such as radiation and viruses. With Supplement 6 (IARC, 1987a), the title of the series was modified from *IARC Monographs on the Evaluation of the Carcinogenic Risk of Chemicals to Humans* to *IARC Monographs on the Evaluation of Carcinogenic Risks to Humans*, in order to reflect the widened scope of the programme.

The criteria established in 1971 to evaluate carcinogenic risk to humans were adopted by the working groups whose deliberations resulted in the first 16 volumes of the *IARC Monographs* series. Those criteria were subsequently updated by further ad-hoc working groups (IARC, 1977, 1978, 1979, 1982, 1983, 1987b, 1988, 1991a; Vainio *et al.*, 1992).

### 2. OBJECTIVE AND SCOPE

The objective of the programme is to prepare, with the help of international working groups of experts, and to publish in the form of monographs, critical reviews and evaluations of evidence on the carcinogenicity of a wide range of human exposures. The *Monographs* may also indicate where additional research efforts are needed.

The *Monographs* represent the first step in carcinogenic risk assessment, which involves examination of all relevant information in order to assess the strength of the available evidence that certain exposures could alter the incidence of cancer in humans. The second step is quantitative risk estimation. Detailed, quantitative evaluations of epidemiological data may be made in the *Monographs*, but without extrapolation beyond the range of the data available. Quantitative extrapolation from experimental data to the human situation is not undertaken.

The term 'carcinogen' is used in these monographs to denote an exposure that is capable of increasing the incidence of malignant neoplasms; the induction of benign neoplasms may in some circumstances (see p. 19) contribute to the judgement that the exposure is carcinogenic. The terms 'neoplasm' and 'tumour' are used interchangeably.

Some epidemiological and experimental studies indicate that different agents may act at different stages in the carcinogenic process, and several mechanisms may be involved. The aim of the *Monographs* has been, from their inception, to evaluate evidence of carcinogenicity at any stage in the carcinogenesis process, independently of the underlying mechanisms. Information on mechanisms may, however, be used in making the overall evaluation (IARC, 1991a; Vainio *et al.*, 1992; see also pp. 25–27).

The *Monographs* may assist national and international authorities in making risk assessments and in formulating decisions concerning any necessary preventive measures. The evaluations of IARC working groups are scientific, qualitative judgements about the evidence for or against carcinogenicity provided by the available data. These evaluations represent only one part of the body of information on which regulatory measures may be based. Other components of regulatory decisions vary from one situation to another and from country to country, responding to different socioeconomic and national priorities. **Therefore, no recommendation is given with regard to regulation or legislation, which are the responsibility of individual governments and/or other international organizations.**

The *IARC Monographs* are recognized as an authoritative source of information on the carcinogenicity of a wide range of human exposures. A survey of users in 1988 indicated that the *Monographs* are consulted by various agencies in 57 countries. About 2500 copies of each volume are printed, for distribution to governments, regulatory bodies and interested scientists. The Monographs are also available from IARC*Press* in Lyon and via the Marketing and Dissemination (MDI) of the World Health Organization in Geneva.

## 3. SELECTION OF TOPICS FOR MONOGRAPHS

Topics are selected on the basis of two main criteria: (a) there is evidence of human exposure, and (b) there is some evidence or suspicion of carcinogenicity. The term 'agent' is used to include individual chemical compounds, groups of related chemical compounds, physical agents (such as radiation) and biological factors (such as viruses). Exposures to mixtures of agents may occur in occupational exposures and as a result of personal and cultural habits (like smoking and dietary practices). Chemical analogues and compounds with biological or physical characteristics similar to those of suspected carcinogens may also be considered, even in the absence of data on a possible carcinogenic effect in humans or experimental animals.

The scientific literature is surveyed for published data relevant to an assessment of carcinogenicity. The IARC information bulletins on agents being tested for carcinogenicity (IARC, 1973–1996) and directories of on-going research in cancer epidemiology (IARC, 1976–1996) often indicate exposures that may be scheduled for future meetings. Ad-hoc working groups convened by IARC in 1984, 1989, 1991, 1993 and

# PREAMBLE

1998 gave recommendations as to which agents should be evaluated in the IARC Monographs series (IARC, 1984, 1989, 1991b, 1993, 1998a,b).

As significant new data on subjects on which monographs have already been prepared become available, re-evaluations are made at subsequent meetings, and revised monographs are published.

## 4. DATA FOR MONOGRAPHS

The *Monographs* do not necessarily cite all the literature concerning the subject of an evaluation. Only those data considered by the Working Group to be relevant to making the evaluation are included.

With regard to biological and epidemiological data, only reports that have been published or accepted for publication in the openly available scientific literature are reviewed by the working groups. In certain instances, government agency reports that have undergone peer review and are widely available are considered. Exceptions may be made on an ad-hoc basis to include unpublished reports that are in their final form and publicly available, if their inclusion is considered pertinent to making a final evaluation (see pp. 25–27). In the sections on chemical and physical properties, on analysis, on production and use and on occurrence, unpublished sources of information may be used.

## 5. THE WORKING GROUP

Reviews and evaluations are formulated by a working group of experts. The tasks of the group are: (i) to ascertain that all appropriate data have been collected; (ii) to select the data relevant for the evaluation on the basis of scientific merit; (iii) to prepare accurate summaries of the data to enable the reader to follow the reasoning of the Working Group; (iv) to evaluate the results of epidemiological and experimental studies on cancer; (v) to evaluate data relevant to the understanding of mechanism of action; and (vi) to make an overall evaluation of the carcinogenicity of the exposure to humans.

Working Group participants who contributed to the considerations and evaluations within a particular volume are listed, with their addresses, at the beginning of each publication. Each participant who is a member of a working group serves as an individual scientist and not as a representative of any organization, government or industry. In addition, nominees of national and international agencies and industrial associations may be invited as observers.

## 6. WORKING PROCEDURES

Approximately one year in advance of a meeting of a working group, the topics of the monographs are announced and participants are selected by IARC staff in consultation with other experts. Subsequently, relevant biological and epidemiological data are collected by the Carcinogen Identification and Evaluation Unit of IARC from recognized sources of information on carcinogenesis, including data storage and retrieval systems such as MEDLINE and TOXLINE.

For chemicals and some complex mixtures, the major collection of data and the preparation of first drafts of the sections on chemical and physical properties, on analysis, on production and use and on occurrence are carried out under a separate contract funded by the United States National Cancer Institute. Representatives from industrial associations may assist in the preparation of sections on production and use. Information on production and trade is obtained from governmental and trade publications and, in some cases, by direct contact with industries. Separate production data on some agents may not be available because their publication could disclose confidential information. Information on uses may be obtained from published sources but is often complemented by direct contact with manufacturers. Efforts are made to supplement this information with data from other national and international sources.

Six months before the meeting, the material obtained is sent to meeting participants, or is used by IARC staff, to prepare sections for the first drafts of monographs. The first drafts are compiled by IARC staff and sent before the meeting to all participants of the Working Group for review.

The Working Group meets in Lyon for seven to eight days to discuss and finalize the texts of the monographs and to formulate the evaluations. After the meeting, the master copy of each monograph is verified by consulting the original literature, edited and prepared for publication. The aim is to publish monographs within six months of the Working Group meeting.

The available studies are summarized by the Working Group, with particular regard to the qualitative aspects discussed below. In general, numerical findings are indicated as they appear in the original report; units are converted when necessary for easier comparison. The Working Group may conduct additional analyses of the published data and use them in their assessment of the evidence; the results of such supplementary analyses are given in square brackets. When an important aspect of a study, directly impinging on its interpretation, should be brought to the attention of the reader, a comment is given in square brackets.

## 7. EXPOSURE DATA

Sections that indicate the extent of past and present human exposure, the sources of exposure, the people most likely to be exposed and the factors that contribute to the exposure are included at the beginning of each monograph.

Most monographs on individual chemicals, groups of chemicals or complex mixtures include sections on chemical and physical data, on analysis, on production and use and on occurrence. In monographs on, for example, physical agents, occupational exposures and cultural habits, other sections may be included, such as: historical perspectives, description of an industry or habit, chemistry of the complex mixture or taxonomy. Monographs on biological agents have sections on structure and biology, methods of detection, epidemiology of infection and clinical disease other than cancer.

For chemical exposures, the Chemical Abstracts Services Registry Number, the latest Chemical Abstracts primary name and the IUPAC systematic name are recorded; other synonyms are given, but the list is not necessarily comprehensive. For biological agents, taxonomy and structure are described, and the degree of variability is given, when applicable.

Information on chemical and physical properties and, in particular, data relevant to identification, occurrence and biological activity are included. For biological agents, mode of replication, life cycle, target cells, persistence and latency and host response are given. A description of technical products of chemicals includes trade names, relevant specifications and available information on composition and impurities. Some of the trade names given may be those of mixtures in which the agent being evaluated is only one of the ingredients.

The purpose of the section on analysis or detection is to give the reader an overview of current methods, with emphasis on those widely used for regulatory purposes. Methods for monitoring human exposure are also given, when available. No critical evaluation or recommendation of any of the methods is meant or implied. The IARC published a series of volumes, *Environmental Carcinogens: Methods of Analysis and Exposure Measurement* (IARC, 1978–93), that describe validated methods for analysing a wide variety of chemicals and mixtures. For biological agents, methods of detection and exposure assessment are described, including their sensitivity, specificity and reproducibility.

The dates of first synthesis and of first commercial production of a chemical or mixture are provided; for agents which do not occur naturally, this information may allow a reasonable estimate to be made of the date before which no human exposure to the agent could have occurred. The dates of first reported occurrence of an exposure are also provided. In addition, methods of synthesis used in past and present commercial production and different methods of production which may give rise to different impurities are described.

Data on production, international trade and uses are obtained for representative regions, which usually include Europe, Japan and the United States of America. It should not, however, be inferred that those areas or nations are necessarily the sole or major sources or users of the agent. Some identified uses may not be current or major applications, and the coverage is not necessarily comprehensive. In the case of drugs, mention of their therapeutic uses does not necessarily represent current practice, nor does it imply judgement as to their therapeutic efficacy.

Information on the occurrence of an agent or mixture in the environment is obtained from data derived from the monitoring and surveillance of levels in occupational environments, air, water, soil, foods and animal and human tissues. When available, data on the generation, persistence and bioaccumulation of the agent are also included. In the case of mixtures, industries, occupations or processes, information is given about all agents present. For processes, industries and occupations, a historical description is also given, noting variations in chemical composition, physical properties and levels of occupational exposure with time and place. For biological agents, the epidemiology of infection is described.

Statements concerning regulations and guidelines (e.g., pesticide registrations, maximal levels permitted in foods, occupational exposure limits) are included for some countries as indications of potential exposures, but they may not reflect the most recent situation, since such limits are continuously reviewed and modified. The absence of information on regulatory status for a country should not be taken to imply that that country does not have regulations with regard to the exposure. For biological agents, legislation and control, including vaccines and therapy, are described.

## 8. STUDIES OF CANCER IN HUMANS

### (a) Types of studies considered

Three types of epidemiological studies of cancer contribute to the assessment of carcinogenicity in humans — cohort studies, case–control studies and correlation (or ecological) studies. Rarely, results from randomized trials may be available. Case series and case reports of cancer in humans may also be reviewed.

Cohort and case–control studies relate the exposures under study to the occurrence of cancer in individuals and provide an estimate of relative risk (ratio of incidence or mortality in those exposed to incidence or mortality in those not exposed) as the main measure of association.

In correlation studies, the units of investigation are usually whole populations (e.g. in particular geographical areas or at particular times), and cancer frequency is related to a summary measure of the exposure of the population to the agent, mixture or exposure circumstance under study. Because individual exposure is not documented, however, a causal relationship is less easy to infer from correlation studies than from cohort and case–control studies. Case reports generally arise from a suspicion, based on clinical experience, that the concurrence of two events — that is, a particular exposure and occurrence of a cancer — has happened rather more frequently than would be expected by chance. Case reports usually lack complete ascertainment of cases in any population, definition or enumeration of the population at risk and estimation of the expected number of cases in the absence of exposure. The uncertainties surrounding interpretation of case reports and correlation studies make them inadequate, except in rare instances, to form the sole basis for inferring a causal relationship. When taken together with case–control and cohort studies, however, relevant case reports or correlation studies may add materially to the judgement that a causal relationship is present.

Epidemiological studies of benign neoplasms, presumed preneoplastic lesions and other end-points thought to be relevant to cancer are also reviewed by working groups. They may, in some instances, strengthen inferences drawn from studies of cancer itself.

## (b) Quality of studies considered

The Monographs are not intended to summarize all published studies. Those that are judged to be inadequate or irrelevant to the evaluation are generally omitted. They may be mentioned briefly, particularly when the information is considered to be a useful supplement to that in other reports or when they provide the only data available. Their inclusion does not imply acceptance of the adequacy of the study design or of the analysis and interpretation of the results, and limitations are clearly outlined in square brackets at the end of the study description.

It is necessary to take into account the possible roles of bias, confounding and chance in the interpretation of epidemiological studies. By 'bias' is meant the operation of factors in study design or execution that lead erroneously to a stronger or weaker association than in fact exists between disease and an agent, mixture or exposure circumstance. By 'confounding' is meant a situation in which the relationship with disease is made to appear stronger or weaker than it truly is as a result of an association between the apparent causal factor and another factor that is associated with either an increase or decrease in the incidence of the disease. In evaluating the extent to which these factors have been minimized in an individual study, working groups consider a number of aspects of design and analysis as described in the report of the study. Most of these considerations apply equally to case–control, cohort and correlation studies. Lack of clarity of any of these aspects in the reporting of a study can decrease its credibility and the weight given to it in the final evaluation of the exposure.

Firstly, the study population, disease (or diseases) and exposure should have been well defined by the authors. Cases of disease in the study population should have been identified in a way that was independent of the exposure of interest, and exposure should have been assessed in a way that was not related to disease status.

Secondly, the authors should have taken account in the study design and analysis of other variables that can influence the risk of disease and may have been related to the exposure of interest. Potential confounding by such variables should have been dealt with either in the design of the study, such as by matching, or in the analysis, by statistical adjustment. In cohort studies, comparisons with local rates of disease may be more appropriate than those with national rates. Internal comparisons of disease frequency among individuals at different levels of exposure should also have been made in the study.

Thirdly, the authors should have reported the basic data on which the conclusions are founded, even if sophisticated statistical analyses were employed. At the very least, they should have given the numbers of exposed and unexposed cases and controls in a case–control study and the numbers of cases observed and expected in a cohort study. Further tabulations by time since exposure began and other temporal factors are also important. In a cohort study, data on all cancer sites and all causes of death should have been given, to reveal the possibility of reporting bias. In a case–control study, the effects of investigated factors other than the exposure of interest should have been reported.

Finally, the statistical methods used to obtain estimates of relative risk, absolute rates of cancer, confidence intervals and significance tests, and to adjust for confounding should have been clearly stated by the authors. The methods used should preferably have been the generally accepted techniques that have been refined since the mid-1970s. These methods have been reviewed for case–control studies (Breslow & Day, 1980) and for cohort studies (Breslow & Day, 1987).

### (c) Inferences about mechanism of action

Detailed analyses of both relative and absolute risks in relation to temporal variables, such as age at first exposure, time since first exposure, duration of exposure, cumulative exposure and time since exposure ceased, are reviewed and summarized when available. The analysis of temporal relationships can be useful in formulating models of carcinogenesis. In particular, such analyses may suggest whether a carcinogen acts early or late in the process of carcinogenesis, although at best they allow only indirect inferences about the mechanism of action. Special attention is given to measurements of biological markers of carcinogen exposure or action, such as DNA or protein adducts, as well as markers of early steps in the carcinogenic process, such as proto-oncogene mutation, when these are incorporated into epidemiological studies focused on cancer incidence or mortality. Such measurements may allow inferences to be made about putative mechanisms of action (IARC, 1991a; Vainio et al., 1992).

### (d) Criteria for causality

After the individual epidemiological studies of cancer have been summarized and the quality assessed, a judgement is made concerning the strength of evidence that the agent, mixture or exposure circumstance in question is carcinogenic for humans. In making its judgement, the Working Group considers several criteria for causality. A strong association (a large relative risk) is more likely to indicate causality than a weak association, although it is recognized that relative risks of small magnitude do not imply lack of causality and may be important if the disease is common. Associations that are replicated in several studies of the same design or using different epidemiological approaches or under different circumstances of exposure are more likely to represent a causal relationship than isolated observations from single studies. If there are inconsistent results among investigations, possible reasons are sought (such as differences in amount of exposure), and results of studies judged to be of high quality are given more weight than those of studies judged to be methodologically less sound. When suspicion of carcinogenicity arises largely from a single study, these data are not combined with those from later studies in any subsequent reassessment of the strength of the evidence.

If the risk of the disease in question increases with the amount of exposure, this is considered to be a strong indication of causality, although absence of a graded response is not necessarily evidence against a causal relationship. Demonstration of a decline in risk after cessation of or reduction in exposure in individuals or in whole populations also supports a causal interpretation of the findings.

Although a carcinogen may act upon more than one target, the specificity of an association (an increased occurrence of cancer at one anatomical site or of one morphological type) adds plausibility to a causal relationship, particularly when excess cancer occurrence is limited to one morphological type within the same organ.

Although rarely available, results from randomized trials showing different rates among exposed and unexposed individuals provide particularly strong evidence for causality.

When several epidemiological studies show little or no indication of an association between an exposure and cancer, the judgement may be made that, in the aggregate, they show evidence of lack of carcinogenicity. Such a judgement requires first of all that the studies giving rise to it meet, to a sufficient degree, the standards of design and analysis described above. Specifically, the possibility that bias, confounding or misclassification of exposure or outcome could explain the observed results should be considered and excluded with reasonable certainty. In addition, all studies that are judged to be methodologically sound should be consistent with a relative risk of unity for any observed level of exposure and, when considered together, should provide a pooled estimate of relative risk which is at or near unity and has a narrow confidence interval, due to sufficient population size. Moreover, no individual study nor the pooled results of all the studies should show any consistent tendency for the relative risk of cancer to increase with increasing level of exposure. It is important to note that evidence of lack of carcinogenicity obtained in this way from several epidemiological studies can apply only to the type(s) of cancer studied and to dose levels and intervals between first exposure and observation of disease that are the same as or less than those observed in all the studies. Experience with human cancer indicates that, in some cases, the period from first exposure to the development of clinical cancer is seldom less than 20 years; studies with latent periods substantially shorter than 30 years cannot provide evidence for lack of carcinogenicity.

## 9. STUDIES OF CANCER IN EXPERIMENTAL ANIMALS

All known human carcinogens that have been studied adequately in experimental animals have produced positive results in one or more animal species (Wilbourn *et al.*, 1986; Tomatis *et al.*, 1989). For several agents (aflatoxins, 4-aminobiphenyl, azathioprine, betel quid with tobacco, bischloromethyl ether and chloromethyl methyl ether (technical grade), chlorambucil, chlornaphazine, ciclosporin, coal-tar pitches, coal-tars, combined oral contraceptives, cyclophosphamide, diethylstilboestrol, melphalan, 8-methoxypsoralen plus ultraviolet A radiation, mustard gas, myleran, 2-naphthylamine, nonsteroidal estrogens, estrogen replacement therapy/steroidal estrogens, solar radiation, thiotepa and vinyl chloride), carcinogenicity in experimental animals was established or highly suspected before epidemiological studies confirmed their carcinogenicity in humans (Vainio *et al.*, 1995). Although this association cannot establish that all agents and mixtures that cause cancer in experimental animals also cause cancer in humans, nevertheless, **in the absence of adequate data on humans, it is biologically plausible and prudent to regard agents and mixtures for which there is** *sufficient evidence* **(see p. 24) of carcinogenicity in experimental animals as if they presented a carcinogenic risk to humans**. The possibility that a given agent may cause cancer through a species-specific mechanism which does not operate in humans (see p. 27) should also be taken into consideration.

The nature and extent of impurities or contaminants present in the chemical or mixture being evaluated are given when available. Animal strain, sex, numbers per group, age at start of treatment and survival are reported.

Other types of studies summarized include: experiments in which the agent or mixture was administered in conjunction with known carcinogens or factors that modify carcinogenic effects; studies in which the end-point was not cancer but a defined precancerous lesion; and experiments on the carcinogenicity of known metabolites and derivatives.

For experimental studies of mixtures, consideration is given to the possibility of changes in the physicochemical properties of the test substance during collection, storage, extraction, concentration and delivery. Chemical and toxicological interactions of the components of mixtures may result in nonlinear dose–response relationships.

An assessment is made as to the relevance to human exposure of samples tested in experimental animals, which may involve consideration of: (i) physical and chemical characteristics, (ii) constituent substances that indicate the presence of a class of substances, (iii) the results of tests for genetic and related effects, including studies on DNA adduct formation, proto-oncogene mutation and expression and suppressor gene inactivation. The relevance of results obtained, for example, with animal viruses analogous to the virus being evaluated in the monograph must also be considered. They may provide biological and mechanistic information relevant to the understanding of the process of carcinogenesis in humans and may strengthen the plausibility of a conclusion that the biological agent under evaluation is carcinogenic in humans.

(a) *Qualitative aspects*

An assessment of carcinogenicity involves several considerations of qualitative importance, including (i) the experimental conditions under which the test was performed, including route and schedule of exposure, species, strain, sex, age, duration of follow-up; (ii) the consistency of the results, for example, across species and target organ(s); (iii) the spectrum of neoplastic response, from preneoplastic lesions and benign tumours to malignant neoplasms; and (iv) the possible role of modifying factors.

As mentioned earlier (p. 11), the *Monographs* are not intended to summarize all published studies. Those studies in experimental animals that are inadequate (e.g., too short a duration, too few animals, poor survival; see below) or are judged irrelevant to the evaluation are generally omitted. Guidelines for conducting adequate long-term carcinogenicity experiments have been outlined (e.g. Montesano *et al.*, 1986).

Considerations of importance to the Working Group in the interpretation and evaluation of a particular study include: (i) how clearly the agent was defined and, in the case of mixtures, how adequately the sample characterization was reported; (ii) whether the dose was adequately monitored, particularly in inhalation experiments; (iii) whether the doses and duration of treatment were appropriate and whether the survival of treated animals was similar to that of controls; (iv) whether there were adequate numbers of animals per group; (v) whether animals of each sex were used; (vi) whether animals were allocated randomly to groups; (vii) whether the duration of observation was adequate; and (viii) whether the data were adequately reported. If available, recent data on the incidence of specific tumours in historical controls, as well as in concurrent controls, should be taken into account in the evaluation of tumour response.

When benign tumours occur together with and originate from the same cell type in an organ or tissue as malignant tumours in a particular study and appear to represent a stage in the progression to malignancy, it may be valid to combine them in assessing tumour incidence (Huff *et al.*, 1989). The occurrence of lesions presumed to be preneoplastic may in certain instances aid in assessing the biological plausibility of any neoplastic response observed. If an agent or mixture induces only benign neoplasms that appear to be end-points that do not readily progress to malignancy, it should nevertheless be suspected of being a carcinogen and requires further investigation.

### (b) Quantitative aspects

The probability that tumours will occur may depend on the species, sex, strain and age of the animal, the dose of the carcinogen and the route and length of exposure. Evidence of an increased incidence of neoplasms with increased level of exposure strengthens the inference of a causal association between the exposure and the development of neoplasms.

The form of the dose–response relationship can vary widely, depending on the particular agent under study and the target organ. Both DNA damage and increased cell division are important aspects of carcinogenesis, and cell proliferation is a strong determinant of dose–response relationships for some carcinogens (Cohen & Ellwein, 1990). Since many chemicals require metabolic activation before being converted into their reactive intermediates, both metabolic and pharmacokinetic aspects are important in determining the dose–response pattern. Saturation of steps such as absorption, activation, inactivation and elimination may produce nonlinearity in the dose–response relationship, as could saturation of processes such as DNA repair (Hoel *et al.*, 1983; Gart *et al.*, 1986).

(c) *Statistical analysis of long-term experiments in animals*

Factors considered by the Working Group include the adequacy of the information given for each treatment group: (i) the number of animals studied and the number examined histologically, (ii) the number of animals with a given tumour type and (iii) length of survival. The statistical methods used should be clearly stated and should be the generally accepted techniques refined for this purpose (Peto *et al.*, 1980; Gart *et al.*, 1986). When there is no difference in survival between control and treatment groups, the Working Group usually compares the proportions of animals developing each tumour type in each of the groups. Otherwise, consideration is given as to whether or not appropriate adjustments have been made for differences in survival. These adjustments can include: comparisons of the proportions of tumour-bearing animals among the effective number of animals (alive at the time the first tumour is discovered), in the case where most differences in survival occur before tumours appear; life-table methods, when tumours are visible or when they may be considered 'fatal' because mortality rapidly follows tumour development; and the Mantel-Haenszel test or logistic regression, when occult tumours do not affect the animals' risk of dying but are 'incidental' findings at autopsy.

In practice, classifying tumours as fatal or incidental may be difficult. Several survival-adjusted methods have been developed that do not require this distinction (Gart *et al.*, 1986), although they have not been fully evaluated.

## 10. OTHER DATA RELEVANT TO AN EVALUATION OF CARCINOGENICITY AND ITS MECHANISMS

In coming to an overall evaluation of carcinogenicity in humans (see pp. 25–27), the Working Group also considers related data. The nature of the information selected for the summary depends on the agent being considered.

For chemicals and complex mixtures of chemicals such as those in some occupational situations or involving cultural habits (e.g. tobacco smoking), the other data considered to be relevant are divided into those on absorption, distribution, metabolism and excretion; toxic effects; reproductive and developmental effects; and genetic and related effects.

Concise information is given on absorption, distribution (including placental transfer) and excretion in both humans and experimental animals. Kinetic factors that may affect the dose–response relationship, such as saturation of uptake, protein binding, metabolic activation, detoxification and DNA repair processes, are mentioned. Studies that indicate the metabolic fate of the agent in humans and in experimental animals are summarized briefly, and comparisons of data on humans and on animals are made when possible. Comparative information on the relationship between exposure and the dose that reaches the target site may be of particular importance for extrapolation between species. Data are given on acute and chronic toxic effects (other than cancer), such as organ toxicity, increased cell proliferation, immunotoxicity and endocrine effects. The presence and toxicological significance of cellular receptors is described. Effects on reproduction, teratogenicity, fetotoxicity and embryotoxicity are also summarized briefly.

Tests of genetic and related effects are described in view of the relevance of gene mutation and chromosomal damage to carcinogenesis (Vainio et al., 1992; McGregor et al., 1999). The adequacy of the reporting of sample characterization is considered and, where necessary, commented upon; with regard to complex mixtures, such comments are similar to those described for animal carcinogenicity tests on p. 18. The available data are interpreted critically by phylogenetic group according to the end-points detected, which may include DNA damage, gene mutation, sister chromatid exchange, micronucleus formation, chromosomal aberrations, aneuploidy and cell transformation. The concentrations employed are given, and mention is made of whether use of an exogenous metabolic system *in vitro* affected the test result. These data are given as listings of test systems, data and references. The data on genetic and related effects presented in the *Monographs* are also available in the form of genetic activity profiles (GAP) prepared in collaboration with the United States Environmental Protection Agency (EPA) (see also Waters et al., 1987) using software for personal computers that are Microsoft Windows® compatible. The EPA/IARC GAP software and database may be downloaded free of charge from *www.epa.gov/gapdb*.

Positive results in tests using prokaryotes, lower eukaryotes, plants, insects and cultured mammalian cells suggest that genetic and related effects could occur in mammals. Results from such tests may also give information about the types of genetic effect produced and about the involvement of metabolic activation. Some end-points described are clearly genetic in nature (e.g., gene mutations and chromosomal aberrations), while others are to a greater or lesser degree associated with genetic effects (e.g. unscheduled DNA synthesis). In-vitro tests for tumour-promoting activity and for cell transformation may be sensitive to changes that are not necessarily the result of genetic alterations but that may have specific relevance to the process of carcinogenesis. A critical appraisal of these tests has been published (Montesano et al., 1986).

Genetic or other activity detected in experimental mammals and humans is regarded as being of greater relevance than that in other organisms. The demonstration that an agent or mixture can induce gene and chromosomal mutations in whole mammals indicates that it may have carcinogenic activity, although this activity may not be detectably expressed in any or all species. Relative potency in tests for mutagenicity and related effects is not a reliable indicator of carcinogenic potency. Negative results in tests for mutagenicity in selected tissues from animals treated *in vivo* provide less weight, partly because they do not exclude the possibility of an effect in tissues other than those examined. Moreover, negative results in short-term tests with genetic end-points cannot be considered to provide evidence to rule out carcinogenicity of agents or mixtures that act through other mechanisms (e.g. receptor-mediated effects, cellular toxicity with regenerative proliferation, peroxisome proliferation) (Vainio et al., 1992). Factors that may lead to misleading results in short-term tests have been discussed in detail elsewhere (Montesano et al., 1986).

When available, data relevant to mechanisms of carcinogenesis that do not involve structural changes at the level of the gene are also described.

The adequacy of epidemiological studies of reproductive outcome and genetic and related effects in humans is evaluated by the same criteria as are applied to epidemiological studies of cancer.

Structure–activity relationships that may be relevant to an evaluation of the carcinogenicity of an agent are also described.

For biological agents — viruses, bacteria and parasites — other data relevant to carcinogenicity include descriptions of the pathology of infection, molecular biology (integration and expression of viruses, and any genetic alterations seen in human tumours) and other observations, which might include cellular and tissue responses to infection, immune response and the presence of tumour markers.

## 11. SUMMARY OF DATA REPORTED

In this section, the relevant epidemiological and experimental data are summarized. Only reports, other than in abstract form, that meet the criteria outlined on p. 11 are considered for evaluating carcinogenicity. Inadequate studies are generally not summarized: such studies are usually identified by a square-bracketed comment in the preceding text.

### (a) Exposure

Human exposure to chemicals and complex mixtures is summarized on the basis of elements such as production, use, occurrence in the environment and determinations in human tissues and body fluids. Quantitative data are given when available. Exposure to biological agents is described in terms of transmission and prevalence of infection.

### (b) Carcinogenicity in humans

Results of epidemiological studies that are considered to be pertinent to an assessment of human carcinogenicity are summarized. When relevant, case reports and correlation studies are also summarized.

### (c) Carcinogenicity in experimental animals

Data relevant to an evaluation of carcinogenicity in animals are summarized. For each animal species and route of administration, it is stated whether an increased incidence of neoplasms or preneoplastic lesions was observed, and the tumour sites are indicated. If the agent or mixture produced tumours after prenatal exposure or in single-dose experiments, this is also indicated. Negative findings are also summarized. Dose–response and other quantitative data may be given when available.

*(d)   Other data relevant to an evaluation of carcinogenicity and its mechanisms*

Data on biological effects in humans that are of particular relevance are summarized. These may include toxicological, kinetic and metabolic considerations and evidence of DNA binding, persistence of DNA lesions or genetic damage in exposed humans. Toxicological information, such as that on cytotoxicity and regeneration, receptor binding and hormonal and immunological effects, and data on kinetics and metabolism in experimental animals are given when considered relevant to the possible mechanism of the carcinogenic action of the agent. The results of tests for genetic and related effects are summarized for whole mammals, cultured mammalian cells and nonmammalian systems.

When available, comparisons of such data for humans and for animals, and particularly animals that have developed cancer, are described.

Structure–activity relationships are mentioned when relevant.

For the agent, mixture or exposure circumstance being evaluated, the available data on end-points or other phenomena relevant to mechanisms of carcinogenesis from studies in humans, experimental animals and tissue and cell test systems are summarized within one or more of the following descriptive dimensions:

(i) Evidence of genotoxicity (structural changes at the level of the gene): for example, structure–activity considerations, adduct formation, mutagenicity (effect on specific genes), chromosomal mutation/aneuploidy

(ii) Evidence of effects on the expression of relevant genes (functional changes at the intracellular level): for example, alterations to the structure or quantity of the product of a proto-oncogene or tumour-suppressor gene, alterations to metabolic activation/inactivation/DNA repair

(iii) Evidence of relevant effects on cell behaviour (morphological or behavioural changes at the cellular or tissue level): for example, induction of mitogenesis, compensatory cell proliferation, preoplasia and hyperplasia, survival of premalignant or malignant cells (immortalization, immunosuppression), effects on metastatic potential

(iv) Evidence from dose and time relationships of carcinogenic effects and interactions between agents: for example, early/late stage, as inferred from epidemiological studies; initiation/promotion/progression/malignant conversion, as defined in animal carcinogenicity experiments; toxicokinetics

These dimensions are not mutually exclusive, and an agent may fall within more than one of them. Thus, for example, the action of an agent on the expression of relevant genes could be summarized under both the first and second dimensions, even if it were known with reasonable certainty that those effects resulted from genotoxicity.

## 12.   EVALUATION

Evaluations of the strength of the evidence for carcinogenicity arising from human and experimental animal data are made, using standard terms.

It is recognized that the criteria for these evaluations, described below, cannot encompass all of the factors that may be relevant to an evaluation of carcinogenicity. In considering all of the relevant scientific data, the Working Group may assign the agent, mixture or exposure circumstance to a higher or lower category than a strict interpretation of these criteria would indicate.

(a) *Degrees of evidence for carcinogenicity in humans and in experimental animals and supporting evidence*

These categories refer only to the strength of the evidence that an exposure is carcinogenic and not to the extent of its carcinogenic activity (potency) nor to the mechanisms involved. A classification may change as new information becomes available.

An evaluation of degree of evidence, whether for a single agent or a mixture, is limited to the materials tested, as defined physically, chemically or biologically. When the agents evaluated are considered by the Working Group to be sufficiently closely related, they may be grouped together for the purpose of a single evaluation of degree of evidence.

(i) *Carcinogenicity in humans*

The applicability of an evaluation of the carcinogenicity of a mixture, process, occupation or industry on the basis of evidence from epidemiological studies depends on the variability over time and place of the mixtures, processes, occupations and industries. The Working Group seeks to identify the specific exposure, process or activity which is considered most likely to be responsible for any excess risk. The evaluation is focused as narrowly as the available data on exposure and other aspects permit.

The evidence relevant to carcinogenicity from studies in humans is classified into one of the following categories:

*Sufficient evidence of carcinogenicity*: The Working Group considers that a causal relationship has been established between exposure to the agent, mixture or exposure circumstance and human cancer. That is, a positive relationship has been observed between the exposure and cancer in studies in which chance, bias and confounding could be ruled out with reasonable confidence.

*Limited evidence of carcinogenicity*: A positive association has been observed between exposure to the agent, mixture or exposure circumstance and cancer for which a causal interpretation is considered by the Working Group to be credible, but chance, bias or confounding could not be ruled out with reasonable confidence.

*Inadequate evidence of carcinogenicity*: The available studies are of insufficient quality, consistency or statistical power to permit a conclusion regarding the presence or absence of a causal association between exposure and cancer, or no data on cancer in humans are available.

*Evidence suggesting lack of carcinogenicity*: There are several adequate studies covering the full range of levels of exposure that human beings are known to encounter, which are mutually consistent in not showing a positive association between exposure to the agent, mixture or exposure circumstance and any studied cancer at any observed level of exposure. A conclusion of 'evidence suggesting lack of carcinogenicity' is inevitably limited to the cancer sites, conditions and levels of exposure and length of observation covered by the available studies. In addition, the possibility of a very small risk at the levels of exposure studied can never be excluded.

In some instances, the above categories may be used to classify the degree of evidence related to carcinogenicity in specific organs or tissues.

(ii) *Carcinogenicity in experimental animals*

The evidence relevant to carcinogenicity in experimental animals is classified into one of the following categories:

*Sufficient evidence of carcinogenicity*: The Working Group considers that a causal relationship has been established between the agent or mixture and an increased incidence of malignant neoplasms or of an appropriate combination of benign and malignant neoplasms in (a) two or more species of animals or (b) in two or more independent studies in one species carried out at different times or in different laboratories or under different protocols.

Exceptionally, a single study in one species might be considered to provide sufficient evidence of carcinogenicity when malignant neoplasms occur to an unusual degree with regard to incidence, site, type of tumour or age at onset.

*Limited evidence of carcinogenicity*: The data suggest a carcinogenic effect but are limited for making a definitive evaluation because, e.g. (a) the evidence of carcinogenicity is restricted to a single experiment; or (b) there are unresolved questions regarding the adequacy of the design, conduct or interpretation of the study; or (c) the agent or mixture increases the incidence only of benign neoplasms or lesions of uncertain neoplastic potential, or of certain neoplasms which may occur spontaneously in high incidences in certain strains.

*Inadequate evidence of carcinogenicity*: The studies cannot be interpreted as showing either the presence or absence of a carcinogenic effect because of major qualitative or quantitative limitations, or no data on cancer in experimental animals are available.

*Evidence suggesting lack of carcinogenicity*: Adequate studies involving at least two species are available which show that, within the limits of the tests used, the agent or mixture is not carcinogenic. A conclusion of evidence suggesting lack of carcinogenicity is inevitably limited to the species, tumour sites and levels of exposure studied.

(b) *Other data relevant to the evaluation of carcinogenicity and its mechanisms*

Other evidence judged to be relevant to an evaluation of carcinogenicity and of sufficient importance to affect the overall evaluation is then described. This may include data on preneoplastic lesions, tumour pathology, genetic and related effects, structure–activity relationships, metabolism and pharmacokinetics, physicochemical parameters and analogous biological agents.

Data relevant to mechanisms of the carcinogenic action are also evaluated. The strength of the evidence that any carcinogenic effect observed is due to a particular mechanism is assessed, using terms such as weak, moderate or strong. Then, the Working Group assesses if that particular mechanism is likely to be operative in humans. The strongest indications that a particular mechanism operates in humans come from data on humans or biological specimens obtained from exposed humans. The data may be considered to be especially relevant if they show that the agent in question has caused changes in exposed humans that are on the causal pathway to carcinogenesis. Such data may, however, never become available, because it is at least conceivable that certain compounds may be kept from human use solely on the basis of evidence of their toxicity and/or carcinogenicity in experimental systems.

For complex exposures, including occupational and industrial exposures, the chemical composition and the potential contribution of carcinogens known to be present are considered by the Working Group in its overall evaluation of human carcinogenicity. The Working Group also determines the extent to which the materials tested in experimental systems are related to those to which humans are exposed.

(c) Overall evaluation

Finally, the body of evidence is considered as a whole, in order to reach an overall evaluation of the carcinogenicity to humans of an agent, mixture or circumstance of exposure.

An evaluation may be made for a group of chemical compounds that have been evaluated by the Working Group. In addition, when supporting data indicate that other, related compounds for which there is no direct evidence of capacity to induce cancer in humans or in animals may also be carcinogenic, a statement describing the rationale for this conclusion is added to the evaluation narrative; an additional evaluation may be made for this broader group of compounds if the strength of the evidence warrants it.

The agent, mixture or exposure circumstance is described according to the wording of one of the following categories, and the designated group is given. The categorization of an agent, mixture or exposure circumstance is a matter of scientific judgement, reflecting the strength of the evidence derived from studies in humans and in experimental animals and from other relevant data.

*Group 1 — The agent (mixture) is carcinogenic to humans.*
*The exposure circumstance entails exposures that are carcinogenic to humans.*

This category is used when there is *sufficient evidence* of carcinogenicity in humans. Exceptionally, an agent (mixture) may be placed in this category when evidence of carcinogenicity in humans is less than sufficient but there is *sufficient evidence* of carcinogenicity in experimental animals and strong evidence in exposed humans that the agent (mixture) acts through a relevant mechanism of carcinogenicity.

*Group 2*

This category includes agents, mixtures and exposure circumstances for which, at one extreme, the degree of evidence of carcinogenicity in humans is almost sufficient, as well as those for which, at the other extreme, there are no human data but for which there is evidence of carcinogenicity in experimental animals. Agents, mixtures and exposure circumstances are assigned to either group 2A (probably carcinogenic to humans) or group 2B (possibly carcinogenic to humans) on the basis of epidemiological and experimental evidence of carcinogenicity and other relevant data.

*Group 2A — The agent (mixture) is probably carcinogenic to humans.*
*The exposure circumstance entails exposures that are probably carcinogenic to humans.*

This category is used when there is *limited evidence* of carcinogenicity in humans and *sufficient evidence* of carcinogenicity in experimental animals. In some cases, an agent (mixture) may be classified in this category when there is *inadequate evidence* of carcinogenicity in humans, *sufficient evidence* of carcinogenicity in experimental animals and strong evidence that the carcinogenesis is mediated by a mechanism that also operates in humans. Exceptionally, an agent, mixture or exposure circumstance may be classified in this category solely on the basis of *limited evidence* of carcinogenicity in humans.

*Group 2B — The agent (mixture) is possibly carcinogenic to humans.*
*The exposure circumstance entails exposures that are possibly carcinogenic to humans.*

This category is used for agents, mixtures and exposure circumstances for which there is *limited evidence* of carcinogenicity in humans and less than *sufficient evidence* of carcinogenicity in experimental animals. It may also be used when there is *inadequate evidence* of carcinogenicity in humans but there is *sufficient evidence* of carcinogenicity in experimental animals. In some instances, an agent, mixture or exposure circumstance for which there is *inadequate evidence* of carcinogenicity in humans but *limited evidence* of carcinogenicity in experimental animals together with supporting evidence from other relevant data may be placed in this group.

*Group 3 — The agent (mixture or exposure circumstance) is not classifiable as to its carcinogenicity to humans.*

This category is used most commonly for agents, mixtures and exposure circumstances for which the *evidence of carcinogenicity* is *inadequate* in humans and *inadequate* or *limited* in experimental animals.

Exceptionally, agents (mixtures) for which the *evidence of carcinogenicity* is *inadequate* in humans but *sufficient* in experimental animals may be placed in this category when there is strong evidence that the mechanism of carcinogenicity in experimental animals does not operate in humans.

Agents, mixtures and exposure circumstances that do not fall into any other group are also placed in this category.

*Group 4 — The agent (mixture) is probably not carcinogenic to humans.*

This category is used for agents or mixtures for which there is *evidence suggesting lack of carcinogenicity* in humans and in experimental animals. In some instances, agents or mixtures for which there is *inadequate evidence* of carcinogenicity in humans but *evidence suggesting lack of carcinogenicity* in experimental animals, consistently and strongly supported by a broad range of other relevant data, may be classified in this group.

## 13. REFERENCES

Breslow, N.E. & Day, N.E. (1980) *Statistical Methods in Cancer Research*, Vol. 1, *The Analysis of Case–Control Studies* (IARC Scientific Publications No. 32), Lyon, IARC*Press*

Breslow, N.E. & Day, N.E. (1987) *Statistical Methods in Cancer Research*, Vol. 2, *The Design and Analysis of Cohort Studies* (IARC Scientific Publications No. 82), Lyon, IARC*Press*

Cohen, S.M. & Ellwein, L.B. (1990) Cell proliferation in carcinogenesis. *Science*, **249**, 1007–1011

Gart, J.J., Krewski, D., Lee, P.N., Tarone, R.E. & Wahrendorf, J. (1986) *Statistical Methods in Cancer Research*, Vol. 3, *The Design and Analysis of Long-term Animal Experiments* (IARC Scientific Publications No. 79), Lyon, IARC*Press*

Hoel, D.G., Kaplan, N.L. & Anderson, M.W. (1983) Implication of nonlinear kinetics on risk estimation in carcinogenesis. *Science*, **219**, 1032–1037

Huff, J.E., Eustis, S.L. & Haseman, J.K. (1989) Occurrence and relevance of chemically induced benign neoplasms in long-term carcinogenicity studies. *Cancer Metastasis Rev.*, **8**, 1–21

IARC (1973–1996) *Information Bulletin on the Survey of Chemicals Being Tested for Carcinogenicity/Directory of Agents Being Tested for Carcinogenicity*, Numbers 1–17, Lyon, IARC*Press*

IARC (1976–1996), Lyon, IARC*Press*

  *Directory of On-going Research in Cancer Epidemiology 1976.* Edited by C.S. Muir & G. Wagner

  *Directory of On-going Research in Cancer Epidemiology 1977* (IARC Scientific Publications No. 17). Edited by C.S. Muir & G. Wagner

  *Directory of On-going Research in Cancer Epidemiology 1978* (IARC Scientific Publications No. 26). Edited by C.S. Muir & G. Wagner

  *Directory of On-going Research in Cancer Epidemiology 1979* (IARC Scientific Publications No. 28). Edited by C.S. Muir & G. Wagner

  *Directory of On-going Research in Cancer Epidemiology 1980* (IARC Scientific Publications No. 35). Edited by C.S. Muir & G. Wagner

  *Directory of On-going Research in Cancer Epidemiology 1981* (IARC Scientific Publications No. 38). Edited by C.S. Muir & G. Wagner

*Directory of On-going Research in Cancer Epidemiology 1982* (IARC Scientific Publications No. 46). Edited by C.S. Muir & G. Wagner

*Directory of On-going Research in Cancer Epidemiology 1983* (IARC Scientific Publications No. 50). Edited by C.S. Muir & G. Wagner

*Directory of On-going Research in Cancer Epidemiology 1984* (IARC Scientific Publications No. 62). Edited by C.S. Muir & G. Wagner

*Directory of On-going Research in Cancer Epidemiology 1985* (IARC Scientific Publications No. 69). Edited by C.S. Muir & G. Wagner

*Directory of On-going Research in Cancer Epidemiology 1986* (IARC Scientific Publications No. 80). Edited by C.S. Muir & G. Wagner

*Directory of On-going Research in Cancer Epidemiology 1987* (IARC Scientific Publications No. 86). Edited by D.M. Parkin & J. Wahrendorf

*Directory of On-going Research in Cancer Epidemiology 1988* (IARC Scientific Publications No. 93). Edited by M. Coleman & J. Wahrendorf

*Directory of On-going Research in Cancer Epidemiology 1989/90* (IARC Scientific Publications No. 101). Edited by M. Coleman & J. Wahrendorf

*Directory of On-going Research in Cancer Epidemiology 1991* (IARC Scientific Publications No.110). Edited by M. Coleman & J. Wahrendorf

*Directory of On-going Research in Cancer Epidemiology 1992* (IARC Scientific Publications No. 117). Edited by M. Coleman, J. Wahrendorf & E. Démaret

*Directory of On-going Research in Cancer Epidemiology 1994* (IARC Scientific Publications No. 130). Edited by R. Sankaranarayanan, J. Wahrendorf & E. Démaret

*Directory of On-going Research in Cancer Epidemiology 1996* (IARC Scientific Publications No. 137). Edited by R. Sankaranarayanan, J. Wahrendorf & E. Démaret

IARC (1977) *IARC Monographs Programme on the Evaluation of the Carcinogenic Risk of Chemicals to Humans*. Preamble (IARC intern. tech. Rep. No. 77/002)

IARC (1978) *Chemicals with Sufficient Evidence of Carcinogenicity in Experimental Animals —* IARC Monographs *Volumes 1–17* (IARC intern. tech. Rep. No. 78/003)

IARC (1978–1993) *Environmental Carcinogens. Methods of Analysis and Exposure Measurement*, Lyon, IARCPress

*Vol. 1. Analysis of Volatile Nitrosamines in Food* (IARC Scientific Publications No. 18). Edited by R. Preussmann, M. Castegnaro, E.A. Walker & A.E. Wasserman (1978)

*Vol. 2. Methods for the Measurement of Vinyl Chloride in Poly(vinyl chloride), Air, Water and Foodstuffs* (IARC Scientific Publications No. 22). Edited by D.C.M. Squirrell & W. Thain (1978)

*Vol. 3. Analysis of Polycyclic Aromatic Hydrocarbons in Environmental Samples* (IARC Scientific Publications No. 29). Edited by M. Castegnaro, P. Bogovski, H. Kunte & E.A. Walker (1979)

*Vol. 4. Some Aromatic Amines and Azo Dyes in the General and Industrial Environment* (IARC Scientific Publications No. 40). Edited by L. Fishbein, M. Castegnaro, I.K. O'Neill & H. Bartsch (1981)

*Vol. 5. Some Mycotoxins (IARC Scientific Publications No. 44)*. Edited by L. Stoloff, M. Castegnaro, P. Scott, I.K. O'Neill & H. Bartsch (1983)

*Vol. 6. N-Nitroso Compounds (IARC Scientific Publications No. 45)*. Edited by R. Preussmann, I.K. O'Neill, G. Eisenbrand, B. Spiegelhalder & H. Bartsch (1983)

*Vol. 7. Some Volatile Halogenated Hydrocarbons* (IARC Scientific Publications No. 68). Edited by L. Fishbein & I.K. O'Neill (1985)

*Vol. 8. Some Metals: As, Be, Cd, Cr, Ni, Pb, Se, Zn* (IARC Scientific Publications No. 71). Edited by I.K. O'Neill, P. Schuller & L. Fishbein (1986)

*Vol. 9. Passive Smoking (IARC Scientific Publications No. 81).* Edited by I.K. O'Neill, K.D. Brunnemann, B. Dodet & D. Hoffmann (1987)

*Vol. 10. Benzene and Alkylated Benzenes (*IARC Scientific Publications No. 85). Edited by L. Fishbein & I.K. O'Neill (1988)

*Vol. 11. Polychlorinated Dioxins and Dibenzofurans* (IARC Scientific Publications No. 108). Edited by C. Rappe, H.R. Buser, B. Dodet & I.K. O'Neill (1991)

*Vol. 12. Indoor Air* (IARC Scientific Publications No. 109). Edited by B. Seifert, H. van de Wiel, B. Dodet & I.K. O'Neill (1993)

IARC (1979) *Criteria to Select Chemicals for* IARC Monographs (IARC intern. tech. Rep. No. 79/003)

IARC (1982) *IARC Monographs on the Evaluation of the Carcinogenic Risk of Chemicals to Humans*, Supplement 4, *Chemicals, Industrial Processes and Industries Associated with Cancer in Humans* (IARC Monographs, Volumes 1 to 29), Lyon, IARC*Press*

IARC (1983) *Approaches to Classifying Chemical Carcinogens According to Mechanism of Action* (IARC intern. tech. Rep. No. 83/001)

IARC (1984) *Chemicals and Exposures to Complex Mixtures Recommended for Evaluation in IARC Monographs and Chemicals and Complex Mixtures Recommended for Long-term Carcinogenicity Testing* (IARC intern. tech. Rep. No. 84/002)

IARC (1987a) *IARC Monographs on the Evaluation of Carcinogenic Risks to Humans*, Supplement 6, *Genetic and Related Effects: An Updating of Selected* IARC Monographs *from Volumes 1 to 42*, Lyon, IARC*Press*

IARC (1987b) *IARC Monographs on the Evaluation of Carcinogenic Risks to Humans*, Supplement 7, *Overall Evaluations of Carcinogenicity: An Updating of* IARC Monographs *Volumes 1 to 42*, Lyon, IARC*Press*

IARC (1988) *Report of an IARC Working Group to Review the Approaches and Processes Used to Evaluate the Carcinogenicity of Mixtures and Groups of Chemicals* (IARC intern. tech. Rep. No. 88/002)

IARC (1989) *Chemicals, Groups of Chemicals, Mixtures and Exposure Circumstances to be Evaluated in Future IARC Monographs, Report of an ad hoc Working Group* (IARC intern. tech. Rep. No. 89/004)

IARC (1991a) *A Consensus Report of an IARC Monographs Working Group on the Use of Mechanisms of Carcinogenesis in Risk Identification* (IARC intern. tech. Rep. No. 91/002)

IARC (1991b) *Report of an ad-hoc* IARC Monographs *Advisory Group on Viruses and Other Biological Agents Such as Parasites* (IARC intern. tech. Rep. No. 91/001)

IARC (1993) *Chemicals, Groups of Chemicals, Complex Mixtures, Physical and Biological Agents and Exposure Circumstances to be Evaluated in Future* IARC Monographs, *Report of an ad-hoc Working Group* (IARC intern. Rep. No. 93/005)

IARC (1998a) *Report of an ad-hoc* IARC Monographs *Advisory Group on Physical Agents* (IARC Internal Report No. 98/002)

IARC (1998b) *Report of an ad-hoc* IARC Monographs *Advisory Group on Priorities for Future Evaluations* (IARC Internal Report No. 98/004)

McGregor, D.B., Rice, J.M. & Venitt, S., eds (1999) *The Use of Short and Medium-term Tests for Carcinogens and Data on Genetic Effects in Carcinogenic Hazard Evaluation* (IARC Scientific Publications No. 146), Lyon, IARC*Press*

Montesano, R., Bartsch, H., Vainio, H., Wilbourn, J. & Yamasaki, H., eds (1986) *Long-term and Short-term Assays for Carcinogenesis — A Critical Appraisal* (IARC Scientific Publications No. 83), Lyon, IARC*Press*

Peto, R., Pike, M.C., Day, N.E., Gray, R.G., Lee, P.N., Parish, S., Peto, J., Richards, S. & Wahrendorf, J. (1980) Guidelines for simple, sensitive significance tests for carcinogenic effects in long-term animal experiments. In: *IARC Monographs on the Evaluation of the Carcinogenic Risk of Chemicals to Humans*, Supplement 2, *Long-term and Short-term Screening Assays for Carcinogens: A Critical Appraisal*, Lyon, IARC*Press*, pp. 311–426

Tomatis, L., Aitio, A., Wilbourn, J. & Shuker, L. (1989) Human carcinogens so far identified. *Jpn. J. Cancer Res.*, **80**, 795–807

Vainio, H., Magee, P.N., McGregor, D.B. & McMichael, A.J., eds (1992) *Mechanisms of Carcinogenesis in Risk Identification* (IARC Scientific Publications No. 116), Lyon, IARC*Press*

Vainio, H., Wilbourn, J.D., Sasco, A.J., Partensky, C., Gaudin, N., Heseltine, E. & Eragne, I. (1995) Identification of human carcinogenic risk in IARC Monographs. *Bull. Cancer*, **82**, 339–348 (in French)

Waters, M.D., Stack, H.F., Brady, A.L., Lohman, P.H.M., Haroun, L. & Vainio, H. (1987) Appendix 1. Activity profiles for genetic and related tests. In: *IARC Monographs on the Evaluation of Carcinogenic Risks to Humans*, Suppl. 6, *Genetic and Related Effects: An Updating of Selected IARC Monographs from Volumes 1 to 42*, Lyon, IARC*Press*, pp. 687–696

Wilbourn, J., Haroun, L., Heseltine, E., Kaldor, J., Partensky, C. & Vainio, H. (1986) Response of experimental animals to human carcinogens: an analysis based upon the IARC Monographs Programme. *Carcinogenesis*, **7**, 1853–1863

# GENERAL REMARKS

The eighty-fifth volume of *IARC Monographs* considers betel-quid and areca-nut chewing, and some areca-nut-derived nitrosamines. Betel quid generally consists of betel leaf (from the *Piper betle* L. vine), areca nut (from the *Areca catechu* tree) and slaked lime (calcium hydroxide), to which tobacco is often added. Other ingredients and flavouring agents can be included according to local preferences and practices. Betel-quid and areca-nut chewing are widely prevalent in many parts of Asia and in Asian-migrant communities elsewhere in the world. Global reports estimate 600 million users (Trivedy, 2001), making areca-nut chewing the fourth most common habit after consumption of tobacco, alcohol and caffeine-containing beverages (Marshall, 1987; Sullivan & Hagen, 2002). Betel quid is chewed for many reasons, including for its psychostimulating effects, to induce euphoria, to satisfy hunger, to sweeten the breath and as a social and cultural practice that is strongly entrenched in people's day-to-day life.

The chewing of areca nut is a habit of great antiquity. In one study, dentitions of 31 individuals excavated from the Bronze Age site of Nui Nap, Thanh Hoa province, Viet Nam, were examined for the presence of areca-nut residues. The teeth appeared to be stained by betel-quid use (Oxenham *et al.*, 2001). Also, the chewing of areca nut is mentioned in Sanskrit manuscripts, *Sushruta Samhita,* believed to have been written around 600 BC near Benares (Bhishagratna, 1907). The Sanskrit name for the leaf of the betel vine, '*tambula*', persists in modern Hindi (Gode, 1961), as '*tambuli*', and is unchanged in Arabic and Persian (Muir & Kirk, 1960).

There seems to be general agreement that the first mention of betel quid as such dates from 504 BC when it was recorded in the 'Mahawamsa', a register of events in Ceylan written in Pali, that a princess made a gift of betel to her nurse (Krenger, 1942). A story is told about the wife of a Singhalese minister who, in about AD 56, learning of a conspiracy against her husband, sent his 'betel, etc., for mastication, omitting the chunam [slaked lime] hoping that, in coming to search for this missing ingredient, he might escape his impending fate' (see Tennent, 1860). Masudi, the traveller from Baghdad who wrote an account of his voyages in AD 916, stated that the chewing of betel then prevailed along the southern coast of Arabia, and reached as far as Yemen and Mecca (Krenger, 1942). In 1298, Marco Polo (Raghavan & Baruah, 1958) wrote in his travelogues 'the people of India have a habit of keeping in their mouth a certain leaf called the 'tembul'' (Krenger, 1942). The habit is known to have reached the Zanzibar coast between AD 1200 and 1400, and mention is made in Dutch archives from 1664 of a tax on betel leaf imported from India to Malacca (West Malaysia). In 1703, the importation was forbidden, presumably to protect local growers rather than to prevent a well-established habit (Muir & Kirk, 1960).

Tobacco was introduced into India by Europeans in the sixteenth century as a smoking substance. With acceptance and widespread use in royal courts, it found an acceptance in the general population and was mixed with betel quid. As betel quid chewing was a socially accepted practice, the use of betel quid containing tobacco became a widespread habit.

The first reference to betel chewers' cancer was made by Tennent (1860). He mentions in a footnote that 'Dr Elliot of Colombo observed several cases of cancer in the cheek, which from its peculiar characteristics, he designated the 'betel chewer's cancer''. Other early references include those of Bala Ram (1902), Niblock (1902), and Boak (1906), writing from Malabar, Madras, the Sulu Archipelago and British Borneo, respectively, about the chewing of betel quid alone or with tobacco.

While in the Americas, Europe and Oceania, the leading cancers are those of the lung, breast, prostate and colorectum, in India and many other countries in South-East Asia, oral cancer is a leading type of malignancy. In South Central Asia, cancer of the oral cavity is the cancer with the highest incidence among men and the third highest among women (after the cervix and breast) in 1975 (IARC, 1985), and this still held true in 2002 (IARC, 2003).

Betel-quid chewing, with and without tobacco, was considered in the thirty-seventh volume of the *IARC Monographs* (IARC, 1985). Sufficient evidence of carcinogenicity was found for betel quid with tobacco, but the evidence then available was inadequate for betel quid without tobacco. Since that time, several epidemiological studies have become available from areas of the world where tobacco generally is not added to the betel quid. In addition, some recent epidemiological studies in India and Pakistan have been able to separate the effects of betel quid with and without tobacco.

In addition, a large body of evidence has arisen from studies in experimental animals and in-vitro studies that investigated the effects of areca nut alone, as well as those of betel quid with or without tobacco.

In recent years, a variety of mass-produced, prepackaged areca-nut products have become available in many countries around the world. Aggressive advertising, targeted at the middle class and at children, has enhanced the sales of these products. The commercial value of the market for these prepackaged products in India alone is estimated at several hundred million US dollars annually. These products have led to serious public health problems in terms of increasing incidence of oral submucous fibrosis among younger age groups. As a result, several governmental agencies have put regulatory restrictions on these products.

**References**

Bala Ram, A.P. (1902) The use of betelnut as a cause of cancer in Malabar. *Indian med. Gaz.*, **37**, 414

Bhishagratna, K.K. (1907) *Sushrata* [An English Translation of the Sushrata Samhita, based on the Original Sanskrit Text], Calcutta, Bhishagratna, p. iii

Boak, S.D. (1906) Betel-nut chewing. *J. dent. Sci.*, **49**, 1006–1010

Gode, P.K. (1961) *Studies in Indian Cultural History*, Vol. 1, Hoshiarpur, Vishveshvaranand Vedic Research Institute, pp. 113–114

IARC (1985) *IARC Monographs on the Evaluation of the Carcinogenic Risk of Chemicals to Humans*, Vol. 37, *Tobacco Habits Other than Smoking; Betel Quid and Areca-nut Chewing; and Some Related Nitrosamines*, Lyon, IARC*Press*

IARC (2003) *World Cancer Report*, Lyon, IARC*Press*

Krenger, W. (1942) [History and culture of betel chewing. Synthesis and preparation of betel.] *Ciba Z.*, **84**, 2922–2941 (in German)

Marshall, M. (1987) An overview of drugs in Oceania. In: Lindstrom, L., ed., *Drugs in Western Pacific Societies: Relations of Substance (ASAO Monograph No. 11)*, Boston, MA, University Press of America, pp. 1–49

Muir, C.S. & Kirk, R. (1960) Betel, tobacco, and cancer of the mouth. *Br. J. Cancer*, **14**, 597–608

Niblock, W.J. (1902) Cancer in India. *Indian med. Gaz.*, **37**, 161–165

Oxenham, M.F., Locher, C., Nguyen, L.C. & Nguyen, K.T. (2001) Identification of *Areca catechu* (betel nut) residues on the dentitions of Bronze Age inhabitants of Nui Nap, northern Vietnam. *J. archeol. Sci.*, **29**, 909–915

Raghavan, V. & Baruah, H.K. (1958) Arecanut: India's popular masticatory — History, chemistry and utilization. *Econom. Bot.*, **12**, 315–325

Sullivan, R.J. & Hagen, E.H. (2002) Psychotropic substance-seeking: Evolutionary pathology or adaptation? *Addiction*, **97**, 389–400

Tennent, J.E. (1860) *Ceylon. An Account on the Island, Physical, Historical, and Topographical .../with Notices of its Natural History, Antiquities and Productions*, Vol. 1, 5th rev., London, Longman, Green, Longman & Roberts, pp. 112–115, 438–439

Trivedy, C.R. (2001) The legislative issues related to the sale and consumption of areca (betel) nut products in the UK: Current status and objectives for the future. *J. Indian med. Assoc.*, **1**, 10–16

# THE MONOGRAPHS

# BETEL-QUID AND ARECA-NUT CHEWING

# BETEL-QUID AND ARECA-NUT CHEWING

## 1. Exposure Data

### 1.1 Composition of betel quid

Areca-nut/betel-leaf/tobacco chewing habits are widely prevalent in many parts of Asia and in migrant communities arising therefrom. Many betel-quid products in different parts of the world are not actually chewed; rather, they are placed in the mouth or applied to the oral cavity and remain in contact with the oral mucosa. Nevertheless, it is recommended that they all be considered as part of the betel-quid chewing habit. Given the varied ingredients and combinations used in different parts of the world, an accurate description of terms is essential (see Glossary A for definitions and synonyms).

#### 1.1.1 *Betel quid*

The term 'betel quid' is often used with insufficient attention given to its varied contents and practices in different parts of the world. A 'betel quid' (synonymous with '*pan*' or '*paan*') generally contains betel leaf, areca nut and slaked lime, and may contain tobacco. Other substances, particularly spices, including cardamom, saffron, cloves, aniseed, turmeric, mustard or sweeteners, are added according to local preferences. In addition, some of the main ingredients (tobacco, areca nut) can be used by themselves or in various combinations without the use of betel leaf. Numerous commercially produced mixtures containing some or all of these ingredients are also available in various parts of the world. A consensus workshop held in 1996 (Zain *et al*., 1999) recommended that the term 'quid' should be defined as 'a substance, or mixture of substances, placed in the mouth [...], usually containing at least one of the two basic ingredients, tobacco or areca nut, in raw or any manufactured or processed form.'

A chewing substance may primarily consist of (Table 1):
- areca nut alone, without any betel leaf, slaked lime or tobacco
- chewing tobacco without any areca nut
- areca nut with components of betel vine and any other ingredients except tobacco (betel quid without tobacco)
- areca nut with components of betel vine and any other ingredients including tobacco (betel quid with tobacco).

## Table 1. Composition of the different types of chewing substances

| | Areca nut[a] | Betel[b] | | | Catechu[d] | Tobacco[e] | Slaked lime |
|---|---|---|---|---|---|---|---|
| | | Leaf | Inflo-rescence | Stem[c] | | | |
| Areca | X | | | | | | |
| Betel quid without tobacco | X | X | | | (X)[f] | | X |
| Betel quid with tobacco | X | X | | | (X)[f] | X | X |
| Gutka | X | | | | X | X | X |
| *Pan masala*[g] | X | | | | X | | X |
| Khaini | | | | | | X | X |
| Mawa | X | | | | | X | X |
| *Mainpuri* tobacco | X | | | | | X | X |
| *Lao-hwa* (Taiwan) | X[g] | | X | | | | X |
| Betel quid (Taiwan) | X[g] | X | | | | | X |
| Stem quid (Taiwan) | X[g] | | | X | | | X |
| *Naswar* | | | | | | X | X |
| *Zarda* | | | | | | X | X |

[a] May be used unripe, raw or processed by baking, roasting or baking with sweetening, flavouring and decorative agents (see Table 2).
[b] In place of the leaf, the inflorescence or its stem may also be used (see Table 2).
[c] Stem of inflorescence
[d] In powdered or paste form (see Table 2)
[e] In flaked, powdered or paste form, with or without processing, with or without sweetening (see Table 2)
[f] ( ) means optional
[g] Used in unripe form

It is recommended that, when the term 'betel quid' is used, other ingredients used to make up the quid be specified. A betel quid is often formulated to an individual's wishes with selected ingredients. In many countries, ready-made, mass-produced packets of the above products are now available as proprietary mixtures known as *pan masala* or *gutka* (see Section 1.2). The major constituents of a betel quid are listed in Table 2 and are outlined below.

### 1.1.2 *Areca nut*

Areca nut is the seed of the fruit of the oriental palm *Areca catechu*. It is the basic ingredient of a variety of widely used chewed products. Use of the term 'betel nut' is not botanically correct; it has caused considerable confusion in the scientific literature and should be avoided.

Areca nut is an important agricultural product in many regions of the world. The world's largest producers of areca nut, as estimated by the Food and Agriculture Organiza-

**Table 2. Constituents of betel quid**

| Constituent | Origin/preparation |
|---|---|
| Areca nut | Unripe/ripe<br>Whole/sliced<br>Raw/roasted/sun dried<br>Boiled/soaked in water<br>Fermented (under mud) |
| *Piper betle* L. | Fresh leaf<br>Inflorescence<br>Stem |
| Slaked lime | From coral<br>From shell fish<br>From quarried lime stone |
| Tobacco | Sun dried<br>Fermented<br>Boiled with molasses<br>Perfumed<br>Concentrated extract (kiwam) |
| Catechu (extracted from) | • Heartwood of *Acacia catechu* or *A. suma*<br>• Leaves of *Uncaria gambier*<br>• Bark of *Lithocarpus polystachya* (*nang ko*) |
| Spices | Cloves<br>Cardamom<br>Aniseed (± sugar coat) |
| Sweeteners | Coconut<br>Dried dates |
| Essences | Rose essence<br>Menthol<br>Mint<br>Rose petals |

Updated from Gupta & Warnakulasuriya (2002)

tion (FAO), are listed in Table 3. The FAO has estimated that world production of areca nut is increasing (FAO, 2003). In most South Asian countries where information is available, the production of areca nut has increased several fold over the past four decades. In India, production of the nut has risen nearly threefold and may reflect the commercialization of areca products since the early 1980s. Notably, Bangladesh is a significant contributor to the agricultural base of areca-nut production, but its use by the Bangladeshi population is not well documented (see Section 1.3.3).

There are several palms under the genus *Areca* that are native to South and South-East Asia and the Pacific islands. An annotated list of the *Areca* species according to their geo-

Table 3. Production of areca nut by country since 1961 (in millions of tonnes)

| Country | 1961 | 1971 | 1981 | 1991 | 2001 |
|---|---|---|---|---|---|
| Bangladesh | 62 995 | 23 369 | 25 051 | 24 120 | 47 000 |
| India | 120 000 | 141 000 | 195 900 | 238 500 | 330 000 |
| Indonesia | 13 000 | 15 000 | 18 000 | 22 812 | 36 200 |
| Kenya | NA | NA | NA | 100 | 90 |
| Malaysia | 6 500 | 3000 | 2 500 | 4000 | 2500 |
| Maldives | 1 | 1 | 5 | 16 | 37 |
| Myanmar | 8000 | 19 203 | 25 807 | 32 270 | 51 463 |
| Taiwan, China[a] | 3718 | 10 075 | 24 358 | 111 090 | 165 076 |
| Thailand | NA | NA | NA | 13 250 | 20 500 |
| World | 428 428 | 423 296 | 583 242 | 892 316 | 1 305 732 |

From FAO (2003)
NA, not available
[a] From Council of Agriculture, ROC (2003)

graphical cultivation in South and South-East Asia and in the Pacific basin was given by Furatado (1933). Areca nut for chewing is obtained exclusively from *Areca catechu*, which is believed to be native to Sri Lanka, West Malaysia and Melanesia (IARC, 1985a). This tropical palm tree bears fruit all year, which are ovoid or oblong with a pointed apex, measuring 3–5 cm in length and 2–4 cm in diameter. The outer surface is green when unripe and orange-yellow when ripe. The seed (endosperm) is separated from a fibrous pericarp, is rounded with a truncated base and is opaque and buff-coloured with dark wavy lines. It has a characteristic astringent and slightly bitter taste and is consumed at different stages of maturity according to preference. An individual may consume the whole nut or thin slices of the nut, in its natural state or after processing in many forms.

The nut may be used fresh or it may be dried and cured before use, by sun-drying, baking or roasting (Table 2). Areca fruit may also be boiled and fermented (in eastern parts of India, Sri Lanka) by covering it with mud to soften the nut for consumption. These treatments change the flavour of the nut and its astringency. In Taiwan, China, areca nut is most often used in the unripe stage when it is green, like a small olive.

Areca nut is known colloquially in Hindi and other languages in India as *supari*; it is called *puwak* in Sri Lanka, *gua* in Sylheti (Bangladesh), *mak* in Thailand, *pinang* in Malaysia, *daka* in Papua New Guinea, *pugua* in Guam and *Kun-ywet* in Myanmar (IARC, 1985a).

**Chemical constituents**

Comprehensive analyses of the chemical composition of areca nut have been reported and reviewed (Raghavan & Baruah, 1958; Shivashankar *et al.*, 1969; Arjungi, 1976; Jayalakshmi & Mathew, 1982). The major constituents of the nut are carbohydrates, fats, proteins, crude fibre, polyphenols (flavonols and tannins), alkaloids and mineral matter. The ranges in concentration of the chemical constituents of areca nut are given in Tables 4 and 5. Variations in the concentrations of the various constituents may occur in nuts from different geographical locations and according to the degree of maturity of the nut. Of the chemical ingredients, tannins, alkaloids and some minerals that may have biological activity and adverse effects on tissues have been subjected to detailed study.

*Polyphenols (flavonols, tannins)* constitute a large proportion of the dry weight of the nut. The ranges in concentration of polyphenols in unprocessed and processed nuts are shown in Tables 4 and 5. The polyphenol content of a nut may vary depending on the region where *Areca catechu* is grown, its degree of maturity and its processing method. The tannin content is highest in unripe areca nuts and decreases substantially with increasing maturity (Raghavan & Baruah, 1958). The roasted nut possesses the highest average content of tannins, ranging from 5 to 41% (mean, 21.4%); the average tannin content of sun-dried nuts is 25%; and the lowest levels are seen in boiled nuts, which contain 17% (Awang, 1987).

Polyphenols are responsible for the astringent taste of the nut (Raghavan & Baruah, 1958).

*Alkaloids*: Among the chemical constituents, alkaloids are the most important biologically. The nut has been shown to contain at least six related alkaloids, of which four (arecoline, arecaidine, guvacine and guvacoline) (Figure 1) have been conclusively identified in biochemical studies (Raghavan & Baruah, 1958; Huang & McLeish, 1989; Lord *et al.*, 2002). Arecoline is generally the main alkaloid. The ranges in concentration of arecoline in unprocessed and processed nuts are given in Tables 4 and 5.

The contents in the four major alkaloids of fresh areca nuts obtained from Darwin, Australia, have been determined by high-performance liquid chromatography (Table 6).

**Table 4. Ranges in concentration[a] of the chemical constituents of a variety of unprocessed green and ripe areca nuts**

| Constituents | Green (unripe) nut | Ripe nut |
|---|---|---|
| Moisture content | 69.4–74.1 | 38.9–56.7 |
| Total polysaccharides | 17.3–23.0 | 17.8–25.7 |
| Crude protein | 6.7–9.4 | 6.2–7.5 |
| Fat | 8.1–12.0 | 9.5–15.1 |
| Crude fibre | 8.2–9.8 | 11.4–15.4 |
| Polyphenols | 17.2–29.8 | 11.1–17.8 |
| Arecoline | 0.11–0.14 | 0.12–0.24 |
| Ash | 1.2–2.5 | 1.1–1.5 |

From Jayalakshmi & Mathew (1982)
[a] Percentage based on dry weight (except moisture)

**Table 5. Ranges in concentration[a] of some chemical constituents of a variety of processed areca nuts in India**

| Type/trade name | No. of samples analysed | Poly-phenols (%) | Arecoline (%) | Fat (%) | Crude fibre (%) | Total poly-saccharides (%) |
|---|---|---|---|---|---|---|
| Chali | 65 | 7.3–34.9 | 0.1–0.7 | 4.9–24.4 | 7.1–17.4 | 14.3–26.3 |
| Parcha | 18 | 11.7–25.0 | 0.1–0.5 | 12.3–18.1 | 8.0–14.3 | 13.0–27.3 |
| Lyon | 25 | 19.6–45.9 | 0.1–0.7 | 6.8–18.1 | 5.4–13.3 | 13.5–28.2 |
| Api | 54 | 15.2–41.3 | 0.2–0.9 | 5.3–18.5 | 5.4–18.5 | 9.2–28.2 |
| Batlu | 31 | 22.4–55.2 | 0.1–0.9 | 4.3–17.9 | 3.1–12.3 | 14.2–27.0 |
| Choor | 33 | 24.9–43.7 | 0.1–0.9 | 5.9–17.8 | 5.1–15.2 | 11.1–28.1 |
| Erazel | 9 | 16.9–38.0 | 0.2–0.8 | 5.5–12.3 | 5.9–8.7 | 13.1–26.6 |
| Chalakudi | 3 | 32.0–39.3 | 0.4–0.9 | 7.1–10.5 | 5.3–14.9 | 22.1–26.9 |
| Nuli | 6 | 39.0–47.9 | 0.6–0.9 | 3.7–13.8 | 3.8–6.0 | 16.4–22.7 |

From Shivashankar et al. (1969)
[a] Percentages based on dry weight

**Figure 1. Chemical structure of areca alkaloids**

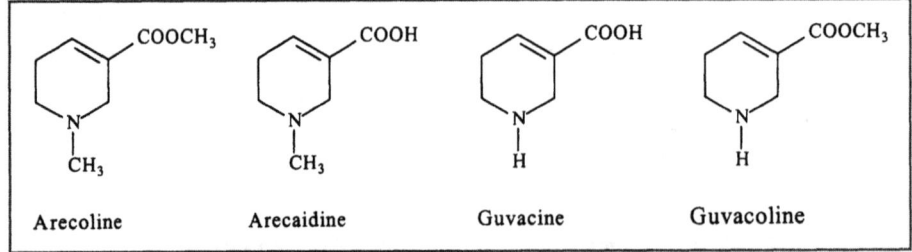

From Mujumdar et al. (1982)

**Table 6. Alkaloid content of fresh areca nuts from Darwin, Australia**

| Alkaloid | % Nut[a] |
|---|---|
| Arecoline | 0.30–0.63 |
| Arecaidine | 0.31–0.66 |
| Guvacoline | 0.03–0.06 |
| Guvacine | 0.19–0.72 |

From Huang & McLeish (1989)
[a] [Percentage not specified, probably based on dry weight]

The levels were slightly higher than those observed for Indian and Papua New Guinean nuts. The authors concluded that this difference may result from seasonal and geographical variations (Huang & McLeish, 1989).

In an aqueous extract of Taiwanese betel quid composed of fresh areca nut, betel inflorescence and red lime paste (80.5:12.5:7 by weight), arecaidine was the most abundant alkaloid (7.53 mg/g dry wt) and guvacoline the least abundant (0.26 mg/g dry wt). No change in the levels of alkaloids was observed during cold storage or during the process of freeze-drying (Wang et al., 1999).

Examining volatile alkaloids in areca nut [source unspecified] by gas chromatography–mass spectrometry, Holdsworth et al. (1998) and Self et al. (1999) described the presence of at least six other related alkaloids in addition to arecoline and guvacoline. These were identified as nicotine (~0.02%), methyl nicotinate, ethyl nicotinate, methyl- and ethyl-*N*-methyl piperidine-3-carboxylate and ethyl-*N*-methyl-1,2,5,6-tetrahydro-pyridine-3-carboxylate.

Wide variations in the arecoline content of areca nut have been demonstrated in commercially available nuts, ranging between 0 and 1.4% (Table 5; Awang, 1986; Canniff et al., 1986). Arecoline content is reduced following processing of the nut (Awang, 1988). The content is reduced from 1.4% to 1.35% by sun-drying, to 1.29% by roasting, to 0.7% by soaking in water and to 0.1% by boiling in water (Awang, 1988). The practice of boiling the nut in a liquor obtained from the previous year's boiling is designed to increase the alkaloid content of treated nuts (Canniff et al., 1986).

*Elemental composition*: Concentrations of sodium, magnesium, chlorine calcium, vanadium, manganese, copper and bromine were measured in areca nut, *pan masala* and other chewing materials available in the United Kingdom (Ridge et al., 2001). The values obtained for areca nut were lower than those reported in areca nut from Taiwan, China (Wei & Chung, 1997), but generally showed good consistency. Mean concentrations of 36 elements in areca nut, betel leaf, slaked lime and catechu are shown in Table 7 and Figure 2 (Zaidi et al., 2002).

In view of possible fibrogenic, mutagenic and toxic effects of areca nut, the copper content in samples of raw and processed areca nut was analysed and reported to be much higher than that found most frequently in other nuts consumed by humans (Trivedy et al., 1997). The mean concentration of copper in samples of processed, commercially available areca nut was $18 \pm 8.7$ µg/g (Trivedy et al., 1999). In an Indian Food Report, the copper content of processed areca nut was found to be 2.5 times that of the raw nut (Gopalan et al., 1989).

*Areca-nut-derived nitrosamines*: No study has been undertaken to determine areca-nut-derived nitrosamines in any variety of areca nut (J. Nair, personal communication).

**Table 7. Concentration[a] of trace elements in betel-quid ingredients**

| Element[b] | Areca nut | Betel leaf | Slaked lime | Catechu |
|---|---|---|---|---|
| Cr (µg/g) | 0.50 ± 0.06 | 0.46 ± 0.06 | 19.2 ± 2.9 | 7.3 ± 1.2 |
| Mn (µg/g) | 47 ± 6 | 380 ± 38 | 57.1 ± 8.6 | 170 ± 20 |
| Fe (µg/g) | 75 ± 8 | 171 ± 21 | 190 ± 29 | 5156 ± 774 |
| Co | 27 ± 4 | 132 ± 16 | 66 ± 9 | 2250 ± 360 |
| Zn (µg/g) | 5 ± 1 | 16.6 ± 2.2 | 1.24 ± 0.19 | 1.77 ± 0.27 |
| Mg (µg/g) | 2.8 ± 0.4 | 6.2 ± 0.9 | 1.30 ± 0.06 | 19.4 ± 2.9 |
| Na (µg/g) | 127 ± 14 | 793 ± 95 | 67 ± 7 | 6424 ± 964 |
| K (% wt) | 0.43 ± 0.04 | 4.42 ± 0.44 | 0.013 ± 0.002 | 0.46 ± 0.07 |
| Ba (µg/g) | 1.7 ± 0.3 | 15.4 ± 1.8 | 16.0 ± 2.4 | 7.7 ± 1.2 |
| Ca (µg/g) | 1.2 ± 0.2 | 4.8 ± 0.7 | NA | 12.6 ± 1.2 |
| Ga | 9 ± 1 | 16 ± 3 | 5 ± 1 | 58 ± 9 |
| Al (µg/g) | 2.9 ± 0.5 | 5.7 ± 0.8 | 7.2 ± 1.2 | 18.4 ± 0.2 |
| V | 12 ± 2 | 26 ± 4 | 15 ± 2 | 67 ± 10 |
| Ti | 14 ± 2 | 36 ± 6 | 48 ± 7 | 73 ± 12 |
| In | 18 ± 3 | 26 ± 4 | 31 ± 5 | 89 ± 13 |
| Sn (µg/g) | 1.4 ± 0.2 | 7.2 ± 1.1 | 9.4 ± 1.4 | 23.1 ± 3.4 |
| Sb | 13 ± 2 | 46 ± 5 | 404 ± 60 | 1100 ± 200 |
| As (µg/g) | 0.34 ± 0.04 | 18.3 ± 2.2 | 0.28 ± 0.04 | 5.96 ± 0.89 |
| Se | 120 ± 20 | 38 ± 5 | 70 ± 8 | 1045 ± 158 |
| Hg | 6 ± 1 | 9 ± 1 | 8 ± 1 | 12 ± 2 |
| Cl (% wt) | 0.15 ± 0.02 | 0.55 ± 0.1 | ND | 0.064 ± 0.01 |
| Br (µg/g) | 7.2 ± 0.9 | 7.1 ± 0.9 | 0.46 ± 0.07 | 0.61 ± 0.01 |
| Cs | 250 ± 40 | 7 ± 1 | 6 ± 1 | 14 100 ± 2100 |
| Sc | 18 ± 2 | 33 ± 4 | 274 ± 41 | 2490 ± 398 |
| Rb (µg/g) | 57 ± 7 | 225 ± 27 | 20.2 ± 2.8 | 232 ± 37 |
| Ta | 7 ± 1 | 9 ± 2 | 38 ± 6 | 1100 ± 180 |
| La | 44 ± 4 | 37 ± 4 | 2958 ± 473 | 7300 ± 1022 |
| Ce (µg/g) | 0.24 ± 0.04 | 1.14 ± 0.20 | 8.5 ± 1.3 | 20.6 ± 3.1 |
| Nd | 10 ± 2 | 18 ± 2 | 16 ± 2 | 21 ± 3 |
| Sm | 23 ± 4 | 35 ± 5 | 19 ± 3 | 51 ± 8 |
| Eu | 5 ± 1 | 7 ± 1 | 120 ± 20 | 296 ± 44 |
| Gd | 21 ± 5 | 12 ± 2 | 38 ± 6 | 49 ± 7 |
| Tb | 10 ± 2 | 9 ± 1 | 90 ± 10 | 121 ± 18 |
| Dy | 12 ± 2 | 10 ± 2 | 26 ± 3 | 38 ± 4 |
| Yb | 8 ± 1 | 78 ± 13 | 347 ± 56 | 2142 ± 343 |
| Hf | 18 ± 2 | 98 ± 12 | 78 ± 12 | 1200 ± 200 |

From Zaidi *et al.* (2002)
NA, not applicable; ND, not detected
[a] Mean ± standard deviation of five determinations
[b] Values expressed in ng/g dry weight, unless otherwise specified

**Figure 2. Trace elements found in the main ingredients of betel quid**

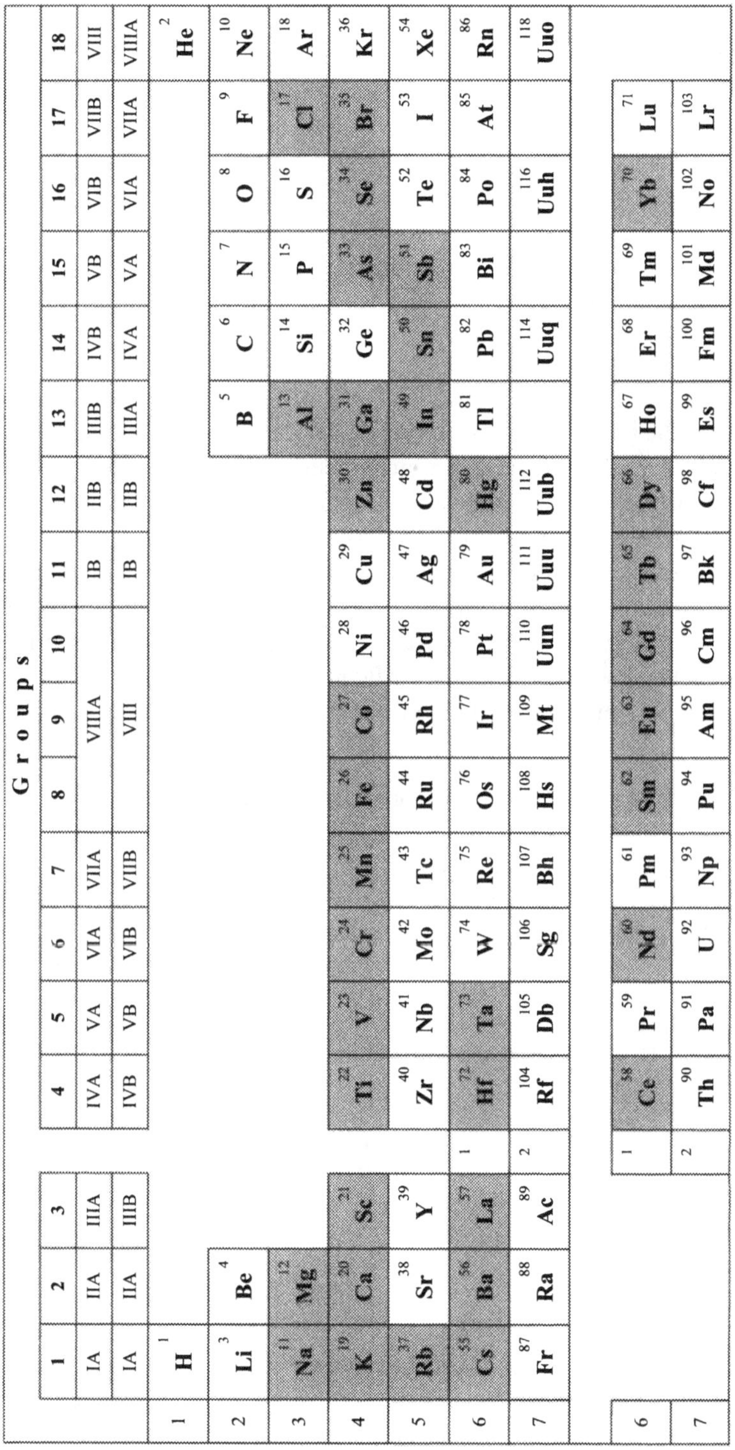

## 1.1.3 Betel leaf

The most common accompaniment for chewing areca nut globally is the leaf of *Piper betle*. This has led to areca nut being labelled 'betel nut' in the English literature, but the Working Group does recommend this nomenclature.

Betel leaves contain betel oil, a volatile liquid, which contains several phenols including hydroxychavicol, eugenol, betel phenol and chavicol. Vitamin C (1.9 mg/g) and a large amount of carotenes (80.5 mg/g) have also been reported (Wang & Wu, 1996).

Mean concentrations of 36 trace elements in betel leaf are listed in Table 7 and Figure 2 (Zaidi *et al.*, 2002).

## 1.1.4 Betel inflorescence

Apart from the leaf, other parts of the vine such as the stem, inflorescence (also called flower or pods) or catkins are also consumed with areca nut (Tables 1 and 2). Consumption of the inflorescence is common in Melanesia and in parts of Taiwan, China, and it is mostly added to the quid for its aromatic flavour.

Betel inflorescence contains a high concentration of phenolic compounds including hydroxychavicol, eugenol, isoeugenol, eugenol methyl ester and safrole (Hwang *et al.*, 1992; Wang & Hwang, 1993). Concentrations of phenolic compounds in fresh *Piper betle* flower, determined by high-performance liquid chromatographic analysis, are listed in Table 8. Safrole, the major phenolic compound, is a possible human carcinogen (IARC, 1976).

**Table 8. Concentrations of phenolic compounds in fresh *Piper betle* flower by high-performance liquid chromatographic analysis**

| Phenolic compound | Molecular weight (g) | Concentration (mg/g fresh wt) |
|---|---|---|
| Safrole | 162 | 15.35 |
| Hydroxychavicol | 151 | 9.74 |
| Eugenol | 164 | 2.51 |
| Eugenol methyl ester | 178 | 1.81 |
| Isoeugenol | 164 | 1.81 |
| Quercetin | 338 | 1.11 |

From Hwang *et al.* (1992)

## 1.1.5 Slaked lime

Slaked lime (calcium hydroxide) is often combined with areca nut (Table 1). In coastal areas, it is obtained by heating the covering of shell fish (sea shells) or is harvested from corals. In central parts of a country, it is quarried from limestone (Table 2). In the

Asian markets, slaked lime is sold as a paste mixed with water, which is white or pink. In Papua New Guinea, slaked lime is available in the powdered form and stored in air-tight containers.

Free calcium hydroxide, iron(II) and magnesium(II) were measured in 25 samples of slaked lime from Papua New Guinea, and large variations in their concentrations were found (Nair *et al.*, 1990). Mean concentrations of 35 trace elements measured in slaked lime are listed in Table 7 and Figure 2 (Zaidi *et al.*, 2002).

### 1.1.6  *Catechu*

Catechu is an astringent, reddish-brown substance which is often smeared on the betel leaf used to wrap the ingredients of betel quid. Two main types of catechu may be used depending on the tree or shrub from which the catechu has been extracted (Table 2). One type of catechu is prepared by decoction and extraction from the heartwood of *Acacia catechu*, Willd. (N.O. Leguminosae), a tree indigenous to India and Myanmar. It is sometimes referred to as black catechu or cutch. The main constituents are catechu-tannic acid (25–35%), acacatechin (2–10%), quercetin and catechu red. Another type of catechu is an aqueous extract prepared from the leaves and young shoots of *Uncaria Gambier*, Roxb. (N.O. Rubiaceae), a climbing shrub indigenous to the Malay Archipelago. It is sometimes referred to as pale catechu or *gambir*. The main constituents are catechin (7–33%), catechu-tannic acid (22–50%), quercetin and catechu red (Council of the Pharmaceutical Society of Great Britain, 1911). In addition, in Northern Thailand, catechu may be derived from the sun-dried pounded bark of *Lithocarpus polystachya*. It is referred to as *nang ko* (Mougne *et al.*, 1982).

Mean concentrations of 35 trace elements measured in catechu are listed in Table 7 and Figure 2 (Zaidi *et al.*, 2002).

### 1.1.7  *Tobacco*

Tobacco is often added to the quid mixture. Chewing tobacco in the Indian subcontinent is prepared from sun-dried and partly fermented, coarsely cut leaves of *Nicotiana rustica* and *Nicotiana tabacum* without further processing. Sometimes tobacco is powdered and combined with molasses or boiled before use (Table 2).

### 1.1.8  *Miscellaneous additives and contaminants*

Some of the most common additives are listed in Table 2.

Sago palm nut is sometimes used as an adulterant in packages of sun-dried or processed areca nut. Sweet potato and tapioca are other adulterants (Jayalakshmi & Mathew, 1982).

Areca nut can be contaminated with fungi such as *Aspergillus flavus*, *A. niger* and *Rhizopus sp.* (Borle & Gupta, 1987). Almost 40% (12/32) of samples of areca nut from India analysed using thin-layer chromatography contained aflatoxins (IARC, 2002). The mean concentration of aflatoxin $B_1$ in the analysed samples was 94 μg/kg (range,

18–208 µg/kg), largely exceeding the commonly accepted food limit of 5 µg/kg. Nine samples contained concentrations of aflatoxin $B_1$ higher than 50 µg/kg (Raisuddin & Misra, 1991). All 10 samples of raw areca nut analysed in a South African study contained aflatoxin $B_1$, with a mean concentration of 5 µg/kg (range, 2.1–10.2 µg/kg) (Van der Bijl *et al*., 1996).

## 1.2 Areca nut-based industrial packaged products

A variety of packaged areca products are now available in several countries. Based on labelling, these packaged products may fall into any one of the four categories described in Section 1.1.1, depending on the substances included (see Table 1).

Two main products are *gutka* and *pan masala*. *Gutka* is a dry, relatively non-perishable commercial preparation containing areca nut, slaked lime, catechu, condiments and powdered tobacco. The same mixture without tobacco is called *pan masala*. The products arrived on the market in the late 1960s and early 1970s. Both *gutka* and *pan masala* come in attractive foil packets (sachets) and tins which can be stored and carried conveniently. Aggressive advertising, targeted at the middle class and adolescents since the early 1980s, has enhanced the sales of these products. In advertisements, *pan masala* is depicted as implying hospitality and equality, as is betel quid. *Pan masala* and *gutka* are very popular in urban areas of India and Pakistan, especially among adolescents, and their popularity is growing fast in rural areas (Gupta & Ray, 2002). Although the actual prevalence of this habit is unknown, its popularity can be gauged by current commercial estimates valuing the Indian market for *pan masala* and *gutka* at several hundred million US dollars. These products are exported to all countries where Asian migrants live (see Section 1.3.20).

## 1.3 Consumption by geographical region

Global estimates report up to 600 million chewers (Gupta & Warnakulasuriya, 2002). This section reviews patterns and prevalence of consumption in different countries. For the sake of clarity, the nomenclature has been made uniform throughout the section (see Glossary A for definitions).

### 1.3.1 *India*

Countrywide surveys on the use of areca nut have not been conducted, nor have any other surveys been conducted to investigate specifically the use of areca nut. Surveys of habits have been conducted on the use of tobacco and other chewing habits, especially betel-quid chewing, in limited populations. Studies of adults are presented first, followed by those of children and adolescents. Within these categories, rural studies are presented first, followed by available urban studies.

The tobacco included in betel quid varies from region to region. In Uttar Pradesh, *mainpuri* tobacco, which is a mixture of tobacco with slaked lime, finely cut areca nut and powdered cloves or camphor, is commonly used (Wahi, 1968).

(a) *Adults*

(i) *Rural studies*

Several studies have investigated the prevalence of betel-quid chewing in limited population samples.

The prevalence of all chewing habits, with and without areca nut and with and without tobacco, was recorded in house-to-house surveys among villagers in various parts of India (Mehta *et al.*, 1971, 1972). There were marked differences between localities and some differences between sexes (Table 9).

In Ernakulam District, Kerala, information on smoking and chewing habits was collected during a survey of oral lesions in a sample of 5099 persons aged 15 years and older (Daftary *et al.*, 1980). Betel-quid chewing, mostly with tobacco, was practiced by 23.7%, smoking by 21.5% and both habits by 9.8% (Table 10). Overall, 34.7% of men and 32.4% of women indulged in the habit, and only about 0.7% chewed betel quid without consuming any form of tobacco.

In another house-to-house survey during 1977–78 in Ernakulam District, 12 212 tobacco users aged 15 years or older were identified in a rural population of about 48 000 (Gupta *et al.*, 1986, 1989). Of these, 11 412 were interviewed. Among tobacco users, 37.7% were chewers only, mostly of betel quid, and 14.3% both chewed and smoked (Table 11). Thus, approximately 50% of tobacco users chewed betel quid. Among tobacco users, 95.5% of women and 33.6% of men (of whom more than half also smoked) chewed. Betel-quid chewing was most common in the group aged 35 years and above.

Table 9. Prevalence of chewing habits (with and without smoking) in house-to-house surveys among villagers in India[a]

| Location (state) | Sample size | Prevalence of chewing habits (%) | |
|---|---|---|---|
| | | With tobacco | Without tobacco |
| Andhra Pradesh | 10 169 | 2.3 | 0.5 |
| Bihar, Darbhanga | 10 340 | 15 | 1.3 |
| Bihar, Singhbhum | 10 048 | 13 | 0.4 |
| Gujarat | 10 071 | 3 | 1.5 |
| Kerala | 10 287 | 26 | 0.4 |
| Maharashtra | 101 761[b] | 28 | 0.6 |

[a] From Mehta *et al.* (1971), unless otherwise specified
[b] From Mehta *et al.* (1972)

**Table 10. Prevalence of tobacco and areca-nut habits in a population ≥ 15 years old in Ernakulam District, Kerala, India**

| Habit | Men | | Women | | All | |
|---|---|---|---|---|---|---|
| | No. | % | No. | % | No. | % |
| No habit | 467 | 19.6 | 1828 | 67.2 | 2295 | 45.0 |
| Smoking only | 1087 | 45.6 | 11 | 0.4 | 1098 | 21.5 |
| Chewing only | 338 | 14.2 | 868 | 31.9 | 1206 | 23.7 |
| With tobacco | | | | | 1170 | 23.0 |
| Without tobacco | | | | | 36 | 0.7 |
| Both habits | 487 | 20.5 | 13 | 0.5 | 500 | 9.8 |
| Total | 2379 | 100.0 | 2720 | 100.0 | 5099 | 100.0 |

From Daftary et al. (1980)

**Table 11. Prevalence of tobacco and areca-nut habits among tobacco users ≥ 15 years old in Ernakulam District, Kerala, India**

| Tobacco habit | Men | | Women | | All | |
|---|---|---|---|---|---|---|
| | No. | % | No. | % | No. | % |
| Smoking only | 5330 | 66.5 | 150 | 4.4 | 5480 | 48.0 |
| Chewing only[a] | 1137 | 14.2 | 3162 | 93.2 | 4299 | 37.7 |
| Both habits | 1554 | 19.4 | 79 | 2.3 | 1633 | 14.3 |
| Total | 8021 | 100.0 | 3391 | 100.0 | 11 412 | 100.0 |

From Gupta et al. (1986)
[a] Tobacco was chewed mostly in the form of betel quid.

In 1986, a house-to-house survey of tobacco habits was conducted among 30 544 villagers of all ages in 373 villages in three areas of Kolar District, Karnataka, to gather baseline information for an intervention study (Anantha et al., 1995). About 8–16% of men and 29–39% of women had chewing habits (Table 12). While the content of the substances chewed was not defined in this study, a case–control study carried out in Karnataka by one of the authors identified the chewing habits of women as including tobacco, betel leaf, areca nut and slaked lime and as being the only tobacco habit of women (Carley et al., 1994).

*Mawa* is popular in Gujarat, India, especially among the young. The prevalence of this habit increased tremendously in the 1970s and 1980s (Sinor et al., 1990).

Table 12. Prevalence of tobacco and areca-nut habits among villagers in Kolar District, Karnataka, India

| Habit | Dibbur | Malur | Gudiband |
|---|---|---|---|
| *Men* | | | |
| No. | 5464 | 5369 | 4893 |
| Tobacco smoking | 17.7% | 21.0% | 21.7% |
| Tobacco chewing | 16.4% | 7.7% | 8.4% |
| *Women* | | | |
| No. | 5236 | 4905 | 4677 |
| Tobacco smoking | 0% | 0% | 0% |
| Tobacco chewing[a] | 38.5% | 28.7% | 30.4% |

From Anantha *et al.* (1995)
[a] Inferred as betel quid with tobacco from Carley *et al.* (1994)

The distribution of areca-nut use and tobacco smoking and chewing habits was assessed through a house-to-house survey in Bhavnagar District, Gujarat. Of 21 842 villagers aged 15 years and above (Gupta *et al.*, 1998), 2298 men (20.4% of all men) were chewing only and used areca nut in the form of *mawa* or betel quid with tobacco (Table 13).

Table 13. Prevalence of tobacco and areca-nut habits among villagers in Bhavnagar District, Gujarat, India

| Habit | Men | | Women | |
|---|---|---|---|---|
| | No. | % | No. | % |
| No habit | 3 648 | 32.4 | 9 325 | 88.1 |
| Smoking only (any) | 3 942 | 35.0 | 16 | 0.2 |
| Chewing only (any) | 3 124 | 27.7 | 1 242 | 11.7 |
| *Mawa* | 2 127 | 18.9 | 7 | 0.1 |
| Betel quid with tobacco | 171 | 1.5 | 2 | – |
| Tobacco | 799 | 7.1 | 2 | – |
| *Bajar*[a] | 27 | 0.2 | 1 231 | 11.6 |
| Mixed habits | 544 | 4.8 | 1 | – |
| Total | 11 258 | 100.00 | 10 584 | 100.0 |

From Gupta *et al.* (1998)
[a] Dry snuff

In West Bengal, 1990 women aged 16–60 years attending rural cancer detection clinics attached to a Calcutta-based cancer institute were interviewed about their tobacco and areca-nut habits (Chakrabarti et al., 1990). The habit usually consisted of chewing betel leaf, areca nut, slaked lime, catechu and a few flavouring agents. Sometimes women added *zarda*. A total of 23.3% reported chewing betel quid, half of whom used tobacco in the quid (Table 14).

**Table 14. Prevalence of tobacco and areca-nut habits in women attending rural cancer detection clinics in West Bengal, India**

| Habit | No. | % |
|---|---|---|
| No habit | 1502 | 75.5 |
| Betel quid without tobacco | 226 | 11.4 |
| Betel quid with tobacco | 236 | 11.9 |
| Other habits[a] | 26 | 1.3 |
| Total | 1990 | 100.0 |

From Chakrabarti et al. (1990)
[a] Other habits included drinking and chewing of anise seeds and cloves.

A study of chewing and smoking habits among 259 rural school teachers (230 men and 29 women) aged 28–63 years was conducted in Hoogly District, West Bengal (Pandey et al., 2001). In this population, 51% were current tobacco users and 16.2% were former users. Among the current users, 72% were predominantly smokers, while 28% preferred smokeless forms of tobacco. Some 12% of all teachers chewed betel leaves with tobacco (Table 15). A small fraction used manufactured areca-nut products such as *gutka* and *pan masala*.

(ii) *Urban studies*

The most detailed account of chewing habits was reported among 10 000 persons admitted to the clinic of the dental school in Lucknow, Uttar Pradesh. No less than 22 different betel-chewing habits were reported (Pindborg et al., 1967).

Dayal et al. (1978) presented a detailed report on chewing habits without a simultaneous smoking habit among 57 518 textile-mill workers aged 35 years and above in Ahmedabad, Gujarat (Table 16). Of all workers, 8710 (15.2%) had no oral habit, 2212 (3.8%) had a current chewing habit and 475 (0.8%) had a past chewing habit, all of them without a simultaneous smoking habit. The data show that the practice of a single chewing habit is rare.

A survey on issues pertaining to the control of oral cancer was conducted among 120 health professionals in the field of oncology from all over India, 85% of whom were men

Table 15. Prevalence of smoking and chewing habits in rural school teachers of Hoogly District, West Bengal, India

| Habit | No. | %[a] |
|---|---|---|
| No habit | 127 | 49.0 |
| Smoking | | |
|   Filter-tipped cigarettes | 82 | [31.7] |
|   Untipped cigarettes | 75 | [29.0] |
| Chewing | | |
|   Betel leaves with tobacco | 32 | [12.4] |
|   Others[b] | 17 | [6.6] |

From Pandey et al. (2001)
[a] Percentages do not add up because 66 respondents used more than one form of tobacco.
[b] Including tobacco quid (khaini), snuff, tobacco paste (gudaku), pan masala and gutka

Table 16. Prevalence of current chewing habits among 57 518 textile-mill workers in Ahmedabad, Gujarat, India

| Chewing habit | No. | % |
|---|---|---|
| Betel quid with slaked lime, catechu, areca nut and tobacco | 1335 | [2.3] |
| Betel quid with slaked lime, catechu and areca nut | 737 | [1.3] |
| Betel quid with slaked lime | 2 | [0.003] |
| Betel quid with areca nut | 3 | [0.005] |
| Areca nut | 113 | [0.2] |
| Others | 22 | [0.04] |

From Dayal et al. (1978)

and 28% of whom were under 35 years of age (Stanley & Stjernsward, 1986). Among those surveyed, 8% currently chewed betel quid with tobacco, 4% were previous regular chewers and 22% reported occasional chewing (Table 17). The prevalence of chewing was similar among men and women.

In 1992–94, a baseline survey on tobacco and areca-nut habits was conducted among 99 598 permanent residents of Mumbai, aged 35 years and above, belonging to the lower socioeconomic strata (Gupta, 1996). The prevalence of smokeless habits was high among both women and men (Table 18). Overall, areca nut in all forms was used by 29.7% of women and 37.8% of men, and betel quid without tobacco by 0.4% of men and 0.5% of women. Ten per cent of men practised both smokeless (including areca-nut habits) and smoking habits.

## Table 17. Prevalence of tobacco and areca-nut habits of 120 health professionals in the field of oncology in India

| Habit | Prevalence (%) | | | | |
|---|---|---|---|---|---|
| | Current | Occasional | Past[a] | Never | Total |
| Cigarette | 10 | 9 | 14 | 66 | 100 |
| Bidi | 0 | 1 | 1 | 97 | 100 |
| Betel quid with tobacco | 8 | 22 | 4 | 66 | 100 |

From Stanley & Stjernsward (1986)
[a] Past habit was defined as those having quit for at least 1 month.

## Table 18. Prevalence of tobacco and areca-nut habits among permanent residents of Mumbai, India, of lower socioeconomic status

| Habit | Men | | Women | | All | |
|---|---|---|---|---|---|---|
| | No. | % | No. | % | No. | % |
| No current habit[a] | [12 280] | [30.7] | [25 268] | [42.5] | [37 548] | [37.7] |
| Smokeless tobacco | 18 322 | 45.7 | 34 019 | 57.1 | 52 341 | 52.5 |
| Smoking | 5 494 | 13.7 | 146 | 0.2 | 5 640 | 5.7 |
| Smokeless tobacco and smoking | 3 975 | 9.9 | 94 | 0.2 | 4 069 | 4.1 |
| Total | 40 071 | 100.0 | 59 527 | 100.0 | 99 598 | 100.0 |
| *Use of smokeless tobacco* | | | | | | |
| *Mishri* | [4 140] | 10.3 | 15 740 | 26.5 | 19 880 | 20.0 |
| *Mishri* + betel quid with tobacco | 4 976 | 12.4 | 10 687 | 18.0 | 15 663 | 15.7 |
| Betel quid with tobacco | 5 871 | 14.7 | 3 527 | 5.9 | 9 398 | 9.4 |
| Tobacco + slaked lime | 2 997 | 7.5 | 640 | 1.1 | 3 637 | 3.7 |
| Others with tobacco | 1 144 | 2.9 | 1 200 | 2.0 | 2 344 | 2.4 |
| Multiple practices | 2 993 | 7.4 | 2 013 | 3.3 | 5 006 | 5.0 |
| Areca nut[b] | 176 | 0.4 | 306 | 0.5 | 482 | 0.5 |
| No smokeless tobacco use (no habit + smoking only) | 17 774 | 44.4 | 25 414 | 42.7 | 43 188 | 43.4 |
| Total | 40 071 | 100.0 | 59 527 | 100.0 | 99 598 | 100.0 |

From Gupta (1996)
[a] Includes about [14%] of men and [5%] of women who were former users of tobacco, mostly in the form of smokeless tobacco.
[b] Areca-nut chewing, most often as betel quid without tobacco

In a northern suburb of Trivandrum City, Kerala, two groups of men and women, 35 years of age or older, mostly of lower socioeconomic status, were interviewed in 1995–98 (Sankaranarayanan et al., 2000). Chewing habits, consisting mainly of betel quid with tobacco, were practised by 26.8% of men and 26.4% of women in one group and 20.5% of men and 17.6% of women in the other group (Table 19). Chewing habits were more common in low-income, low-education participants and in individuals with a manual occupation or retirees (Hashibe et al., 2003). Among those for whom information was available, 89% chewed betel quid with tobacco, 11% chewed betel quid without tobacco and 0.4% chewed tobacco only (Thomas et al., 2003).

Table 19. Prevalence[a] of tobacco and areca-nut habits among urban residents in Trivandrum, Kerala, India

| Habit | Men (%) | | Women (%) | |
|---|---|---|---|---|
| | Group I | Group II | Group I | Group II |
| No. | 25 453 | 23 356 | 34 441 | 31 351 |
| No habit | 31.4 | 44.1 | 72.3 | 81.8 |
| Chewing[b] | 26.8 | 20.5 | 26.4 | 17.6 |
| Smoking | 55.8 | 43.9 | 2.4 | 1.0 |

From Sankaranarayanan et al. (2000)
[a] Percentages do not add up to 100% possibly because some residents reported multiple habits.
[b] Mostly betel quid with tobacco

(b) *Children and adolescents*

In 1992, a survey of 146 children and teenagers (84 boys and 62 girls) between the ages of 5 and 20 years was conducted in the coastal fishing community of Mariyanad, Kerala (George et al., 1994). Chewing of betel quid with tobacco was by far the most prevalent habit in both boys and girls, and was inversely related to level of education (Table 20). Two boys both chewed betel quid with tobacco and drank alcohol. One boy, 17 years of age, chewed betel quid with tobacco and smoked.

A survey conducted in 1998 among 400 male medical students revealed that about 12.5% were regular users of *gutka* (Table 21) and 27.5% were occasional users of areca-nut products without tobacco (Sinha & Gupta, 2001). Among those with a regular habit, about half had smokeless habits, consisting of chewing *gutka* and *khaini*. Occasional users mainly chewed areca-nut products not containing tobacco, e.g. *pan masala*.

A number of surveys conducted in households in India have shown that *pan masala* and *gutka* are commonly chewed by children and adolescents, especially in Gujarat, Maharashtra and Bihar. In a survey of 1200 students from junior and degree colleges of Maharastra, 9.9% chewed *pan masala* and 9.6% chewed *gutka*. In a survey of 95 boys and girls in the 8th and 9th grades (13–14 years old) of a small-town private school in Anand, Gujarat, 16% used *gutka*. In a village community of Kheda District, Gujarat, 72% of men and 50% of women under 26 years of age used tobacco products. Men favoured bidis and *gutka* while women preferred *gutka* and tobacco toothpaste. Among high school students in classes 10–12 (15–17 years old) in Patna, Bihar, approximately 12% used *pan masala* (Gupta & Ray, 2002).

Table 20. Prevalence of tobacco and areca-nut habits of children and teenagers aged 5–20 years in a coastal fishing village in Kerala, India

| Habit | Boys | | Girls | | All | |
|---|---|---|---|---|---|---|
| | No. | % | No. | % | No. | % |
| No habit | [44] | [52.3] | [52] | [83.9] | [96] | [65.8] |
| Betel quid with tobacco chewing | | | | | | |
| Occasionally | 12 | 14.3 | 7 | 11.3 | 19 | 13.0 |
| Regularly | 23 | 27.4 | 1 | 1.6 | 24 | 16.4 |
| Bidi smoking | | | | | | |
| Occasionally | – | – | 2 | 3.2 | 2 | 1.4 |
| Regularly | 1 | 1.2 | – | – | 1 | 0.7 |
| Alcohol drinking | | | | | | |
| Occasionally | 4 | 4.8 | – | – | 4 | 2.7 |
| Regularly | – | | – | | – | – |
| Total | 84 | 100.0 | 62 | 100.0 | 146 | 100.0 |

From George *et al.* (1994)

Table 21. Prevalence of tobacco and areca-nut habits of medical students in Patna, Bihar, India

| Habit | No. | % |
|---|---|---|
| No habit | [78] | 18.8 |
| Tobacco (smoking and chewing) | | |
| Regular | 172 | 43.0 |
| Smoking | | 20.7 |
| Chewing | | 20.2 |
| *Gutka* | | 12.5 |
| Occasional | 37 | 9.3 |
| Areca-nut products without tobacco | | |
| Regular | 3 | 0.8 |
| Occasional | 110 | 27.5 |
| Total | 400 | 100.0 |

From Sinha & Gupta (2001)

## 1.3.2 Pakistan

In a study on dietary and chewing/smoking habits, data on 10 749 persons of low and middle socioeconomic status, aged 20 years and over, were collected from various districts of Karachi (Mahmood et al., 1974). Overall, 27.9% of men and 37.8% of women chewed areca nut in the form of betel quid (Table 22). Of this group, 47.5% of men and 31.9% of women chewed betel quid without tobacco (Table 23).

**Table 22. Prevalence of tobacco and areca-nut habits in a population sample in Karachi, Pakistan, 1967–72**

| Habit | Men (%) | Women (%) | Total (%) |
|---|---|---|---|
| No. | 5802 | 4947 | 10 749 |
| No habit | 36.9 | 56.8 | 46.0 |
| Pan | 4.2 | 11.5 | 7.6 |
| Tobacco chewing | 2.6 | 1.9 | 2.2 |
| Smoking | 30.3 | 2.2 | 17.4 |
| *Pan* + tobacco chewing | 6.1 | 25.0 | 14.8 |
| *Pan* + smoking | 8.9 | 0.4 | 5.0 |
| Tobacco chewing + smoking | 0.7 | 0.1 | 0.5 |
| All three habits | 8.7 | 0.9 | 5.1 |
| Unknown | 1.6 | 1.2 | 1.4 |
| Total | 100 | 100 | 100 |

From Mahmood et al. (1974)

**Table 23. Prevalence of *pan*-chewing habits in a population sample in Karachi, Pakistan, 1967–72**

| Habit | Men (%) | Women (%) | Total (%) |
|---|---|---|---|
| No *pan* habit | 70.9 | 61.2 | 66.5 |
| Without tobacco | 13.3 | 12.0 | 12.7 |
| With tobacco *qiwam*[a] | 2.1 | 2.6 | 2.3 |
| With tobacco leaf | 12.3 | 22.5 | 17.0 |
| With tobacco leaf + *qiwam*[a] | 0.3 | 0.6 | 0.5 |
| Other types | 0.2 | 0.3 | 0.3 |
| Unknown | 0.9 | 0.9 | 0.9 |
| Total | 100.0 | 100.0 | 100.0 |

From Mahmood et al. (1974)
[a] *Qiwam* (also spelt *kiwam*): paste prepared from processed tobacco leaves, from which the stalks and stems have been removed, that are soaked and boiled in water with flavourings and spices, macerated and strained. The paste is chewed.

A survey was conducted in a sample of 160 primary school students aged 4–16 years (98% were < 12 years) in a fishing community on Baba Island of Karachi, Pakistan (Shah et al., 2002). Of the 159 respondents, 118 (74.2%) used areca-nut products in the form of sweetened areca nut or betel quid (Table 24).

Table 24. Prevalence of areca-nut habits among primary school children (4–16 years of age) on Baba Island, Karachi Harbor, Pakistan

| Habit | No. | % |
|---|---|---|
| No habit | 41 | 25.8 |
| Sweetened areca nut only | 63 | 39.6 |
| Betel quid only | 4 | 2.5 |
| Sweetened areca nut and betel quid | 51 | 32.1 |
|    Betel quid[a] with tobacco | 10 | [6.2] |
|    Betel quid without tobacco | 46 | [28.9] |
| Total | 159 | 100.0 |

From Shah et al. (2002)
[a] Alone or in conjunction with sweetened areca nut
[The Working Group noted small inconsistencies between the text and table in the percentage of users of sweetened areca nut and the number of betel-quid users.]

### 1.3.3 Bangladesh

Prevalence patterns of use of tobacco and areca nut by Bangladeshi populations have not been published in the English language literature. Extrapolating from migrant populations originating from Bangladesh and living in the United Kingdom, it is clear that the habit of chewing areca nut with and without tobacco is very prevalent in this population (see Section 1.3.6) and may therefore be taken as evidence for the existence of the habit in the home country.

### 1.3.4 Sri Lanka

In Sri Lanka, the quid consists of fresh areca nut, slaked lime from seashells, fresh betel leaf and slightly dried (or processed) tobacco (Chiba et al., 1998). Studies in the early 1970s (Senewiratne & Uragoda, 1973) indicated that, among a group of healthy people, 55.6% of the men and 42.7% of the women added tobacco to the quid.

In rural Sri Lanka, the habit of betel-quid chewing is widely practised. Stephen and Uragoda (1970) reported that 30.1% of 1088 persons (men, 27.9%; women, 32.3 %) chewed betel quid with tobacco. In a large-scale study in rural Sri Lanka, it was shown that [57%] of men and women were chewers, about half of whom included tobacco in their quid (Warnakulasuriya, 1992). In a nationwide survey conducted between 1994 and 1995 (Ministry of Health, 1998), approximately 4000 adults over the age of 35 years were interviewed on their betel-quid chewing habits. The prevalence of betel-quid chewing was [33.8%] among those aged 35–44 years and [47.7%] among those aged 65–74 years. In another study, the average number of quids used per day was 5.5 (Topcu et al., 2002).

### 1.3.5 Maldives

In a study of 344 schoolchildren aged 5–15 years, 31% chewed 'betel' daily, 48% chewed occasionally and 21% did not chew. The prevalence of daily chewing for ages 5–6, 10 and 15 years was 15, 27 and 51%, respectively (Knudsen et al., 1985). [The habit was not described in detail.]

### 1.3.6 People's Republic of China

Betel-quid chewing is popular in the south-eastern part of China, particularly in the Hunan Province and on Hainan Island (Tang et al., 1997). In Xiangtan City, Hunan Province, fresh areca fruit is imported from Hainan Island and is treated with maltose and lime. The nut is cut longitudinally into four or six pieces and is usually chewed with a few drops of cassia twig oil (Tang et al., 1997). On Hainan Island, the fruit is chewed fresh with lime and wrapped in betel leaf (Pindborg et al., 1984). In neither region is tobacco added to the quid.

An epidemiological survey was conducted in Xiangtan City in over 10 000 randomly selected subjects (Tang et al., 1997). Just over one third of the population sample chewed betel quid (Table 25). Among the chewers, 32% of the men and 97% of the women did not have a smoking habit.

Of 100 betel-quid chewers in the Linshui district of Hainan, 42 chewed betel quid alone, 31 chewed betel quid and smoked cigarettes, 21 chewed betel quid and smoked a

Table 25. Prevalence of tobacco and areca-nut habits among randomly selected subjects in Xiangtan City, Hunan Province, China

| Habit | Men (%) | Women (%) | Total (%) |
|---|---|---|---|
| No habit | 50.6 | 69.2 | 59.0 |
| Areca nut | 12.6 | 29.6 | 20.3 |
| Smoking | 10.0 | 0.3 | 5.6 |
| Areca nut + smoking | 26.8 | 0.9 | 15.1 |
| Total | 100 | 100 | 100 |

From Tang et al. (1997)

waterpipe and one chewed betel quid, and smoked cigarettes and a waterpipe. Of the 46 women surveyed, 87% chewed areca nut with no additional habit (Pindborg *et al.*, 1984).

### 1.3.7 Taiwan, China

It was estimated that about 10% of the population of 2 million in Taiwan, China, chew betel quid (Ko *et al.*, 1992). The ingredients of a quid vary with the area and ethnic group.

Quids in Taiwan can be classified into three types (see Table 1; Yang *et al.*, 2001): *lao-hwa* quid, betel quid and stem quid. *Lao-hwa* quid prevails in urban districts, and is prepared by inserting a piece of inflorescence of *Piper betle* L. with red lime paste (slaked lime and some local flavouring) into an unripe areca nut. The second most popular quid is betel quid made by wrapping a split unripe areca nut and white slaked lime paste in a piece of betel leaf, and is popular in urban and aboriginal areas. Betel quid is always chewed without tobacco. The third type of quid, stem quid, is similar to lao-hwa quid except that the piece of inflorescence of *Piper betle* L. is replaced by a piece of stem of *Piper betle* L. The use of stem quid is rare and only seen in southern parts of aboriginal areas, primarily in the Paiwan and Yami tribes.

Table 26 summarizes a series of surveys on the prevalence of chewing habits in Taiwan, China.

Inhabitants of Kaohsiung of all ages and individuals from three aboriginal tribes (Paiwan, Rukai and Bunun) over 15 years of age were interviewed in their home in a house-to-house survey (Ko *et al.*, 1992). Among the inhabitants of Kaohsiung, the prevalence of chewers was higher in men, older people, blue-collar workers, smokers, drinkers and less educated people; of the chewers, 86% were smokers and 75% were drinkers. Both men and women had chewed an average of 14 portions a day for an average of over 14 years. Among aboriginal people, prevalences were 42.1% for current betel-quid chewers (46.5% for men; 38.0% for women) and about 1% for former chewers for both men and women. No significant differences with respect to level of education or occupation were found. Of the chewers, 36% were smokers and 55% were drinkers; 55% used betel quid with men having chewed on average 23 portions a day for over 11 years and women 16 portions a day for over 7 years.

Another survey on betel-quid chewing among residents in Kaohsiung aged 15 years and above gave similar findings (Chen & Shaw, 1996).

A population-based survey of an aboriginal community of southern Taiwan, China, was conducted in 1997 and included 312 participants aged 20 years or older (Yang *et al.*, 2001). The lifetime prevalence of chewing was 89.4%, with 69.5% for current chewers. The prevalence in women (78.7%) was higher than that in men (60.6%). The rates in young subjects were similar to those in the elderly. Betel quid was the predominant type (65%), followed by stem quid (57%); only 11% of people used *lao-hwa* quid. The average duration of chewing was 22 years for men and 26 years for women, and the average number of portions per day was 17.3. Almost half of the chewers also had smoking and/or drinking habits.

## Table 26. Surveys on the prevalence of betel-quid chewing in Taiwan, China

| Reference | Study population | Chewing habit[a] | Chewing category | Prevalence (%) | Comments |
|---|---|---|---|---|---|
| Ko et al. (1992) | 1299 residents of Kaohsiung and 827 aborigines from three tribes | Lao-hwa; lao-hwa + smoking; betel quid; betel quid + smoking | Former chewer<br>Current chewer<br><br>Lao-hwa<br>Lao-hwa + smoking<br>Betel quid<br>Betel quid + smoking<br><br>Former chewer<br>Current chewer<br><br>Lao-hwa<br>Lao-hwa + smoking<br>Betel quid<br>Betel quid + smoking | *Kaohsiung inhabitants*<br>4 (6.7 M, 1.3 F)<br>6 (9.8 M, 1.6 F)<br>Among chewers:<br>10.6 M, 40.0 F<br>86.4 M, 60.0 F<br>0 M, 0 F<br>3.0 M, 0 F<br>*Aborigine tribes*<br>1.0 (1.3 M, 0.7 F)<br>42.1 (46.5 M, 38.0 F)<br>Among chewers<br>18.9 M, 33.7 F<br>33.5 M, 3.1 F<br>22.7 M, 55.8 F<br>24.9 M, 7.4 F | Information on intensity and duration available for both groups and both sexes |
| Lu et al. (1993) | 2367 students in junior high school in Changhua | Lao-hwa; betel quid | Chewer<br>Grade (mean age)<br><br><br>Residential area<br><br><br>Achievement level<br><br>Family member chewing<br>Among chewers<br>Lao-hwa<br>Betel quid | 4.7 (9.2 M, 0.7 F)<br>Seventh (12.5): 1.2<br>Eighth (13.6): 4.2<br>Ninth (14.5): 8.7<br>Village: 6.5<br>Town: 3.7<br>City: 3.0<br>Ordinary: 8.4<br>High: 1.6<br>None: 2.4<br>≥ 1: 7.0<br><br>87.5<br>12.5 | 53.6% of students that chewed first experimented with a family member. |
| Chen & Shaw (1996) | 1162 residents (511 M, 651 F) of Kaohsiung aged ≥ 15 years | Betel quid | Casual chewer<br>Daily chewer<br>Ever chewer | 10.5 (21.9 M, 1.4 F)<br>2.8 (6.5 M, 0 F)<br>13.3 (28.4 M, 1.4 F) | |
| Yang et al. (1996) | 3185 students (1581 M, 1604 F) in a junior high school (13–15 years old) and 1325 students (1083 M, 241 F) in a vocational school (16–18 years old) located in southern Taiwan | Betel quid | Current chewer<br>Former chewer<br>Ever chewer<br><br>Current chewer<br>Former chewer<br>Ever chewer | *Junior high school*<br>1.9 (3.4 M, 0.4 F)<br>14.0 (24.4 M, 5.0 F)<br>15.9<br><br>*Vocational high school*<br>10.2 (12.5 M, 0 F)<br>31.0 (36.1 M, 8.3 F)<br>41.2 | Prevalence of betel-quid chewing increased with tobacco use, alcohol use and friendship with other betel-quid chewers |

**Table 26 (contd)**

| Reference | Study population | Chewing habit[a] | Chewing category | Prevalence (%) | Comments |
|---|---|---|---|---|---|
| Chong et al. (1999) | 774 junior high school students (14–16 years old) | Betel quid | Chewer<br>Residential area | 2.2 (4.4 M, 0.3 F)<br>Urban: 1.3<br>Suburban: 1.1<br>Rural: 5.0 | |
| Ho et al. (2000a) | 2572 students in senior high schools (16–18 years old) in southern Taiwan (Kaohsiung and Pingtung areas) | Betel quid | Type of school<br>General<br>Commercial<br>Medical technician<br>Manufacturing<br>Agricultural | *Ever chewer*<br>4.7 (8.0 M, 0.8 F)<br>6.9 (33.3 M, 5.2 F)<br>16.3 (33.3 M, 9.9 F)<br>25.6 (31.2 M, 4.8 F)<br>31.3 (40.1 M, 14.2 F) | |
| Ho et al. (2000b) | 2087 junior high school students (13–15 years old), including 82 students from the aboriginal area in Taichung County | Betel quid | <br>Current chewer<br>Former chewer<br><br>Current chewer<br>Former chewer | *Overall*<br>5.4<br>6.8<br>*Aboriginal area*<br>30.1<br>21.7 | Information on time and location of first chewing experience |
| Chen et al. (2001) | 6318 residents (3188 M, 3130 F) of I-Lan aged 13–35 years | Betel quid | Overall<br>13–15 years<br>16–18 years<br>19–22 years<br>23–35 years<br><br>Aborigines<br>Non-aborigines | 15.5 M, 1.3 F<br>3.0 M, 0.4 F<br>6.8 M, 0.4 F<br>12.1 M, 1.3 F<br>23.9 M, 2.0 F<br>*Ethnic group*<br>23.8 (35.3 M, 12.8 F)<br>7.4 (14.2 M, 0.5 F) | Prevalence of betel-quid chewing increased with tobacco use, alcohol use, illicit drug use and lower education |
| Yang et al. (2001) | 312 randomly selected subjects (119 M, 193 F) aged ≥ 20 years, aboriginal community in southern Taiwan | Betel quid; stem quid; *lao-hwa* | No chewing<br>Chewing only<br>Chewing/drinking<br>Chewing/smoking<br>Chewing/smoking/drinking<br>Current chewer<br><br>Betel quid<br>Stem quid<br>*Lao-hwa* | [9.3]<br>[47.8]<br>[13.1]<br>[17.0]<br>[12.8]<br><br>69.5 (60.6 M, 78.7 F)<br>Among chewers:<br>64.9 (61.9 M, 67.8 F)<br>56.6 (53.7 M, 59.4 F)<br>10.5 (13.1 M, 8.0 F) | See also Section 2 |
| Kuo et al. (2002) | 905 junior high school students (458 M, 447 F) (12–17 years old) in Taipei City | Betel quid | Grade 7<br>Grade 8<br>Grade 9 | 3.1 (3.5 M, 2.8 F)<br>2.7 (2.7 M, 2.7 F)<br>6.6 (12.3 M, 1.2 F) | |

[a] Betel quid is always without tobacco.

## Adolescents

Using a random sampling design that stratified for district (village, town and city), level of achievement (ordinary versus high), sex and grade, another survey selected 2367 students aged between 12 and 15 years (Lu *et al.*, 1993). The overall prevalence for areca-nut chewing was 4.7%. The prevalence was much higher in boys than in girls, increased with age and decreased with increasing achievement level. Students in village districts had the highest prevalence, followed by those in town and city districts. Also, students with at least one family member who chewed areca nut had a higher prevalence than those with none. Of the chewers, 40.5% were smokers and 21.5% were drinkers. Most chewers used *lao-hwa*.

One study aimed at surveying adolescents was conducted by sampling students from a junior high school and a vocational school (Yang *et al.*, 1996). The prevalence of chewing betel quid was higher among students in the vocational school, among boys, and was related to alcohol use, smoking, drug use and low academic achievement. Male students with the habit of drinking (odds ratio, 4.4; 95% confidence interval [CI], 3.0–6.4 for junior high school; odds ratio, 3.2; 95% CI, 2.0–5.4 for vocational school) or smoking (odds ratio, 9.6; 95% CI, 6.7–14.1 for junior high school; odds ratio, 16.0; 95% CI, 9.8–26.1 for vocational school) were more likely to chew betel quid than those who did not. Junior high school students who had classmates or friends who chewed betel quid had a fivefold higher risk (odds ratio, 5.3; 95% CI, 3.2–8.7) and vocational school students had a fourfold higher risk (odds ratio, 3.8; 95% CI, 2.1–6.8) of chewing betel quid compared with those who did not.

A cross-sectional study was designed to estimate the prevalence of betel-quid chewing for students in five types of senior high schools, one general school and four vocational schools (Ho *et al.*, 2000a). The prevalence in the general school was lower than that in all vocational schools. Among the latter, the highest prevalence was found in the agricultural school, followed by the manufacturing school, medical technician school and commercial school.

Ho *et al.* (2000b) conducted a cross-sectional survey to explore the betel-quid chewing behaviour of junior high school students in Taichung County. The prevalences of current chewers among non-aboriginal students from different areas were 4.0–5.0%. Much higher prevalences were found for current and former chewers among aboriginal students.

In I-Lan (Chen *et al.*, 2001), a northern county of Taiwan, China, the prevalence of betel-quid chewing increased significantly ($p < 0.001$) with age, was higher among aboriginal people compared with non-aboriginal people and was higher among those with lower levels of education.

Junior high school students from Taipei City were asked to complete a questionnaire on substance use (Kuo *et al.*, 2002). Alcoholic beverages were the most frequently used, followed by smoking and areca-nut chewing. There was a sharp increase in areca-nut chewing among boys between grade 8 and grade 9. For all subjects, lower levels of parental education and poorer school competence were associated with higher prevalence of use of areca nut.

### 1.3.8  Myanmar

Lay et al. (1982) briefly described a betel quid known as 'kun-ya' or 'kun', as 'containing the betel nut-areca nut and other ingredients'. Sein et al. (1992) stated that 'there are different patterns of chewing among chewers. The most common form is chewing betel quid which usually consists of a leaf of betel-vine, areca nut, slaked lime and some aroma. Many of the chewers used tobacco in betel quid but some chewed without it.'

### 1.3.9  Thailand

The main constituents of betel quid in Thailand are similar to those found elsewhere in South-east Asia. The leaf of *Piper betle* L., areca nut, lime prepared from limestone or seashells, cutch (catechu) and frequently air- and sun-dried tobacco make up a quid (Simarak et al., 1977). There are, however, a number of variations in betel-quid chewing in Thailand (Reichart, 1995).

Mougne et al. (1982) studied smoking, chewing and drinking habits in northern Thailand. These authors confirmed that the main constituents of the betel quid included areca nut, betel vine and slaked lime. Commonly used additives are cutch, *nang ko*, *dok can* — sandalwood or moonflower bark — and tobacco. Only 2.6% of participants reported occasional betel-quid chewing and 6.8% used it daily. Regular, current chewers were almost entirely men and women over the age of 50 years: 22.7% of women and 18.4% of men in that age range chewed betel quid daily. Nearly all regular chewers consumed between one and seven quids per day. All chewers used betel leaf, slaked lime and *nang ko*; 6% did not use areca nut; 83% used tobacco, 65% used cutch and 2% used *dok can* as further additives. Most chewers used dried areca nut and dried betel leaf. However, fresh nut and leaf were accepted by 30% of the betel-quid chewers.

From 1979 to 1984, Reichart et al. (1987) carried out a study among northern Thai hill tribes (Lahu, Karen, Lisu, Meo) and rural Thai. Prevalence of the betel-quid chewing habit was reported to be 5–44% in men and 9–46% in women. The habit was less predominant among rural Thai than among hill tribes. The Meo tribe did not practise betel-quid chewing; instead, the habit of chewing *miang* (fermented wild tea leaves) was preferred.

The habit of betel-quid chewing seems to be on the decline in Thailand. Reichart (1995) observed that only very few villagers below the age of 35 chewed betel quid, once a universal custom among the Thai. Also, the betel-quid chewing habit has almost vanished from large cities such as Bangkok or Chiang Mai. Axéll et al. (1990) reported that only 3/234 (1.3%) individuals attending the Chiang Mai Dental Faculty reported any use of betel quid. A study on 385 Thai dental students' knowledge of the chewing habit in Thailand revealed that only 62.6% considered this habit as typical for Thailand. It was widely accepted that betel-quid chewing is more common in the provinces (83.6%) and that it is a habit of the elderly (92.2%). The decline in the habit was also demonstrated by the fact that 96.1% of the students' parents and 62.3% of their grandparents did not indulge in the habit. Less than 8% of the students themselves had tried betel quid and none indulged in the habit (Reichart et al., 1999).

### 1.3.10  Lao People's Democratic Republic

Asma (1997) reported on smokeless tobacco in the form of betel-quid chewing among women. The betel quid was reported to consist of areca nut, betel leaf, slaked lime and tobacco. In Lao People's Democratic Republic, betel leaf is smeared with slaked lime, and areca nut and finely cut tobacco are added to the quid, a procedure identical to that in neighbouring countries. Interestingly, camphor is used to remove red stains from the teeth after chewing. The report also mentions 'bark of a certain tree' as an ingredient of betel quid. No epidemiological studies on the betel-quid habit in this country are available.

### 1.3.11  Cambodia

Len Meng (1969) described in detail the habit of betel-quid chewing in Cambodia. The betel quid is composed of areca nut, betel leaf and slaked lime; tobacco is frequently added. Ikeda et al. (1995) published a prevalence study of oral mucosal lesions in 1319 individuals (953 women, 366 men) aged 15–99 years: 31.2% were betel-quid chewers, with a prevalence of 40.6% in women and 6.8% in men. A study of 102 rural Cambodian women who chewed betel quid, aged 39–80 years, and their family members revealed that betel-quid chewing is popular mainly among elderly women while younger people do not seem to have taken up this habit (Reichart et al., 1996). This was confirmed in a later study (Reichart et al., 2002). When questioned about betel-quid chewing habits in Cambodia, 95 Khmer medical and dental students, none of whom indulged in this habit, had poor knowledge on the subject. Betel-quid chewing was practised by 5.3% of their parents and 40% of their grandparents, thus indicating a declining prevalence. Most students agreed that betel-quid chewing is a habit of elderly women (Reichart et al., 1997).

### 1.3.12  Malaysia

Chin and Lee (1970) studied the chewing habits of 212 Indian and 84 Malay betel-quid chewers. The betel quid used by 167 Indian subjects consisted of young betel leaf, slaked stone lime, tobacco and powdered or sliced, dried areca nut, while 45 chewed betel quid without tobacco. Among the Malays, 45 used a betel quid consisting of a more mature betel leaf, *gambir*, slaked stone lime and fresh areca nut without tobacco and 39 chewed without *gambir*.

Gan (1998) studied tobacco use and other oral habits among rural Bajau women in Sabah: 80.2% of the women had some type of chewing habit (Table 27); 77% of the

Table 27. Prevalence of tobacco and areca-nut habits among Bajau women in Malaysia

| Habit | No. | % |
|---|---|---|
| No habit | | [16.5] |
| Chewing | | |
|   Tobacco, betel leaf, areca nut, lime, *gambir* | 183 | 42.4 |
|   Tobacco, betel leaf, areca nut, lime | 137 | 31.8 |
|   Tobacco, betel leaf, areca nut | 1 | 0.2 |
|   Tobacco, lime | 3 | 0.7 |
|   Tobacco, areca nut | 2 | 0.5 |
|   Tobacco only | 6 | 1.4 |
|   Various combinations without tobacco | 14 | 3.2 |
| Smoker (daily and occasional) | | 3.3 |
| Total | 431 | 100.0 |

From Gan (1998)

women used smokeless tobacco compared with 4.3% of the men. The prevalence of tobacco in betel quid increased with increasing age.

In a recent study conducted among adults of six Malaysian estates, 114 of 618 subjects were current betel-quid chewers. The habit was more prevalent among women: 76.3% of the chewers were women and 23.7% were men (Tan *et al.*, 2000).

### 1.3.13 *Singapore*

Among Singaporeans, betel-quid chewing is still practised by some of the older Indian people and Malay women (Cheong, 1984). Kuek *et al.* (1990) also reported the tradition of betel-quid chewing among the Indian community, which represents 6.4% of the entire population. The quid consists of areca nut, betel leaf, slaked lime and a variety of seeds (sesame, clover) and aromas. *Pan masala* is also available on the market.

### 1.3.14 *Indonesia*

Möller *et al.* (1977) described the composition of the betel quid in Indonesia as usually comprising areca nut, betel leaf and slaked lime. Catechu may also be added. Spices such as cardamom or clove may be added for flavour. In most parts of Indonesia, tobacco does not constitute an ingredient of the betel quid itself. Rather, after the betel quid has been chewed for several minutes, a lump of fine-cut tobacco is placed in the labial commissure and finally used to clean the teeth (IARC, 1985a). The habit of betel-quid chewing is more common in women than in men, and is more prevalent in women over the age of 35 compared with those under 35 years of age. The habit is usually acquired between the ages of 15 and 20 years. Recently, Budhy *et al.* (2001) speculated that the habit of chewing betel quid may be dying out in Indonesia.

## 1.3.15 *The Philippines*

According to Davis (1915), betel-quid chewing was an almost universal habit in elderly persons in the Philippines around the turn of the last century. The betel quid *buyo* consisted of betel leaves, areca nut, slaked lime and tobacco, or combinations of these constituents. [No recent data were available to the Working Group.]

## 1.3.16 *Papua New Guinea*

Several types of areca palm are recognized in Papua New Guinea, and their nuts differ in appearance, flavour and strength. Areca nuts are used at all stages, from young and green (preferred) to old, dry and germinating. They are chewed raw and are not cured (MacLennan *et al.*, 1985).

One of the earliest reports describing the habit of areca-nut chewing in Papua New Guinea was by Atkinson *et al.* (1964). The method of chewing is relatively uniform throughout the country, with some occasional minor differences. The nut is chewed when it is either ripe or half ripe, and is chewed in association with slaked lime obtained either from shells or from coral. The lime preparation consists of slaked lime and calcium oxide with some traces of calcium carbonate. In addition, in many areas, wild ginger is added together with betel leaf and/or betel inflorescence; these additions are optional. The method of chewing involves first chewing the nut, then adding slaked lime from a hollow gourd container by means of a dipping stick. The slaked lime-coated stick is wiped against the buccal mucosa and the slaked lime is often entirely removed from the stick when the latter is withdrawn from the mouth between the lips. The mixture then becomes deep red in colour. The slaked lime, as well as the betel leaf and other ingredients, are added more or less continually, according to preference. Tobacco is not added to the betel quid at any stage (Atkinson *et al.*, 1964). In a more recent report, MacLennan *et al.* (1985) confirmed that, in contrast to most of Asia, unwrapped betel quids are used and tobacco is never added to the mixture.

The habit of betel-quid chewing begins early in life. In one survey, the average starting age was just under 3 years, although the amounts used were small until the age of about 12. On a different part of the coast, the average starting age was just under 5 years (Atkinson *et al.*, 1964).

Pindborg *et al.* (1968) examined 1226 Papua and New Guinean villagers. Coastal villagers indulged heavily in areca-nut chewing: 81.4% on the south coast and 95.4% on the north coast chewed areca nut, compared with 26.8% in the highlands. In the coastal regions, the same prevalence was found among men and women, whereas among highlanders, the habit was seen almost exclusively among men.

Many subsequent investigations in Papua New Guinea have confirmed the habit of areca-nut chewing with lime described above (Cooke, 1969; Scrimgeour & Jolley, 1983; Jamrozik, 1985; Talonu, 1989; Martin *et al.*, 1992; Thomas & MacLennan, 1992).

De Costa and Griew (1982) studied betel-quid chewing in pregnant women in Papua New Guinea. None of 400 consecutive mothers, each of whom had made at least one antenatal visit, smoked or drank alcohol but all gave an unambiguous history of having chewed betel quid daily throughout pregnancy. It was not possible to quantify the amount of betel quid consumed.

### 1.3.17 Palau

In Palau, areca nut is chewed in the green unripe state. It is split in half and slaked lime from fire-burned coral is placed in the centre portion of one of the halves. Tobacco which, although now imported, used to be grown on the island, and, less frequently, ginger root or other substances may also be added. These combined ingredients are wrapped in a piece of betel leaf. The excessive saliva produced by chewing this concoction is oranged-red in colour and is spat out on the ground or into a spittoon. Throughout Palau, sets of ingredients for a single chew are sold in many retail stores. These sets consist of half an areca nut, some lime, a piece of betel leaf and half a cigarette, all wrapped in aluminium foil (Ysaol et al., 1996).

All residents of Palau aged 90 years or over ($n = 31$) were interviewed about their chewing habits (Jensen & Polloi, 1988). All had chewed areca nut regularly during their lifetime, but three had quit. Edentulous subjects pulverised the nut prior to use. Twenty-one of 28 current chewers included tobacco in their quid (Table 28).

A study was conducted in Palau in 1995 on a sample of 1110 residents aged 5 years or more in Koror and Airai states (Ysaol et al., 1996). The population sample included more than 5% of each age group and represented 7.9% of the entire population. The proportion of chewers did not differ significantly between age groups, except for the 5–14-year-olds (Table 29). Between 58% and 96% of the respondents in the different age groups added tobacco to the quid, with 87% in the youngest age group. The two youngest age groups reported using significantly less betel leaf. The possible explanations were that

Table 28. Areca-nut and tobacco habits among the very old (≥ 90 years) population of Palau

| Habit | No. |
|---|---|
| Betel-quid chewing | |
|   Current user | 28 |
|   Former user | 3 |
| Current user | |
|   With tobacco | 21 |
|   Without tobacco | 7 |
| Cigarette smoking | |
|   Current smoker | 1 |
|   Nonsmoker | 30 |

From Jensen & Polloi (1988)

Table 29. Proportion of betel-quid chewers and of ingredients used among residents of Palau

|  | Proportion chewing (%) | Proportion (%) of chewers using | | |
| --- | --- | --- | --- | --- |
|  |  | Betel leaf | Slaked lime | Tobacco |
| Age (years) |  |  |  |  |
| 5–14 | 55 | 48[a] | 99 | 87 |
| 15–24 | 77 | 51 | 99 | 96 |
| 25–34 | 86 | 84 | 100 | 88 |
| 35–44 | 89 | 94 | 99 | 72 |
| 45–54 | 82 | 96 | 99 | 68[a] |
| 55–64 | 77[a] | 100 | 100 | 58[a] |
| 65–74 | 86[a] | 96 | 100 | 65[a] |
| > 74 | 84[a] | 100 | 100 | 76[a] |
| Men | 72 | 73 | 100 | 81 |
| Women | 80 | 75 | 99 | 84 |
| Total no. | 845 | 624 | 840 | 700 |

From Ysaol et al. (1996)
[a] Maximum error exceeds 9% at $p < 0.05$. All other proportions have a maximum error of less than 9% at $p < 0.05$.

adolescents have less access to the sometimes scarce leaf or they may wish to avoid the reddened saliva and stained teeth caused by chewing the leaf to escape detection of their habit by disapproving authorities and institutions.

### 1.3.18 Guam

Chewing areca nut (*pugua*) is an old tradition in Guam, particularly among the native Chamorro people (Gerry et al., 1952). Islanders prefer the hard reddish variety of nut but citizens of Micronesia prefer a soft (unripe) areca nut that is succulent and gelatinous (Anon., 2003).

Another account of the chewing habits of Guamanians in 1986 reported that indigenous people chewed either the entire fresh green areca fruit (nut, husk and skin) or the areca nut together with betel leaf. Slake lime is not used during chewing, nor is tobacco (Stich et al., 1986). A comparison with previous reports indicated that this practice had not changed over the last 40–50 years.

### 1.3.19 Others

In various countries, including Nepal, Viet Nam, Kenya and the Solomon Islands, the habit of chewing betel quid or areca nut is known, but no reports are available.

### 1.3.20 *Migrant populations*

Population migration brings a wide variety of traditional products into cultures that were hither to unfamiliar with them. Examination of chewing habits among Asian migrants has shown that the use of areca nut alone or in the form of *pan masala* and *gutka* is prevalent in these communities and that the patterns of use are very similar to the local chewing customs prevalent in their country of origin (Warnakulasuriya *et al.*, 2002). Available data on the prevalence of areca-nut chewing among the migrant populations in South Africa and the United Kingdom are reviewed here. The prevalence of areca-nut use by Indian migrants to the Malay peninsula is described in earlier sections under the relevant geographical region.

#### (a) South Africa

The habit of areca-nut chewing was introduced into South Africa by Indian immigrants in 1860 (Choonoo, 1967). The commonest way to prepare the betel quid is similar to that described for India (Schonland & Bradshaw, 1969). However, the nut is often chewed alone, and red, white or black nuts are preferred by different chewers. Roasted areca nut is preferred. Tobacco is added as a small quantity of coarse shreds by a small minority of chewers, mainly men. Other additives include slaked lime, catechu and flavouring agents. Men and women chewers differ little in their chewing preferences (Table 30).

Shear *et al.* (1967) and Dockrat and Shear (1969) examined the habits of chewing areca nut and betel quid (with or without tobacco), the use of tobacco (smoking) and the intake of snuff among Indian residents (729 men, 1471 women) in the Pretoria–Johannesburg area and in metropolitan Durban. Overall, 912 subjects had a chewing habit, of which 13.7% were men and 86.3% were women. The youngest chewer was aged 2.5 years and the oldest was aged 98 years. The chewers of areca nut or betel quid represented 17.1% of the men and 53% of the women in the population sample.

**Table 30. Prevalence of areca-nut and betel-leaf chewing habit among chewers in Durban, South Africa**

| Habit | Men ($n = 77$) | Women ($n = 479$) |
|---|---|---|
| Chewing habit | | |
| Betel leaf only | 5.2 | 2.9 |
| Areca nut only | 29.9 | 28.8 |
| Areca nut + betel leaf | 64.9 | 68.3 |
| Ingredients added | | |
| Lime | 64.9 | 63.4 |
| Tobacco | 7.8 | 2.8 |
| Catechu | 32.5 | 14.2 |

From Schonland & Bradshaw (1969)

Schonland and Bradshaw (1969) undertook a survey amongst Natal Indians with special reference to betel-quid chewing habits. Of 1842 women of all ages, 30.7% were chewers, while of 1836 men, 5.5% were chewers. The percentage of chewers increased with age in both men and women, 71.9% of women and 10.3% of men aged 60 years or more chewed. Although the mean age at which chewing started was between 20 and 24 years, women started marginally earlier than men. Two-fifths of chewers began the habit before the age of 20 years and a negligible number after the age of 40 years. Also, more women were heavy chewers (four or more times a day) and more men were light or occasional chewers (1–6 times a week). No significant age differences were noted in frequency of chewing, and no significant sex differences in the mean duration of the habit.

Seedat (1985) and Seedat and Van Wyk (1988) described chewing habits in a random sample of 2058 Indian residents of Durban: 186 subjects (9%) were chewers, among whom 162 chewed betel quid without tobacco and 67 chewed more than six times per day. Most chewers swallowed the juice after chewing. The ratio of women to men among chewers was 13:1, and women chewers outnumbered men in all age groups.

In a survey among 78 South African Indian chewers (77 women and one man) aged 19–77 years, four used the raw nut, 39 preferred it boiled and 34 preferred it baked. One woman chewed a nut that could not be identified (Van der Bijl & Van Wyk, 1995).

*(b)    United Kingdom*

Commercially prepared, small foil-packaged products — *pan masala* or gutka — and raw areca nut with other ingredients are readily available through small businesses throughout the United Kingdom, mostly where Asians live (Chauhan, 2000). Several population studies conducted among Asian ethnic minority groups resident in the United Kingdom are reviewed below.

The term 'Asians in Britain' refers to people from the subcontinent of India, Pakistan, Bangladesh and Sri Lanka and to people from East Africa whose families originated in the Indian subcontinent. They constitute almost 3% of the total British population. There is a concentration of Asian ethnic minority groups in some areas of Britain, particularly in Inner and Greater London, West Yorkshire and the West Midlands. The majority of the recently reported prevalence studies examining chewing habits among British Asians have originated from these regions. Just under one half of the Asian ethnic minority population as a whole was born in the United Kingdom and some of these studies have examined chewing patterns of adolescents and young people.

Table 31 summarizes the areca-nut and betel-quid chewing habits recorded from several adult Asian migrant communities living in Britain (Summers *et al.*, 1994; Bedi & Gilthorpe, 1995; Atwal *et al.*, 1996; Pearson *et al.*, 1999; Shetty & Johnson, 1999; Mannan *et al.*, 2000; reviewed in Warnakulasuriya, 2002). It is recognized that the sample sizes used for most of these studies are small and many studies interviewed selected community groups that could be labelled as convenient samples, thereby introducing biases related to sampling and data collection. It is clear from the studies that sampled the British Bangladeshi population (Summers *et al.*, 1994; Bedi & Gilthorpe, 1995; Pearson *et al.*,

Table 31. Prevalence of areca-nut and betel-quid chewing among adult Asian migrant ethnic groups resident in the United Kingdom

| Region | No. of samples | Community | Habit | Prevalence (%) |
|---|---|---|---|---|
| Yorkshire | 296 | Bangladeshi, women | Pan masala | 4 |
| | | | Betel quid | 95 |
| | | | Betel leaf | 100 |
| | | | Areca nut | 97 |
| | | | Lime | 90 |
| | | | Tobacco | 69 |
| | | | Zarda | 27 |
| Birmingham | 334 | Bangladeshi, men and women | Betel quid[a] | |
| | 158 | | Men | 92 |
| | | | Women | 96 |
| | | | With tobacco | |
| | | | Men | 37 |
| | | | Women | 81 |
| London, East | 158 | Bangladeshi, men and women | Betel quid[a,b] | 78 |
| | 993 | | Betel quid with tobacco | 75 |
| London, West | 181 | Mixed Asian | Betel quid[a] | 47 |
| | | | With tobacco | |
| | | | Men | 33 |
| | | | Women | 5 |
| London, North-West | 367 | Mixed Asian | Betel quid[a] | 27 |
| | | | Men | 27 |
| | | | Women | 27 |
| Leicester | 519 | Mixed Asian | Betel quid[a] | 33 |

Adapted from Mannan et al. (2000); Warnakulasuriya (2002)
[a] Betel quid with or without tobacco
[b] More women than men added tobacco to the quid.

1999; Mannan et al., 2000) that their betel-quid chewing habits are widespread (75–96%), whereas the prevalence of the habits is lower among mixed Asian groups (27–47%).

Three studies (Osman et al., 1997; Farrand et al., 2001; Prabhu et al., 2001) that examined the betel-quid chewing habits among Asian adolescents living in Britain suggest that the habit is prevalent at a young age (Table 32). The majority of the younger age groups were occasional chewers. However, on reaching school-leaving age, they had become regular users of areca nut and often added chewing tobacco to the quid mixture. Longitudinal studies involving young persons have not been reported.

Comparison of chewing and tobacco habits among first- and second-generation Asian men living in Leicester suggests that betel-quid chewing habits and use of tobacco are continued by cultural bonding long after migration of ethnic groups (Vora et al., 2000).

**Table 32. Prevalence of areca-nut and betel-quid chewing by adolescent Asian ethnic groups resident in the United Kingdom**

| Reference | Region | No. of samples | Age range (years) | Community | Habit | Prevalence (%) |
|---|---|---|---|---|---|---|
| Osman et al. (1997) | Luton | 1058 | 11–16 | Mixed Asian | Betel quid[a] | 44 |
| Farrand et al. (2001) | London, East | 204 | 12–18 | Bangladeshi | Betel quid[a] Men Women With tobacco | 28 30 27 12 |
| Prabhu et al. (2001) | London, East | 704 | 11–15 | 70% Bangladeshi | Areca nut | 77 |

[a] Betel quid with or without tobacco

Examining distinct ethnic groups interviewed in this study, it is clear that Sikhs from either the first or second generation do not indulge in tobacco or betel-quid chewing while the Hindus from both generations continue chewing betel quid or *pan masala* in their country of residence. Muslims and Jains of the second generation, on the other hand, were less likely to chew these products.

(i) *Tobacco in betel quid*

In the three studies of adolescents quoted above, the majority began chewing betel quid without tobacco but some converted to adding tobacco to the quid during senior school ages or used commercially packaged products, which predominantly contained areca nut and tobacco (*gutka*). The social pressures on young Bangladeshi women in the United Kingdom to introduce chewing tobacco to their betel quid are presented by Bedi and Gilthorpe (1995). Among older Asian adults, up to 50% are recorded as adding tobacco to the betel quid when this was made up at home according to their own recipe. For older Bangladeshi women, it may reach close to 90% (Rudat, 1994; Bedi, 1996). A further proportion predominantly chewed sweetened tobacco products such as *zarda*. With the emergence of commercially packaged areca products, it is increasingly difficult to disentangle the effect of tobacco, as these products are often mixtures of sun-dried tobacco and cured areca nut.

(ii) *Determinants of chewing habits among Asians*

Ethnic variations in the chewing of betel quid and tobacco among Asian migrants in the United Kingdom are recognized in several studies. The predominant group retaining chewing habits in Britain are Bangladeshi adults (Williams *et al.*, 2002). Socioeconomic status and education certainly seem to have effects on the prevalence of the habit. Among Indians, people who are educated beyond the age of 16 years are more likely to chew products containing tobacco, while the reverse effect was found in the Bangladeshi group (Khan *et al.*, 2000). Sex differences are small (Shetty & Johnson, 1999) and recent data indicate that chewing practices have extended to second-generation Asians born in Britain (Osman *et al.*, 1997; Vora *et al.*, 2000).

(c)   *Others*

There are no population prevalence studies on areca-nut chewing habits among migrants settled in other western countries.

In North America, reports on chewing areca nut or betel quid are limited. Pickwell *et al.* (1994) reported on 10 women refugees from Cambodia in California indulging in the habit of chewing. One Canadian publication refers to a 4-year-old child who developed oral submucous fibrosis following areca-nut use (Hayes, 1985).

### 1.3.21  *Placement of the quid in the mouth*

The entire oral environment is likely to be exposed to the effects of chewing substances. However, the quid may be in close contact with the oral mucosa for prolonged periods and the site of placement of the quid may correspond to the site of oral lesions.

Areca nut and betel quid are masticatory substances chewed and often retained in the mouth in the lower buccal sulcus and retromolar areas.

In Papua New Guinea, slaked lime is applied to the buccal mucosa and the oral commissure during the chewing of areca nut.

## 1.4   Regulations and legislation

Regulations and legislation on commercial products containing areca nut have largely been overlooked until recently. The ready availability of pre-packaged mixed areca products and free access suggest the desirability of regulation. Raw areca nut available for personal consumption (Croucher & Islam, 2002) and for export in 50–100-kg sacks can be located on the internet.

Areca is usually listed as an edible fruit and is therefore normally sold as a food substance, although its food value is uncertain. It is also claimed to be a mouth freshner. Other minor uses include its supposed medicinal values as an anti-parasitic agent, through a popular belief that the consumption of areca compounds after a meal assists the digestion of food and its traditional use as a toothpaste. In China, areca nut is used in traditional Chinese medicine and is not regulated.

Any regulations related to the import and sale of areca nut in non-producing countries have to be determined by the Food Safety Acts of individual countries. Foods imported from another country that are intended for human consumption must meet the general food safety requirements (e.g. from the Food and Safety Acts in the United Kingdom). In general, these requirements are that any food item must not be: (*a*) rendered injurious to health; (*b*) unfit for human consumption due to contamination and adulteration.

## Regulation of import and sale of areca-containing products

(a)    *India*

On 1 August 2002, the Commissioner for Food and Drug Administration and Food (Health) Authority, Maharashtra State (Sharma, 2002), issued a gazette notification banning the manufacture, sale and storage of *gutka* and *pan masala* or any similar product containing or not containing tobacco. The law was enforced based on the powers conferred by Clause iv of Section 7 of the prevention of Food Adulteration Act of 1954 in the interest of public health, and the prohibition of these food articles will remain in force for a period of 5 years.

In India, a warning label is required on commercial areca-nut and tobacco products, but there are no regulations about the size of the letters. *Gutka* has been banned by several state governments: Tamil Nadu, Adhra Pradesh and Goa. Several other states are at various stages of passing laws to ban *gutka* or are in court after being challenged by the industry. A recommendation that gutka should be banned nationwide has been made to the central government by the Central Committee on Food Safety.

(b)    *North America*

Areca nut figures on the list of herbs that are unacceptable as a non-medicinal ingredient in oral use products (Health Canada, 1995). The sale of areca products has been banned in Canada as a result of the link between arecoline and mutagenic effects (see Section 4.4.2(*a*)(iv)). The US Food and Drug Administration maintains an import alert within the USA, the main concerns being adulteration and addition of unsafe food additives (Croucher & Islam, 2002). In 1976, the US Government announced a ban on interstate traffic of areca nut (Burton-Bradley, 1978).

(c)    *European Union*

Within the European Union (excluding Sweden), there is legislation banning the sale of tobacco products for oral use, particularly those presented in sachet portions or porous sachets, with the exception of those intended to be smoked or chewed. However, there are no specific laws regulating or banning the sale of areca products, even when mixed with smokeless tobacco, as chewing tobacco is excluded from the directive (Council of the European Communities, 2001).

## United Kingdom

In the United Kingdom, there is no law to regulate the import or sale of products containing areca nut and at present numerous areca preparations, with or without tobacco, are commercially available (Bedi, 1996; Vora *et al.*, 2000). The Department of Trade and Industry classifies these products as sweets (Hogan, 2000). Labelling and a list of ingredients on the packaging are sometimes non-existent. Several studies have shown that, in most outlets, sales are unrestricted to minors (Shetty & Johnson, 1999; Warnakulasuriya *et al.*, 2002). A study by Trading Standards Officers in Birmingham revealed that children under the age of 16 were able to purchase *gutka* easily (National Centre for Transcultural Oral Health, 2001). Only a few areca products give specific health warnings on the dangers of chewing areca nut, although most carry the statutory health warning regarding added tobacco. In 20 commercially processed and packaged areca-nut products on sale in the the United Kingdom, only three carried a health warning related to oral cancer; none warned about submucous fibrosis or potential addiction (Trivedy, 2001).

(*d*)   *Limited bans in other countries*

In the late 1970s, the Public Services of Papua New Guinea issued a ban on betel-quid chewing in government offices (Burton-Bradley, 1978). Possession of areca nut in the California public school system is grounds for suspension (Croucher & Islam, 2002). In Singapore, spitting in public places can lead to a fine, indirectly discouraging the practice of betel-quid and areca-nut chewing (Cheong, 1984).

# 2.  Studies of Cancer in Humans

## 2.1  Oral cancer

### 2.1.1  *India, Pakistan and Sri Lanka*

(*a*)   *Descriptive studies and case series*

In this section, the subsites included in oral cancer were rarely specified, but mostly included lip, tongue and mouth. The reports summarized in the previous monograph on betel-quid and areca-nut chewing (IARC, 1985a) are given in Table 33, which shows that the percentage of oral cancer among all cancers diagnosed in hospitals or groups of hospitals in Asia was always much higher than that usually found in western countries (3–5%; Parkin *et al.*, 2003), where the habit of chewing betel quid, with or without tobacco, is virtually unknown.

In many descriptive studies, investigators have obtained histories of chewing betel quid with tobacco from series of patients with oral cancer (Table 34). In most of these studies, the percentage of patients who practise chewing habits is extremely large. Several authors also commented that the cancer generally develops at the place where the quid is kept.

A high incidence of oral, oro- and hypopharyngeal cancer is observed in regions of the world where a high proportion of the population practises betel-quid chewing (Parkin *et al.*, 2003). Of the 267 000 new oral cancers estimated to occur around the year 2000 throughout the world, 128 000 (48%) occur in South and South-East Asia; of the 123 000 cases of oro- and hypopharyngeal cancer estimated to occur globally annually, 63 000 (51.2%) are accounted for in South and South-Easts Asia (Figures 3 and 4).

In India, the age-standardized incidence rates (ASR) of oral cancer (ICD 9: 140–145) per 100 000 population are 12.8 in men and 7.5 in women (Ferlay *et al.*, 2001).

Table 33. Chewing habit and percentage of oral cancer among all cancers

| Location | Habit | All cancers (years) | Oral cancer | Reference |
|---|---|---|---|---|
| Papua New Guinea | Betel quid without tobacco | 1175 (1958–63) | 209 (17.8%) | Atkinson et al. (1964) |
| Papua New Guinea | Betel quid without tobacco | 2300 (1958–65) | (17.1%); 29 (9%) oral cancers were verrucous carcinoma | Cooke (1969) |
| Papua New Guinea | Betel quid without tobacco | 6186 (1958–73) | 890 (14.4%) | Henderson & Aiken (1979) |
| Travancore, South India | Betel quid with tobacco | 1700 (5 years) | 989 (58%)[a] | Bentall (1908) |
| Neyoor, South India | Betel quid with tobacco | 377 epithelial cancers (2 years) | 346 (91.5%)[b] | Fells (1908) |
| Mumbai, India | Betel quid with tobacco | 2880 carcinomas (1941–43) | 1000 (34.7%)[c] | Khanolkar (1944) |
| Mumbai, India (Parsees) | Betel-quid chewing very rare | 1705 (1941–65) | 160 (9.4%)[d] | Paymaster & Gangadharan (1970) |
| Sri Lanka | Betel quid | 2344 (1928–48) | 1130 (48.2%)[e] | Balendra (1949) |
| Thailand | Betel quid | 1100 | 155 (14.1%)[f] | Piyaratn (1959) |
| Malaysia (Indians) | Betel quid with tobacco | – | 219[g] | Marsden (1960) |
| Singapore | Betel quid with tobacco | 7131 | (8%)[h] | Muir (1962) |
| Philippines | Betel leaf, tobacco chewing, reverse cigarette smoking | – (1957–61) | 186 | Tolentino et al. (1963) |
| Malaysia | Betel quid with and without tobacco | 4369 (1961–63) | 476 (10.9%)[i] | Ahluwalia & Duguid (1966) |
| Indians | Betel quid with tobacco | 912 | 306 (33.6%) | |
| Malays | Betel quid without tobacco | 777 | 74 (9.5%) | |
| Bangladesh | Betel quid | 3650 | 672 (18.4%)[j] | Huq (1965) |
| Pakistan | Betel quid with tobacco, cigarette smoking | 14 350 (1960–71) | 2608 (18.2%) | Zaidi et al. (1974) |

[a] Lip, tongue, buccal mucosa
[b] Epithelial cancers of the buccal cavity
[c] Lip, buccal mucosa, alveolus, tongue, palate
[d] Lip, tongue, alveolus, floor of mouth, buccal mucosa, palate
[e] Cheek, tongue, palate and tonsil, jaw, floor of mouth, pahrynx and larynx, lip
[f] Lip, tongue, oral cavity
[g] 'Betel cancers'
[h] Buccal cavity and pharynx
[i] Lip, tongue, floor of mouth, cheek, palate
[j] Buccal cavity

Table 34. Case series of oral cancer and chewing habits

| Location | Habit | All cancers (years) | Oral cancer | Reference |
|---|---|---|---|---|
| South-west Pacific Islands – New Britain | Betel quid without tobacco | 60 (1921–40) | 7 (11.7%) | Eisen (1946) |
| Papua New Guinea | Betel quid without tobacco (98%) | – | 110 | Farago (1963a) |
| Papua New Guinea | Betel quid without tobacco (129/130) | 1160 (1960–61) | 210 (18.1%) | Farago (1963b) |
| Mumbai, India | Tobacco and betel-quid chewing (excessive in 35%) | 3627 intra-oral malignant tumours (1941–47) | 650 (buccal mucosa) | Paymaster (1956) |
| Guntur, India | Betel-quid chewers; 9 (3.6%) Betel-quid + tobacco chewers; 29 (12%) Tobacco chewers; 20 (8%) | – (1957–59) | 250 (17.4%) (oral + pharyngeal) | Padmavathy & Reddy (1960) |
| Mumbai, India | 36.5% chewers (tobacco + betel) 21.9% chewers and smokers 23.2% smokers 18.4% no habit (among oral-cavity tumour patients) | 30 219 carcinomas (1941–55) | 14 162 (46.9%) (oral + pharyngeal) | Paymaster (1962) |
| Mumbai, India | 100% tobacco + betel-quid chewers 55.7% chewers and smokers | 519 | 210 (40.5%) (oropharyngeal) | Agarwal & Arora (1964) |
| Madras, India | 76.7% chewers with tobacco 18.6% without tobacco 4.7% non-chewers | 13 626 (1950–59) | 6728 (49.4%) (oral cavity) | Sidiq et al. (1964) |
| Madras, India | 95% betel-quid chewers (83% with tobacco) 34% smokers | 3529 (1962–63) | 362 (10%) (buccal mucosa) | Singh & von Essen (1966) |
| Mainpuri, India | 26.6% tobacco with lime 15.6% smokers 53.9% both 3.9% no habit 2% betel quid | – (1950–62) | 154 (oral + oropharyngeal) | Wahi et al. (1966) |
| Agra, India | 32.5% tobacco with lime 30.1% smokers 18.1% both 19.3% no habit 12% betel quid | – | 83 (oral + oropharyngeal) | Wahi et al. (1966) |

Table 34 (contd)

| Location | Habit | All cancers (years) | Oral cancer | Reference |
|---|---|---|---|---|
| Agra, India | 85% betel quid with tobacco 51% smokers (85 gingival cancer patients) | 6790 (1957–65) | 3173 (46.7%) (intra-oral), 85 (gingival) | Srivastava & Sharma (1968) |
| Jabalpur, India | 84% (100 oral cancers) tobacco chewers 28% smokers | – (1958–67) | 814 (oral + pharyngeal) (33.8%) | Gandagule & Agarwal (1969) |
| Kanpur, India | 14.8% betel quid without tobacco 22% betel quid with tobacco 49% tobacco + lime 5.4% smoking 5% smoking and chewing | 2332 (1958–66) | 630 (27%) (oral) | Samuel et al. (1969) |
| Philippines | 52 buyo[a] chewers 2 non-chewers 21 uncertain | – | 75 (49 of the cheek) | Davis (1915) |
| Thailand | 100% betel quid + tobacco | 53 (1922–23) | 25 (47%) (oral) | Mendelson & Ellis (1924) |
| Taiwan | 59% betel-quid chewers 82% smokers | – (1953–1963) | 89 | Chang (1964) |
| Sri Lanka | Only 3 (1.5%) betel-quid chewers among cases 38 smokers | – (1945 on) 400 new cases seen during 3 months in 1960 | 508 (buccal mucosa) 214 (53.5%) (buccal mucosa) | Balendra (1965) |

[a] Buyo can consist of betel leaves, areca nut, slaked lime and tobacco or any combination of these constituents.

**Figure 3. Cancer of the oral cavity (ICD-9: 140–145) in (a) men and (b) women**

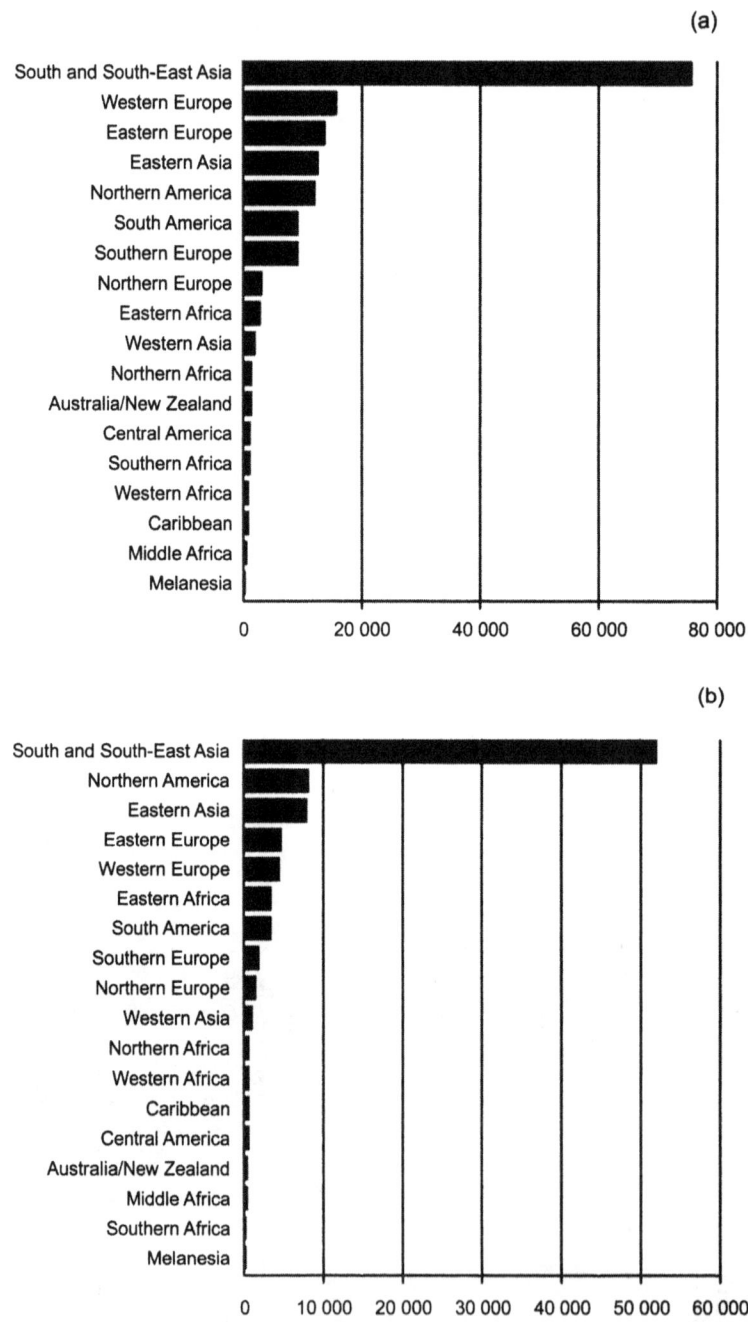

From Ferlay *et al.* (2001) – GLOBOCAN 2000

## Figure 4. Oropharyngeal and hypopharyngeal cancers (ICD-9: 146, 148–149) in (a) men and (b) women

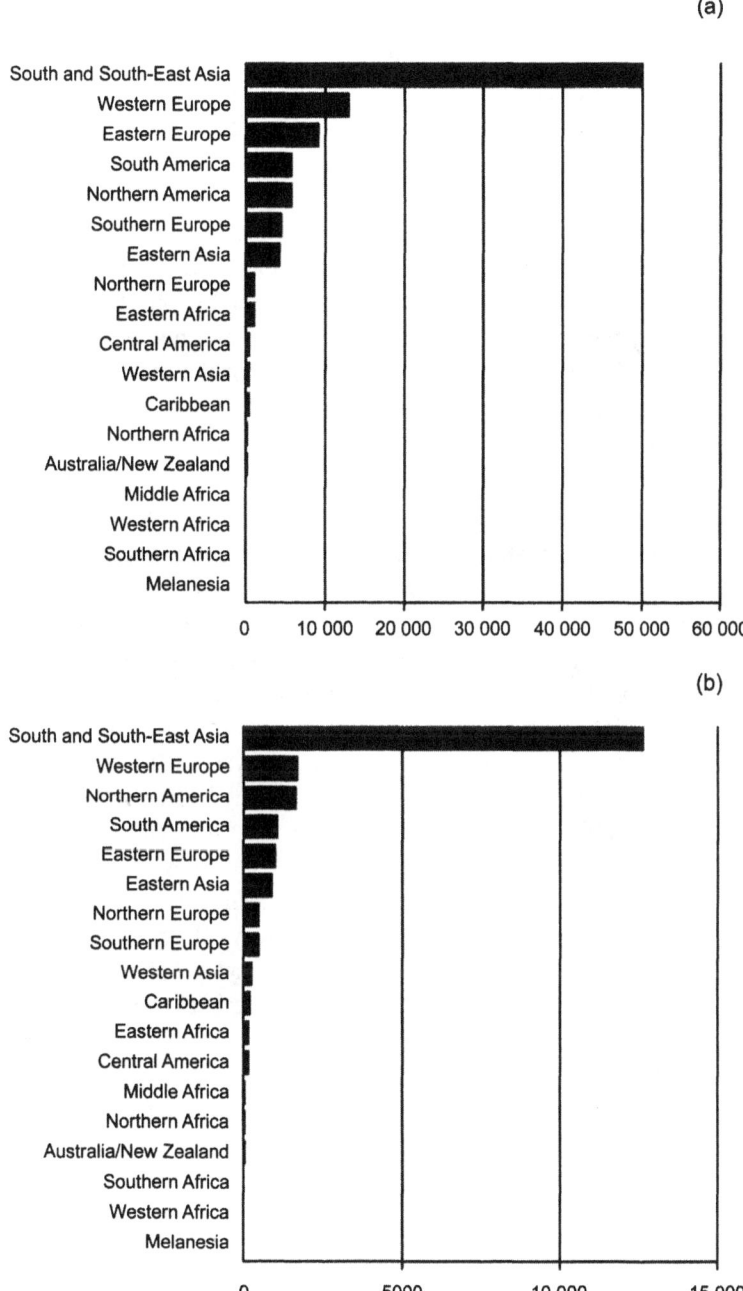

From Ferlay et al. (2001) – GLOBOCAN 2000

A study from Mumbai, India, in 1993–97 compared the incidence rates of oral cancer among Parsi and non-Parsi communities (Yeole et al., 2001). Parsis form a very small subgroup (about 0.8%) of the population of the city of Mumbai; few smoke and very few chew (for religious reasons), whereas chewing and smoking are common in the population of Mumbai as a whole. The annual age-adjusted incidence rates (per 100 000) in 1995 of cancers at several sites were lower among Parsi men than among the male population of Mumbai as a whole: tongue and mouth, 4.5 versus 11.9; pharynx, 2.6 versus 10.6; oesophagus, 2.6 versus 8.7; stomach, 2.8 versus 6.6; larynx, 2.2 versus 7.2; and lung, 4.2 versus 12.6.

Gupta (1999) reported an increase in the incidence rates of mouth cancers (ICD 9: 143–145) in 1995 compared with 1983–87 among inhabitants under the age of 50 years in the city of Ahmedabad, India, which is consistent with the hypothesis of an increase in oral cancer among the young due to increased use of *gutka* and *pan masala*.

In Karachi, Pakistan's largest city, the ASR of cancer of the oral cavity per 100 000 population is 17.9 in men and 16.3 in women (Bhurgri, 2001).

(b) *Cohort studies*

A population-based prospective study was reported by Wahi (1968) from a temporary cancer registration system established in Uttar Pradesh (Mainpuri district), India. Over a period of 30 months (1964–66), a total of 346 cases of oral and oropharyngeal cancer were detected and confirmed histologically. Exposure data were obtained from these patients by questionnaire, and a house-to-house interview survey was conducted on a 10% cluster sample of the district population. The numbers in various exposure categories were then extrapolated to the population as a whole and used as denominators for calculating oral cancer period prevalence. Chewing *Mainpuri* tobacco was distinguished from other chewing habits. Prevalence rates for the two kinds of chewing habits and for combinations of alcohol and smoking habits are summarized in Table 35. Prevalence rates were highest among users of *Mainpuri* tobacco and higher for all other chewing habits than for no chewing habit, after adjusting for smoking and drinking. The strength of the association between chewing and oral cancer was studied in many ways [frequently intercorrelated] (Table 36) and was reported to be positive by every criterion. [The Working Group of *IARC Monographs* Volume 37 noted that differences in age between cancer patients and the population sample do not seem to have been taken into account; it is possible that the prevalence of habits within the population was age-dependent.]

Mehta *et al.* (1972a) examined a cohort of 4734 policemen in Mumbai, India, for oral precancers, at baseline in 1959, and 5 and 10 years later. Of the 3674 policemen followed successfully, 49% chewed (mostly betel quid with tobacco) and 12% chewed and smoked. Oral cancer was found in one man who chewed and smoked.

Of 57 518 textile industry workers in Ahmedabad, India, examined in the first phase of a study conducted in 1967–71, Bhargava *et al.* (1975) re-examined 43 654 workers 2 years later. They diagnosed 13 new cases of oral cancer, all of which had developed among individuals chewing betel quid with tobacco and/or smoking tobacco (Table 37).

Table 35. Numbers of oral cancers and prevalence per 1000 population in a study in Mainpuri district, India[a]

| Habit | No tobacco | | Mainpuri tobacco | | Other kinds of tobacco | |
|---|---|---|---|---|---|---|
| | No. of cases | Prevalence | No. of cases | Prevalence | No. of cases | Prevalence |
| No habit | 27 | 0.18 | 59 | 4.51 | 32 | 0.80 |
| Alcohol drinking | 0 | 0 | 6 | 6.59 | 2 | 1.08 |
| Smoking | 54 | 0.57 | 78 | 8.12 | 47 | 1.76 |
| Drinking and smoking | 9 | 1.56 | 30 | 11.45 | 2 | 0.58 |
| Total | 90 | 0.36 | 173 | 6.60 | 83 | 1.15 |

[a]From Wahi (1968)

Gupta et al. (1980) followed a random sample of 10 287 individuals in Kerala (Ernakulam district) for a period of 10 years (1966–77) in house-to-house surveys, with a follow-up rate of 87%. Chewing betel quid with tobacco was a common habit in that area, and all 13 new cases of oral cancer were diagnosed among either chewers only or chewers who also smoked. The person–years method was used for data analysis and incidence rates were age-adjusted (Table 37).

Apparently healthy subjects aged 35 years or older in rural Kerala were included from 1995–98 in an intervention trial, in which 59 894 individuals formed the screened group and 54 707 formed the non-screened group. Those in the screened group who chewed betel quid with tobacco, smoked or drank alcohol were advised to stop their habit; 31 and 44% of subjects in the screened and non-screened groups, respectively, reported no tobacco (chewing betel quid with tobacco or smoking) or alcohol habit. About 3 years after the start of the study, 47 cases of oral cancer (incidence, 56.1/100 000 person–years) were identified in the screened group and 16 (incidence, 20.3/100 00 person–years) in the non-screened group (Sankaranarayanan et al., 2000).

(c)   Case–control studies

Case–control studies for oral (comprising gum, floor of the mouth, buccal mucosa and palate; the tongue may also be included) and other cancers and their association with chewing betel quid with or without tobacco are described in Table 38 and the dose–response relationships found in these studies are summarized in Table 39. [Data for men and women were combined and relative risks were calculated by the Working Group of IARC Monographs Volume 37 from the data given in the papers published up to 1985, unless provided by the authors]. The derived relative risk estimates for use of betel quid ranged from 0.1 to 45.9 in different studies.

A case–control study was reported by Shanta and Krishnamurthi (1959), consisting of 206 cancers of the buccal mucosa and the floor of the mouth and 278 randomly selected non-cancerous controls. The proportion of betel and areca-nut chewers was 8.7% in the cancer group and 51.8% in the control group. [The percentages of habits given for cases as well as for controls were inconsistent.]

### Table 36. Prevalence of oral cancer by chewing habit

| Chewing habit | Estimated population | No. of cases | Prevalence per 1000 |
|---|---|---|---|
| Total | 349 710 | 346 | 0.99 |
| Non-chewers of tobacco | 251 330 | 90 | 0.36 |
| *Frequency of tobacco chewing* | | | |
| Occasionally | 11 680 | 5 | 0.43 |
| Daily | 86 700 | 251 | 2.90 |
| *Age started chewing (years)* | | | |
| ≥ 30 | 38 290 | 69 | 1.80 |
| 25–29 | 15 000 | 28 | 1.87 |
| 20–24 | 22 230 | 61 | 2.74 |
| 15–19 | 16 030 | 58 | 3.62 |
| 5–14 | 6 870 | 40 | 5.92 |
| *Retention of each quid (min)* | | | |
| 1–20 | 69 030 | 133 | 1.93 |
| 21–30 | 18 680 | 69 | 3.69 |
| ≥ 31 | 9 650 | 53 | 5.49 |
| *Period of exposure (min) per day* | | | |
| Up to 99 | 53 720 | 123 | 2.29 |
| 100–299 | 33 670 | 90 | 2.67 |
| 300–499 | 9 400 | 31 | 3.30 |
| ≥ 500 | 2 230 | 12 | 5.38 |
| *Sleeping with quid in mouth* | | | |
| Never | 85 790 | 175 | 2.04 |
| Occasionally | 10 790 | 58 | 5.38 |
| Daily | 1 740 | 23 | 13.22 |
| *Type of tobacco chewed* | | | |
| *Pattiwala* | 71 610 | 84 | 1.17 |
| *Mainpuri* and *Pattiwala* | 8 950 | 37 | 4.13 |
| *Mainpuri* | 17 160 | 134 | 7.81 |
| Other (*Kapuri, Rampuri, Moradabadi*) | 760 | 1 | 1.32 |
| *Amount of money (paisa)*[a] *spent on tobacco per day* | | | |
| 0–6 | 67 240 | 161 | 2.39 |
| 7–37 | 19 710 | 77 | 3.91 |
| 38–74 | 680 | 4 | 5.88 |
| 75–100 | 260 | 9 | 34.62 |

From Wahi (1968)
[a] 1 paisa = 0.01 rupee

Table 37. Chewing and smoking habits and oral cancer in two cohort studies, India

| Habit | Ahmedabad[a] | | | Ernakulam[b] | | |
|---|---|---|---|---|---|---|
| | Number re-examined[c] | New oral cancers | Incidence per 100 000 | Person–years | New oral cancers | Age-adjusted incidence per 100 000 |
| Chewing | 3 266 | 1 | 31 | 23 416 | 9 | 23 |
| Chewing and smoking | 16 881 | 6 | 36 | 8 476 | 4 | 32 |
| Smoking | 15 378 | 6 | 39 | 20 222 | 0 | 0 |
| None | 7 065 | 0 | 0 | 30 962 | 0 | 0 |

[a] Industrial workers aged 35 years and over; data from Bhargava *et al.* (1975)
[b] House-to-house survey of individuals aged 15 years and over; data from Gupta *et al.* (1980)
[c] Approximately 2 years after the first examination

Chandra (1962) reported a study of 450 cases of cancer of the cheek (287 men, 163 women) and 500 hospital visitor controls (410 men, 90 women) conducted in 1955–59. The proportion of betel-quid chewers was 5.6% and that of chewers of betel quid with tobacco was 23.3% among male cases. Corresponding proportions among male controls were 13.4 and 10.7%, respectively. The proportions among female cases were 18.4 and 43.5% and those among female controls were 16.7 and 18.9%, respectively.

In another case–control study, Shanta and Krishnamurthi (1963) reported on 882 cancer cases (628 men, 254 women) and 400 (300 men, 100 women) controls. Cancer sites included lip (12 men, seven women), buccal mucosa (293 men, 152 women), anterior tongue (69 men, 18 women), posterior tongue (48 men, four women), pharynx (130 men, 25 women), hypopharynx (18 men, 12 women) and oesophagus (57 men, 36 women). For cancer of these different sites, the proportion of male cases who chewed betel quid without tobacco ranged from 8.4 to 38.5% and that among male controls was 49.1%; the proportion of female cases who chewed betel quid without tobacco ranged from 12.4 to 55.5% and that among female controls was 55.5%. [The authors pointed out that most chewers of betel quid without tobacco were occasional chewers and the percentage was high because it was very hard to find Indians who had not chewed betel quid without tobacco at one time or another. They opined that betel-quid and areca-nut chewing was of no statistical significance in etiology and is only a reflection of habit in the general population.]

Hirayama (1966) reported a case–control study of oral and oropharyngeal cancers conducted in India and Sri Lanka. The study included 545 cases of cancer of the buccal mucosa (369 men, 176 women), 143 cases of cancer of the anterior tongue (117 men, 26 women), 37 cases of cancer of the palate (28 men, nine women), 102 cases of cancer of the oropharynx (81 men, 21 women) and 440 controls (277 men, 163 women). The proportion of men who chewed areca nut (reported as betel nut) was 0.8% for cancer of the buccal

Table 38. Case–control studies of oral[a] and other cancers and their association with chewing of betel quid

| Location (years) | Cancer site[b] | No. of cases | Habit | No. of controls | Habit | Relative risk (95% CI) | Reference |
|---|---|---|---|---|---|---|---|
| **Up to 1985** | | | | | | | |
| Travancore, India | Lip | 100 | Q, 98% | 100 | Q, 66% | 25.2 | Orr (1933) |
| Mumbai, India (1952–54) | Base of tongue, oropharynx, hypopharynx, oesophagus | 289 (M + F) (oral) 551 (M + F) (base of tongue, oropharynx, hypopharynx, oesophagus) | Q, 12% Q + S, 39% S, 47% (M) | 400 400 | Q, 9% Q + S, 24% S, 50% (M) | Q, 10.2 Q, 4.0 | Sanghvi et al. (1955) |
| Assam, India (1954–55) | Lip, pharynx, oesophagus, larynx | 238 (108 larynx) | Q, 97% | 3678 | Q, 79% | 7.6 | Sarma (1958) |
| Mumbai, India (1952–54) | Base of tongue, oropharynx, lip | 371 95 (oral) 276 (oropharynx and base of tongue | Q, 12% Q + S, 38% S, 48% Q, 28% Q + S, 42% S, 18% Q, 5% Q + S, 36% S, 58% | 288 288 | Q, 9% Q + S, 24% S, 50% | Q, 8.0 Q, 10.0 | Khanolkar (1959) |
| Madras, India | Only cheek and floor of the mouth | 206 | BQ, 9% BQ + T, 85% S, 26% | 278 | BQ, 52% BQ + T, 13% S, 47% | BQ, 0.1 BQ + T, 39 | Shanta & Krishnamurthi (1959) |

**Table 38 (contd)**

| Location (years) | Cancer site[b] | No. of cases | Habit | No. of controls | Habit | Relative risk (95% CI) | Reference |
|---|---|---|---|---|---|---|---|
| Calcutta, India (1955–59) | Cheek | 450 (M + F) | BQ, 6% (M)<br>BQ + T, 23% (M)<br>T, 6% (M)<br>BQ, 18% (F)<br>BQ + T, 44% (F)<br>T, 3% (F) | 500 | BQ, 13% (M)<br>BQ + T, 11% (M)<br>T, 40% (M)<br>BQ, 17% (F)<br>BQ + T, 19% (F)<br>T, 2% (F) | BQ, 0.8 (M)<br>BQ + T, 2.5 (M)<br>T, 1.5 (M)<br>BQ, 1.1 (F)<br>BQ + T, 3.3 (F)<br>T, 1.4 (F) | Chandra (1962) |
| Madras, India | Lip, oropharynx, hypopharynx, oesophagus, tongue | 882 | BQ, 20% (M)<br>BQ + T, 64% (M)<br>BQ, 50% (F)<br>BQ + T, 71% (F) | 400 | BQ, 40% (M)<br>BQ + T, 9% (M)<br>BQ, 56% (F)<br>BQ + T, 11% (F) | BQ, 0.3 (M)<br>BQ + T, 17.2 (M)<br>BQ, 0.8 (F)<br>BQ + T, 20.1 (F) | Shanta & Krishnamurthi (1963) |
| Agra, India (1950–62) | Lip, tongue, tonsil | 821 | T, 73%<br>T + S, 38%<br>S, 55% | 1916 | T, 12%<br>T + S, 6%<br>S, 28% | T, 41.2 | Wahi et al. (1965) |
| Sri Lanka | Oesophagus only | 111 | Q, 81% | 1088 | Q, 30% | 9.9 | Stephen & Uragoda (1970) |
| Varanasi, India (1966–70) | – | 206 | BQ + T, 39%<br>T, 50% | 100 | Q, 25% | 27.0 | Khanna et al. (1975) |
| Mumbai, India | Anterior two-thirds of tongue, lip | 214 M | Q, 29%<br>Q + S, 32%<br>S, 31% | 230 | Q, 15%<br>Q + S, 20%<br>S, 48% | Q, 4.2 | Notani & Sanghvi (1976) |
| **1985–2003** | | | | | | | |
| Kerala, India (1983–84) | Tongue<br>Floor of mouth | 158 (M)<br>70 (F) | BQ + T, 58% (M)<br>BQ + T, 76% (F) | 314 (M)<br>139 (F) | BQ + T, 30% (M)<br>BQ + T, 39% (F) | BQ + T, 6.1 (3.3–11.4) (M)<br>BQ + T + S, 7.02 (3.6–13.5) (M)<br>S, 4.98 (2.5–9.8) (M) | Sankaranarayanan et al. (1989a) |

## Table 38 (contd)

| Location (years) | Cancer site[b] | No. of cases | Habit | No. of controls | Habit | Relative risk (95% CI) | Reference |
|---|---|---|---|---|---|---|---|
| Kerala, India (1983–84) | Gingiva | 109 (M) 78 (F) | BQ + T, 80% BQ + T, 88% | 546 (M) 349 (F) | BQ + T, 33% (M) BQ + T, 51% (F) | BQ + T, 8.8 (3.6–21.5) (M) BQ + T + S, 16.3 (6.5–40.9) (M) S, 3.8 (1.2–11.7) (M) | Sankaranarayanan et al. (1989b) |
| Kerala, India (1983–84) | Buccal and labial mucosa | 250 (M) 164 (F) | BQ + T, 81% (M) BQ + T, 88% (F) | 546 (M) 349 (F) | BQ + T, 33% (M) BQ + T, 51% (F) | BQ + T, 14.3 (8.2–24.8) (M) BQ + T + S, 21.5 (11.9–38.5) (M) S, 4.2 (2.09–8.5) (M) | Sankaranarayanan et al. (1990a) |
| Bangalore, India (1982–85) | Oral cavity excl. base of tongue | 115 (M) 233 (F) | BQ, 13% (M) BQ + T, 28% (M) BQ, 4% (F) BQ + T, 88% (F) | 115 (M) 233 (F) | BQ, 13% (M) BQ + T, 10% (M) BQ, 13% (F) BQ + T, 25% (F) | Odds ratio not adjusted BQ, 1.5 (0.6–3.8) (M) BQ + T, 4.0 (1.8–8.9) (M) BQ, 2.2 (0.7–6.5) (F) BQ + T, 30.4 (12.6–73.4) (F) | Nandakumar et al. (1990) |
| Mumbai, India (1980–84) | Anterior 2/3 of tongue Posterior 1/3 of tongue | 141 (M) 495 (M) | BQ + T, 54% BQ + T, 35% | 631 (M) | BQ + T, 40% | BQ + T, 1.7 (1.2–2.6) BQ + T, 0.9 (0.7–1.2) | Rao & Desai (1998) |
| Maharashtra, India | Oropharynx | 123 (M + F) | T, 20% Areca, 4% T + areca, 11% BQ, 6% BQ + T, 42% | 246 (M + F) | T, 4% Areca nut, 6% T + areca, 4% BQ, 7% BQ + T, 16% | Odds ratio not adjusted T, 15.9 (6.9–36.7) Areca nut, 2.6 (0.9–7.7) T + areca, 10.2 (4.1–25.5) BQ, 2.8 (1.09–7.4) BQ + T, 9.5 (5.1–17.5) | Wasnik et al. (1998) |
| Bhopal, India (1986–92) | Oral cavity | 148 | BQ, 3% BQ + T, 97% S + T, 33% | 260 | BQ, 10% BQ + T, 90% S + T, 17% | BQ + T, 5.8 (3.6–9.5) BQ, 1.7 (0.9–3.3) | Dikshit & Kanhere (2000) |
| Karachi, Pakistan (1996–98) | Oral cavity | 79 (M + F) | BQ, 33% BQ + T, 52% Naswar, 17% | 149 (M + F) | BQ, 11% BQ + T, 10% Naswar, 7% | BQ, 9.9 (1.8–55.6) BQ + T, 8.4 (2.3–30.6) Naswar, 9.5 (1.7–52.5) | Merchant et al. (2000) |

**Table 38 (contd)**

| Location (years) | Cancer site[b] | No. of cases | Habit | No. of controls | Habit | Relative risk (95% CI) | Reference |
|---|---|---|---|---|---|---|---|
| Chennai, Bangalore & Trivandrum, India (1996–99) | Oral cavity | 309 (M) 282 (F) | BQ, 5% (M) BQ + T, 45% (M) BQ, 5% (F) BQ + T, 79% (F) | 292 (M) 290 (F) | BQ, 2% (M) BQ + T, 13% (M) BQ, 2% (F) BQ + T, 11% (F) | BQ, 4.2 (1.5–11.8) (M) BQ + T, 6.1 (3.8–9.7) (M) BQ, 16.4 (4.8–56.5) (F) BQ + T, 45.9 (25.0–84.1) (F) | Balaram et al. (2002) |
| Chennai & Trivandrum, India (1993–99) | Oral cavity | 1563 (M) | BQ, 6% BQ + T, 48% S, 73% | 3638 (M) | BQ, 5% BQ + T, 10% S, 51% | BQ, 2.2 (1.6–3.0) BQ + T, 5.1 (4.3–6.0) | Znaor et al. (2003) |
| | Tongue | | | | | BQ, 1.7 (1.1–2.6) BQ + T, 2.7 (2.2–3.4) | |
| | Mouth | | | | | BQ, 2.6 (1.8–3.7) BQ + T, 7.0 (5.7–8.5) | |

M, men; F, women; Q, betel quid with or without tobacco; S, smoking only; BQ, betel quid without tobacco; T, tobacco
[a] Usually comprises gum, floor of the mouth, buccal mucosa and palate; the tongue may be also included.
[b] In addition to oral cancer

**Table 39. Dose–response relationship [calculated by the Working Group] between chewing of betel quid with tobacco and oral cancer**

| Frequency of chewing | Relative risk | |
|---|---|---|
| | Hirayama (1966) | Orr (1933) |
| None | 1.0 | 1.0 |
| < 2 times a day | 8.4 | 4.9 |
| 3–5 times a day | 14.2 | 17.7 |
| 6 times or more | 17.6 | 68 |
| Retaining quid in sleep | 63 | 212.5 |

mucosa, 1.7% for cancer of the anterior tongue, 2.5% for oropharyngeal cancer and 2.9% for controls. Among women, the percentage of areca-nut chewers was 4.5% for cancer of the buccal mucosa and 19.6% for controls. Controls were cases of other diseases [not specified] matched for age and sex. [The information on areca-nut use was obtained by interviewing patients and by using hospital records if considered reliable. The proportion of such cases was not mentioned.] A dose–response relationship was calculated by the Working Group of *IARC Monographs* Volume 37 using case–control studies reported by Orr (1933) and Hirayama (1966) and results are given in Table 39. Both studies showed a positive dose–response relationship, the highest relative risk being that of retaining the betel quid during sleep.

The case–control sltudy of Jussawalla & Deshpande (1971) on 2005 cancers of the upper aerodigestive tract also reported increased relative risks for several subsites of oral cancer. These results are described in detail in Section 2.3.

Jafarey *et al.* (1977) reported a case–control study of cancer of the oral cavity and oropharynx conducted in Karachi, Pakistan, in 1967–72, comprising 1192 cases (683 men, 509 women) and 3562 controls (1978 men, 1584 women). Population controls were matched for age, sex and place of birth. Among nonsmokers, the risk for oral cancer of chewing betel quid alone in men and women was 4.2 and 3.2, respectively. When betel quid was chewed with tobacco, the risk among nonsmokers increased to 20.0 in men and 29.9 in women. The joint effect of chewing betel quid with tobacco and smoking was 23 in men and 35.9 in women.

A case–control study on several oral cancer subsites was conducted in Kerala, India. The first part of the study (Sankaranarayanan *et al.*, 1989a) that focused on cancer of the anterior two-thirds of tongue and floor of mouth comprised 228 cases (158 men, 70 women) and 453 hospital non-cancer controls (314 men, 139 women) matched for age, sex and religion. The risk associated with chewing betel quid with tobacco was lower in men than in women. The second part of the study on cancer of the gingiva (Sankaranarayanan *et al.*, 1989b) comprised 187 cases, and the third part on cancer of buccal and labial mucosa comprised

414 cases (Sankaranarayanan et al., 1990a). Hospital controls ($n = 895$) with no cancers were used for both the second and third studies. Attributable risk in men for chewing betel quid with tobacco was estimated at 54% for gingival cancers. Statistically significant dose–response relationships were observed for all oral cancer sites, for duration of chewing betel quid with tobacco and for number of betel quids with tobacco consumed per day (Tables 38 and 40).

Nandakumar et al. (1990) reported a case–control study conducted in Bangalore, India, using cases of cancer of the lip, tongue (excluding base of tongue), alveolus and mouth, registered at the Bangalore population-based cancer registry, and population controls with no evidence of cancer matched by age and area of residence. This study showed increased risk for oral cancer in both genders for chewing betel quid with tobacco (Table 38). Higher risk was seen among those who retained the quid in the mouth while asleep (odds ratio, 17.7; 95% CI, 8.7–36.1) than among those who did not (odds ratio, 8.5; 95% CI, 4.7–15.2). Risk increased with increase in duration of chewing betel quid with tobacco, with the number of tobacco quids consumed per day and with duration (period) of retention of the quid in the mouth (Table 40). Risks for chewing betel quid without tobacco were increased in men (odds ratio, 1.5; 95% CI, 0.6–3.8) and in women (odds ratio, 2.2; 95% CI, 0.7–6.5) and also in the combined analysis of men and women (odds ratio, 1.7; 95% CI, 0.9–3.5); however, these risks were not statistically significant. [The Working Group noted that the results were not adjusted for tobacco smoking. No information was available on other potential confounders.]

A study was conducted in Mumbai, India, of 142 male cases of cancer in the anterior two-thirds of the tongue, 495 male cases of cancer in the posterior third of the tongue and 635 hospital controls without cancer, infection or benign lesion. Information on chewing was available for 141 cases of cancer of the anterior two-thirds of tongue, all cases of cancer of the posterior third of the tongue, and 631 controls. A risk associated with chewing betel quid with tobacco was seen for the anterior two-thirds of the tongue but not for the posterior third (Rao & Desai, 1998) (Table 38).

Wasnik et al. (1998) reported a hospital-based case–control study conducted at three tertiary care centres in Nagpur city, Maharashtra, India, comprising 123 histologically confirmed cases of oropharyngeal cancer (73 men, 50 women), 123 cancer controls (sites other than oropharynx) and 123 non-cancer controls, matched by age and sex. Univariate analysis with both types of controls showed an elevated risk for chewing betel quid without tobacco and for chewing areca nut alone, as well as a more than ninefold risk for chewing tobacco alone or with betel quid. Multivariate analysis adjusting for tobacco smoking and occupation showed an eightfold risk (95% CI, 4.1–13.6) for chewing tobacco. The attributable risk for chewing tobacco was estimated at 87%.

A case–control study conducted on 148 cases of cancer of the oral cavity registered in the population-based Bhopal (India) Cancer Registry and 260 population controls showed a sixfold risk for chewing betel quid with tobacco for cancer of the oral cavity. An increased risk (odds ratio, 1.7; 95% CI, 0.9–3.3) was suggested for chewing betel quid without tobacco. The population attributable risk for developing cancer of the oral cavity

## Table 40. Dose–response relationship associated with chewing habit

|  | Cases | Controls | Odds ratio (95% CI) | p for trend |
|---|---|---|---|---|
| **Kerala Study** | | | | |
| **I. Cancer of anterior 2/3 of tongue and floor of mouth (Sankaranarayanan et al., 1989a)** | | | | |
| **Men** | | | | |
| *Duration of chewing (years)* | | | | |
| Never chewers | 58 | 216 | 1.0 | |
| ≤ 10 | 8 | 8 | 3.9 (1.2–12.8) | |
| 11–20 | 11 | 24 | 1.7 (0.7–3.96) | |
| 21–30 | 29 | 26 | 4.6 (2.4–9.0) | |
| 31–40 | 27 | 23 | 5.2 (2.5–10.7) | |
| > 40 | 17 | 13 | 5.6 (2.3–13.8) | < 0.001 |
| *Average daily amount (no. of quids/day)* | | | | |
| Never chewers | 58 | 216 | 1.0 | |
| < 5 | 32 | 33 | 4.0 (2.2–7.5) | |
| 5–9 | 29 | 43 | 2.9 (1.6–5.3) | |
| ≥ 10 | 31 | 18 | 5.5 (2.9–10.7) | < 0.001 |
| **Women** | | | | |
| *Duration of chewing (years)* | | | | |
| Never chewers | 13 | 84 | 1.0 | |
| ≤ 10 | 8 | 8 | 7.6 (1.97–29.1) | |
| 11–20 | 9 | 11 | 3.5 (1.1–10.8) | |
| 21–30 | 11 | 20 | 4.6 (1.5–13.8) | |
| 31–40 | 10 | 7 | 15.9 (3.6–69.0) | |
| > 40 | 15 | 8 | 18.3 (4.7–71.4) | < 0.001 |
| *Average daily amount (no. of quids/day)* | | | | |
| Never chewers | 13 | 84 | 1.0 | |
| < 5 | 19 | 24 | 5.8 (2.2–15.2) | |
| 5–9 | 20 | 22 | 6.6 (2.5–17.7) | |
| ≥ 10 | 14 | 8 | 9.3 (3.1–27.6) | < 0.001 |
| **II. Cancer of the gingiva (Sankaranarayanan et al., 1989b)** | | | | |
| **Men** | | | | |
| *Duration of chewing (years)* | | | | |
| Never chewers | 19 | 360 | 1.0 | |
| ≤ 10 | 4 | 13 | 5.8 (1.6–20.7) | |
| 11–20 | 9 | 54 | 2.9 (1.2–6.8) | |
| 21–30 | 13 | 49 | 4.95 (2.3–10.8) | |
| 31–40 | 28 | 40 | 13.6 (6.7–27.7) | |
| > 40 | 33 | 25 | 32.1 (13.9–73.8) | < 0.001 |

## Table 40 (contd)

|  | Cases | Controls | Odds ratio (95% CI) | p for trend |
|---|---|---|---|---|
| *Average daily amount (no. of quids/day)* | | | | |
| Never chewers | 19 | 360 | 1.0 | |
| < 5 | 21 | 61 | 5.95 (2.99–11.8) | |
| 5–9 | 30 | 80 | 6.9 (3.7–12.9) | |
| ≥ 10 | 36 | 40 | 15.1 (7.8–29.0) | < 0.001 |
| **Women** | | | | |
| *Duration of chewing (years)* | | | | |
| Never chewers | 6 | 168 | 1.0 | |
| ≤ 10 | 4 | 48 | 2.4 (0.6–9.3) | |
| 11–20 | 10 | 49 | 5.9 (1.97–17.6) | |
| 21–30 | 14 | 48 | 9.3 (3.3–26.6) | |
| 31–40 | 18 | 19 | 32.3 (10.6–98.4) | |
| > 40 | 23 | 13 | 54.2 (16.3–180.4) | < 0.001 |
| *Average daily amount (no. of quids/day)* | | | | |
| Never chewers | 6 | 168 | 1.0 | |
| < 5 | 19 | 92 | 6.6 (2.5–17.7) | |
| 5–9 | 39 | 63 | 18.5 (7.2–47.8) | |
| ≥ 10 | 11 | 22 | 13.7 (4.4–42.5) | < 0.001 |
| **III. Cancer of the buccal and labial mucosa (Sankaranarayanan *et al.*, 1990a)** | | | | |
| **Men** | | | | |
| *Duration of chewing (years)* | | | | |
| Never chewers | 37 | 360 | 1.0 | |
| ≤ 10 | 11 | 13 | 6.9 (2.8–16.8) | |
| 11–20 | 35 | 55 | 5.8 (3.3–10.11) | |
| 21–30 | 39 | 49 | 7.7 (4.4–13.4) | |
| 31–40 | 48 | 40 | 13.2 (7.5–23.3) | |
| > 40 | 70 | 25 | 37.8 (19.5–73.1) | < 0.001 |
| *Average daily amount (no. of quids/day)* | | | | |
| Never chewers | 37 | 360 | 1.0 | |
| < 5 | 59 | 61 | 9.3 (5.6–15.2) | |
| 5–9 | 75 | 80 | 9.04 (5.7–14.5) | |
| ≥ 10 | 69 | 40 | 16.4 (9.7–27.7) | |
| **Women** | | | | |
| *Duration of chewing (years)* | | | | |
| Never chewers | 19 | 168 | 1.0 | |
| ≤ 10 | 11 | 48 | 1.8 (0.8–4.1) | |
| 11–20 | 22 | 49 | 3.8 (1.9–7.8) | |
| 21–30 | 38 | 48 | 7.7 (4.0–15.0) | |
| 31–40 | 33 | 19 | 21.3 (9.6–47.4) | |
| > 40 | 39 | 13 | 54.9 (21.2–142.4) | |

## Table 40 (contd)

|  | Cases | Controls | Odds ratio (95% CI) | $p$ for trend |
|---|---|---|---|---|
| *Average daily amount (no. of quids/day)* | | | | |
| Never chewers | 19 | 168 | 1.0 | |
| < 5 | 36 | 92 | 3.7 (1.99–7.0) | |
| 5–9 | 72 | 63 | 10.8 (6.0–19.6) | |
| ≥ 10 | 35 | 22 | 14.2 (6.9–29.5) | |

### Bangalore study (Nandakumar *et al.*, 1990)

#### Men and women

| | Cases | Controls | Odds ratio (95% CI) | $p$ for trend |
|---|---|---|---|---|
| *Duration of chewing (years)* | | | | |
| Never chewers | 111 | 278 | 1.0 | |
| 1–5 | 4 | 6 | 1.7 (0.3–9.3) | |
| 6–15 | 23 | 7 | 10.3 (3.6–29.6) | |
| 16–25 | 56 | 20 | 12.4 (5.6–27.2) | |
| > 25 | 154 | 37 | 15.95 (8.4–30.2) | |
| *Average daily amount (no. of quids/day)* | | | | |
| Never chewers | 111 | 278 | 1.0 | |
| 1–4 | 82 | 33 | 9.3 (4.9–17.5) | |
| 5–9 | 98 | 28 | 12.8 (6.6–25.0) | |
| ≥ 10 | 35 | 8 | 16.6 (6.3–44.3) | |
| *Chewing period (min)* | | | | |
| Never chewers | 111 | 278 | 1.0 | |
| ≤ 5 | 5 | 3 | 6.4 (0.9–45.1) | |
| 6–10 | 67 | 20 | 9.7 (4.7–19.8) | |
| 11–20 | 59 | 13 | 16.5 (7.2–37.4) | |
| 21–30 | 54 | 17 | 13.2 (5.8–30.0) | |
| > 30 | 11 | 6 | 6.6 (1.6–27.0) | |

### Bhopal study (Dikshit & Kanhere, 2000)

#### Men

| | Cases | Controls | Odds ratio (95% CI) | $p$ for trend |
|---|---|---|---|---|
| *Duration of chewing (years)* | | | | |
| Never chewers | 28 | | 1.0 | |
| 1–20 | 12 | | 1.1 (0.5–2.4) | |
| 21–30 | 32 | | 5.5 (2.9–10.6) | |
| > 30 | 72 | | 23.9 (12.0–47.3) | |
| *Average daily amount (no. of quids/day)* | | | | |
| Never chewers | 28 | | 1.0 | |
| 1–5 | 19 | | 2.0 (1.0–3.8) | |
| 6–10 | 47 | | 6.7 (3.7–12.1) | |
| > 10 | 15 | | 13.9 (7.1–27.2) | |

## Table 40 (contd)

|  | Cases | Controls | Odds ratio (95% CI) | p for trend |
|---|---|---|---|---|

### Multicentre study in South India: Chennai, Bangalore and Trivandrum (Balaram *et al.*, 2002)

**Men**

*Age started chewing (years)*
| | | | | |
|---|---|---|---|---|
| ≥ 25 | 51 | 21 | 1.0 | |
| 20–24 | 42 | 10 | 1.5 (0.6–4.2) | |
| < 20 | 27 | 6 | 1.5 (0.5–5.0) | 0.39 |

*Average daily amount (no. of quids/day)*
| | | | | |
|---|---|---|---|---|
| Never chewers | 127 | 232 | 1.0 | |
| Former chewers | | | | |
| < 5 | 28 | 11 | 4.2 (1.9–9.6) | |
| ≥ 5 | 31 | 9 | 5.8 (2.5–13.2) | |
| Current chewers | | | | |
| < 5 | 40 | 18 | 3.1 (1.6–5.9) | |
| 5–9 | 46 | 12 | 8.2 (3.9–16.9) | |
| ≥ 10 | 34 | 7 | 7.9 (3.2–19.4) | < 0.001 |

**Women**

*Age started chewing (years)*
| | | | | |
|---|---|---|---|---|
| ≥ 25 | 56 | 13 | 1.0 | |
| 20–24 | 74 | 12 | 1.9 (0.7–5.3) | |
| < 20 | 73 | 4 | 5.4 (1.5–19.7) | 0.01 |

*Average daily amount (no. of quids/day)*
| | | | | |
|---|---|---|---|---|
| Never chewers | 29 | 251 | 1.0 | |
| Former chewers | | | | |
| < 5 | 17 | 6 | 20.2 (6.4–63.9) | |
| ≥ 5 | 31 | 3 | 60.4 (15.8–230.7) | |
| Current chewers | | | | |
| < 5 | 51 | 13 | 22.1 (10.1–48.5) | |
| 5–9 | 101 | 13 | 58.6 (26.6–129.0) | |
| ≥ 10 | 51 | 3 | 112.4 (30.9–409.6) | < 0.001 |

### Study in South India: Chennai and Trivandrum (Znaor *et al.*, 2003)

**Men**

| | | | | |
|---|---|---|---|---|
| Never chewing | 711 | 3079 | 1.0 | |

*Duration of chewing (years)*
| | | | | |
|---|---|---|---|---|
| 0–19 | 250 | 286 | 3.1 (2.5–3.9) | |
| 20–39 | 432 | 209 | 5.3 (4.3–6.5) | |
| ≥ 40 | 170 | 64 | 5.2 (3.7–7.3) | |

*Average daily amount (no. of quids/day)*
| | | | | |
|---|---|---|---|---|
| 1–3 | 279 | 343 | 2.06 (1.7–2.5) | |
| 4–5 | 273 | 135 | 6.02 (4.7–7.7) | |
| > 5 | 300 | 800 | 11.9 (8.9–15.96) | |

**Table 40 (contd)**

|  | Cases | Controls | Odds ratio (95% CI) | p for trend |
|---|---|---|---|---|
| *Cumulative exposure to chewing* | | | | |
| < 1000 | 354 | 158 | 3.8 (2.95–4.8) | |
| > 1000 | 211 | 26 | 13.3 (8.5–20.9) | |
| *Time since quitting chewing (years)* | | | | |
| Current chewers | 640 | 460 | 1.0 | |
| 2–4 | 93 | 41 | 1.2 (0.8–1.8) | |
| 5–9 | 59 | 20 | 1.6 (0.9–2.8) | |
| 10–14 | 30 | 19 | 0.7 (0.4–1.4) | |
| ≥ 15 | 30 | 19 | 0.7 (0.4–1.3) | |

CI, confidence interval

was 66% for chewers of betel quid with tobacco (Dikshit & Kanhere, 2000) (Tables 38 and 40).

Merchant *et al.* (2000) reported a case–control study in three hospitals in Karachi, Pakistan, comprising 79 (54 men, 25 women) histologically confirmed cases of oral squamous-cell carcinoma and 149 controls (94 men, 55 women) matched for age, gender, hospital and time of occurrence, without past or present history of cancer. An eight- to ninefold risk for developing oral cancer was associated with ever chewing betel quid with or without tobacco, and ever chewing naswar, after adjustment for oral submucous fibrosis, cigarette smoking, alcohol and other chewing habits where appropriate. A dose–response relationship was observed between tertiles of *pan*–years without tobacco (average number of quids per day × average years of use) and the risk for oral cancer ($p$-value for trend = 0.0008), after adjustment for smoking, oral submucous fibrosis, alcohol drinking, and chewing naswar or pan with tobacco. [Possible limitations of the study are the use of hospital controls without exclusion of betel quid-related diseases and adjustment for oral submucous fibrosis, which is a disease that is strongly related to chewing betel quid.]

Balaram *et al.* (2002) reported a multicentre study conducted in three Indian centres, Bangalore, Chennai and Trivandrum, in 1996–99 on 591 cases of cancer of the oral cavity (309 men, 282 women) and 582 hospital controls (292 men, 290 women). Controls were frequency-matched with cases by centre, age and sex. Controls were identified and interviewed in the same hospital as cases. In Chennai and Bangalore, controls were visitors of patients admitted for cancers other than oral cancer. In Trivandrum, controls were non-cancer patients attending the hospital for diagnosis or treatment. The results showed that 80% of male and female chewers combined chewed quid with tobacco; the odds ratio for chewing betel quid without tobacco versus non-chewers was 4.2 (95% CI, 1.5–11.8) in men and 16.4 (95% CI, 4.8–56.5) in women after adjusting for age, centre and education for men and women and smoking and alcohol drinking for men only. The risk associated with chewing betel quid with or without tobacco was higher among women than among men. A significant dose–response relationship with the number of betel quids with or without tobacco chewed per day was found in both sexes ($p < 0.001$), while early age at starting chewing was significantly associated with the risk for oral cancer in women only ($p = 0.01$). Only 13 (eight cases, five controls) and 11 (six cases, five controls) women in the study were smokers and alcohol drinkers, respectively; therefore, results among women had little chance of being confounded by smoking or alcohol drinking. There was a slight decrease in risk 10 years after quitting the habit of chewing (Tables 38 and 40).

Znaor et al. (2003) reported a study conducted in two centres in South India, Chennai and Trivandrum, on 1563 male oral cancer cases and 3638 controls (1711 male cancer controls from Chennai and Trivandrum and 1927 healthy male hospital visitor controls from Chennai), during the period 1993–99. Although the two centres involved in this study are the same as those in the study of Balaram et al. (2002), different cases and controls were used in the two studies. All cancer cases and cancer controls were histologically confirmed and controls were identified and interviewed in the same hospital as the cases. Odds ratios were adjusted for age, centre, level of education, alcohol consumption and smoking. The risks for chewing betel quid without tobacco were 2.2 (95% CI, 1.6–3.0) for cancer of the oral cavity, 1.7 (95% CI, 1.1–2.6) for cancer of the tongue and 2.6 (95% CI, 1.8–3.7) for cancer of the mouth excluding tongue. The analysis stratified by smoking and alcohol drinking showed the risk for chewing betel quid without tobacco to be 3.4 (95% CI, 2.04–5.7) in nonsmokers and non-drinkers of alcohol. Statistically significant dose–response relationships were observed for duration of the combined habit of chewing betel quid with or without tobacco, average daily amount of betel quid with or without tobacco chewed and cumulative years of chewing betel quid with or without tobacco ($p < 0.001$). The risk associated with oral cancer decreased with duration since quitting the combined habit of chewing betel quid with or without tobacco, but the odds ratios for time since quitting were not statistically significant (Tables 38 and 40).

(d) *Cross-sectional surveys*

Cross-sectional studies summarized in Volume 37 of the *IARC Monographs* (IARC, 1985a) are given in Table 41. These studies provide information on prevalence of oral cancer among persons chewing betel quid with or without tobacco, as well as combined or not with smoking. No new prevalence studies were available to the Working Group of this monograph.

(e) *Synergism*

Jayant et al. (1977) examined the possibility of interaction between chewing and smoking habits in the etiology of cancer of the upper alimentary tract using the data of Jussawalla and Deshpande (1971). It was found that chewing and smoking habits interacted synergistically for cancers of the oral cavity, oropharynx, hypopharynx, larynx and oesophagus.

A significant interaction with the smoking of bidis was observed in the studies from Kerala, India (described in detail in Section 2.1.1(c)). The unadjusted relative risk for chewing betel quid with and without tobacco and smoking bidis in the case–control study

## Table 41. Cross-sectional surveys of oral cancer in India

| Location | Individuals examined | Habit | No. of cancer cases detected | Prevalence per 1000[a] | Reference |
|---|---|---|---|---|---|
| Lucknow | 10 000 in dental clinic | Q and/or S, 33% | 24 | 73 | Pindborg et al. (1965) |
| Ernakulam district, Kerala | 10 000 by random sampling | BQ + T, 25.9%<br>BQ, 0.4%<br>BQ + S, 10.8%<br>S, 22.1% | <br>6<br>6<br>– | <br>2.2<br>5.4<br>– | Mehta et al. (1971) |
| Bhavnagar district, Gujarat | 10 000 | Mishri, 7.1%<br>BQ + T, 3.0%<br>BQ, 1.6%<br>BQ + S, 3.2%<br>S, 29.1% | –<br>–<br>–<br>1<br>2 | –<br>–<br>–<br>3.1<br>0.7 | |
| Darbhanga district, Bihar | 10 000 | BQ, 1.3%<br>BQ + T, 15.2%<br>BQ + S, 14.3%<br>S, 33.2% | –<br>–<br>1<br>– | –<br>–<br>0.7<br>– | |
| Srikakulam district, Andhra Pradesh | 10 000 | BQ, 0.6%<br>BQ + T, 2.8%<br>BQ + S, 7.9%<br>S, 63.0% | –<br>–<br>1<br>9 | –<br>–<br>0.8<br>1.9 | |
| Poona (Pune) district, Maharashtra | 101 761 villagers | BQ, 0.7% (M)<br>BQ + T, 52.1% (M)<br>Mishri, 0.8% (M)<br>BQ + S, 2.4% (M)<br>S, 5.6% (M)<br>BQ, 0.5% (F)<br>BQ + T, 9.5% (F)<br>Mishri, 38.9% (F) | Total of 12 | 0.2 (M)<br>–<br>–<br>1.1<br>0.6<br>0.3 (F) | Mehta et al. (1972b) |
| Ahmedabad, Gujarat | 57 518 industrial workers | Q, 4.7%<br>Q + S, 22.0%<br>S, 35.7%<br>No habit, 15.1% | | –<br>0.9<br>0.6<br>0.2 | Smith et al. (1975) |

Q, betel quid with or without tobacco; S, smoking; BQ, betel quid without tobacco; T, tobacco
[a] Prevalence rates calculated by the Working Group

of oral cancers of the tongue and floor of mouth was 7.02 (95% CI, 3.6–13.5) in men, compared with nonsmokers and non-chewers ($p$ for interaction < 0.01) (Sankaranarayanan et al., 1989a). In the second part of the study on cancer of the gingiva (Sankaranarayanan et al., 1989b), the risk associated with mixed habits of chewing betel quid with tobacco and bidi smoking was 16.5 (95% CI, 7.5–36.1) in men, compared with nonsmokers and non-chewers ($p$ for interaction < 0.05). Risk estimates were not adjusted for age. In the third study on cancer of the buccal and labial mucosa, the risk in men of chewing and smoking bidis was 21.5 (95% CI, 11.9–38.5) compared with nonsmokers and non-chewers ($p$ for interaction < 0.05) (Sankaranarayanan et al., 1990a)

The study by Balaram et al. (2002) conducted in southern India with 591 cases of cancer of the oral cavity and 582 hospital controls (described in Section 2.1.1($c$)) showed a seven-fold risk for developing oral cancer among men who were current chewers of betel quid with or without tobacco and who smoked 20 or more cigarettes/bidis or equivalents per day, and a ninefold risk among those who were current chewers and current drinkers. This study showed a negative interaction between chewing tobacco and smoking (Table 42).

Znaor et al. (2003) reported the results of a study in men conducted in two centres (Chennai and Trivandrum) in South India that included 1563 cases of oral, 636 cases of pharyngeal and 566 cases of oesophageal cancer, 1711 disease controls and 1927 healthy controls (see Section 2.1.1($c$)). Table 43 shows the joint effects of smoking, drinking and chewing habits. Compared with subjects who did not smoke, chew betel quid with or

Table 42. Risk for cancer of the oral cavity among men: interaction between chewing and smoking, and chewing and drinking

|  | Paan chewing | | | |
|---|---|---|---|---|
|  | Never | | Current chewers | |
|  | Cases/ controls | Odds ratio[a] (95% CI) | Cases/ controls | Odds ratio[a] (95% CI) |
| *Tobacco smoking* | | | | |
| Never smokers | 25/106 | 1.0 | 49/16 | 9.2 (4.4–19.3) |
| Current smokers (cig./day) | | | | |
| 1–19 | 33/55 | 1.8 (0.93–3.5) | 35/10 | 8.9 (3.6–21.8) |
| ≥ 20 | 48/35 | 3.7 (1.9–7.2) | 22/8 | 6.7 (2.5–18.3) |
| *Alcohol drinking* | | | | |
| Never drinker | 64/174 | 1.0 | 48/18 | 7.3 (3.8–14.1) |
| Current drinker | 48/38 | 2.8 (1.6–5.1) | 46/13 | 8.6 (4.1–18.1) |

From Balaram et al. (2002)
[a] Unconditional logistic regression adjusted for age, centre, education, oral hygiene, chewing and smoking and drinking habits, as appropriate
CI, confidence interval

**Table 43. Odds ratios for oral cancer and combinations of smoking, chewing and alcohol drinking**

| Habit | | | Oral cavity cancer | | | |
|---|---|---|---|---|---|---|
| Smoking | Chewing | Alcohol | Controls | Cases | Odds ratios | 95% CI |
| No | No | No | 1471 | 122 | 1.0 | – |
| No | Yes T– | No | 83 | 24 | 3.4 | 2.04–5.7 |
| No | Yes T+ | No | 127 | 159 | 9.3 | 6.8–12.7 |
| Yes | No | No | 1084 | 268 | 2.5 | 1.9–3.1 |
| No | No | Yes | 75 | 16 | 2.6 | 1.4–4.6 |
| Yes | Yes T– | No | 49 | 25 | 4.8 | 2.8–8.3 |
| Yes | Yes T+ | No | 102 | 161 | 8.5 | 6.1–11.9 |
| No | Yes T– | Yes | 15 | 6 | 4.4 | 1.6–12.3 |
| No | Yes T+ | Yes | 26 | 95 | 24.3 | 14.9–39.7 |
| Yes | No | Yes | 449 | 287 | 4.8 | 3.7–6.2 |
| Yes | Yes T– | Yes | 34 | 33 | 8.1 | 4.7–14.0 |
| Yes | Yes T+ | Yes | 119 | 342 | 16.3 | 12.1–22.0 |

From Znaor et al. (2003)
Adjusted for age, center and level of education
CI, confidence interval; T+, with tobacco; T–, without tobacco

without tobacco or drink alcohol, the risks were 3.4 (95% CI, 2.04–5.7) for chewing betel quid without tobacco, 9.3 (95% CI, 6.8–12.7) for chewing betel quid with tobacco, 4.8 (95% CI, 2.8–8.3) for both smoking and chewing betel quid without tobacco, 4.4 (95% CI, 1.6–12.3) for both drinking alcohol and chewing quid without tobacco and 8.1 (95% CI, 4.7–14.0) for smoking, drinking alcohol and chewing quid without tobacco. In all estimates related to interaction between two habits, the third habit was controlled for in addition to age, centre and level of education. Likelihood ratio tests were statistically significant ($p < 0.05$) for the combination of the different habits — drinking and smoking, chewing and smoking, but not chewing and drinking.

### 2.1.2 Taiwan, China

(a) *Descriptive study*

One ecological study in Taiwan, China, found that the increase in incidence trends of oropharyngeal cancer parallels the time trend of consumption of areca nut, which almost doubled from 1985 to 1993 and which was much greater than the trend for the consumption of tobacco and alcohol (Ho et al., 2002). As the majority of betel-quid chewers are men, the large increasing trend of these cancers in men also supports the possibility of the cause being consumption of areca nut. Age-standardized incidence rates for men have increased from 5.4 (95% CI, 5.05–5.8) in 1979–83 to 15.95 (95% CI, 15.3–16.6) in 1994–96 and those for women from 1.6 (95% CI, 1.4–1.8) in 1979–83 to 2.1 (95% CI, 1.8–2.4) in 1994–96 (Ho et al., 2002).

(b)   Case–control studies

Kwan (1976) reported a case–control study of oral cancer in Taiwan, China, in which, out of 103 cases, 20 were betel chewers and 35 were betel chewers with other habits. No control subject chewed betel. [Therefore, it was not possible to estimate the relative risk.]

Three recent case–control studies in Taiwan, China, are summarized in Table 44.

Ko et al. (1995) conducted a hospital-based case–control study to assess the effects of betel quid without tobacco, smoking and alcohol on the incidence of oral cancer. A total of 107 oral cancers (104 men, three women) confirmed by histopathology (ICD 140–141, 143–145) between 1992 and 1993 were ascertained from patients at the dental department at Kaohsiung Medical College Hospital, in southern Taiwan, China. Controls were selected from ophtalmology and physical check-up departments in the same period as cases; 93 cases were matched with two controls and 14 cases with one control according to age (± 5 years) and sex. Information on demographic variables, the habit of betel-quid chewing, cigarette smoking and alcohol drinking was collected by a structured questionnaire administered by a trained interviewer. After controlling for education and occupation with a conditional logistic regression model, betel-quid chewing was considered to be the most important risk factor for oral cancer, compared with alcohol drinking and cigarette smoking. The association between chewing betel quid and oral cancer was significant for current chewers, with a sevenfold increase in risk, but was of borderline significance for former chewers, with a fivefold increase. The association between smoking and oral cancer was statistically significant for current smokers (fivefold increase in risk) and of borderline significance for former smokers (fourfold increase). Being a current drinker was also statistically significantly associated with risk for oral cancer, whereas no elevated risk was found for former drinkers. By stratified analysis incorporating the three factors simultaneously, relative risks were estimated at 122.8 (95% CI, 17.1–880.5) for the combination of the three factors, 89.1 (95% CI, 10.0–790.7) for chewing betel quid and smoking, 54.0 (95% CI, 4.4–660) for chewing betel quid and drinking and 28.2 (95% CI, 1.9–414.4) for chewing betel quid only, as compared with participants abstaining from all three habits. The relative risk for combined areca-nut chewing, smoking and alcohol is greater than the risk associated with the three risk factors independently. [A synergistic effect is suggested, but no assessment of interaction was made in this study.] With regard to the type of material chewed, chewers who used *lao-hwa* quid and mixed chewers (*lao-hwa* quid and betel quid) had a 12-fold and ninefold risk, respectively, both of which were statistically significant. Betel-quid chewers with the habit of swallowing the juice had an 11-fold statistically significant risk for oral cancer.

Another matched case–control study was conducted in the central area of Taiwan, China. A total of 40 consecutive histopathologically diagnosed oral cancers (34 men, six women) were ascertained from patients at Changhua Christian Hospital between 1990

Table 44. Case–control studies of betel quid-chewing and oral cancer in Taiwan, China

| Reference, place, period | Characteristics of cases and controls | Oral cancer site | Exposure | Cases/controls | Odds ratio (95% CI) | Comments |
|---|---|---|---|---|---|---|
| Ko et al. (1995), Kaohsiung, 1992–93 | 107 cases (104 men, 3 women) and 200 non-cancer hospital controls (194 men, 6 women) matched on age and sex | ICD 140–141 (lip, tongue), 143–145 (gum, mouth) | Non-drinker | 25/89 | 1.0 | Adjusted for education, occupation and each covariate |
| | | | Former drinker | 14/37 | 1.0 (0.3–3.3) | |
| | | | Current drinker | 68/74 | 2.2 (1.0–4.9) | |
| | | | Non-smoker | 11/72 | 1.0 | |
| | | | Former smoker | 11/30 | 3.6 (0.9–14.6) | |
| | | | Current smoker | 85/98 | 4.6 (1.5–14.0) | |
| | | | Non-chewer | 31/153 | 1.0 | |
| | | | Former chewer | 5/5 | 4.7 (0.9–22.7) | |
| | | | Current chewer | 71/42 | 6.9 (3.1–15.2) | |
| | | | Non-chewer | 31/60 | 1.0 | Adjusted for education, occupation, smoking and drinking |
| | | | Betel quid | 1/7 | 0.1 (0.0–6.3) | |
| | | | Lao-hwa quid | 41/13 | 11.6 (3.7–36.9) | |
| | | | Betel + *lao-hwa* | 34/25 | 8.5 (2.7–26.3) | |
| | | | Not swallowing juice | 3/15 | 0.2 (0.0–2.9) | |
| | | | Swallowing juice | 73/31 | 11.4 (4.0–32.0) | |
| | | | Multivariate analysis | | | Adjusted for education and occupation; reference category: no habit |
| | | | D + S + BQ | 58/34 | 122.8 (17.1–880.5) | |
| | | | D + BQ | 3/2 | 54.0 (4.4–660.0) | |
| | | | S + BQ | 12/9 | 89.1 (10.0–790.7) | |
| | | | S + D | 18/56 | 22.3 (3.2–153.8) | |
| | | | BQ | 3/2 | 28.2 (1.9–414.4) | |
| | | | S | 8/29 | 18.0 (2.4–135.8) | |
| | | | D | 3/19 | 10.2 (1.2–86.4) | |

**Table 44 (contd)**

| Reference, place, period | Characteristics of cases and controls | Oral cancer site | Exposure | Cases/ controls | Odds ratio (95% CI) | Comments |
|---|---|---|---|---|---|---|
| Lu et al. (1996), Changhua, 1990–92 | 40 cases (34 men, 6 women) and 160 population controls with no cancer (136 men, 24 women) matched on age, gender, residence and education | [subsite not specified] | Betel quid | | | Adjusted for age, gender, residence, education and other covariates |
| | | | Non-chewers | 7/122 | 1.0 | |
| | | | Chewers | 33/38 | 58.4 (7.6–447.6) | |
| | | | Tobacco smoking | | | |
| | | | Nonsmokers | 8/59 | 1.0 | |
| | | | Smokers | 32/101 | 2.7 (0.4–19.6) | |
| | | | Alcohol drinking | | | |
| | | | Non-drinkers | 22/111 | 1.0 | |
| | | | Drinkers | 18/49 | 0.7 (0.3–2.2) | |
| | | | Duration of betel-quid chewing (years) | | | Adjusted for age, gender, residence, education, alcohol consumption and tobacco smoking |
| | | | Never | 7/122 | 1.0 | |
| | | | 1–20 | 6/24 | 12.9 (1.3–128.1) | |
| | | | 21–40 | 19/10 | 93.7 (10.1–868.0) | |
| | | | > 40 | 8/4 | 397.5 (19.5–8120.2) | |
| | | | Number of quids/day | | | |
| | | | 0 | 7/122 | 1.0 | |
| | | | 1–9 | 8/27 | 26.4 (2.9–239.7) | |
| | | | 10–20 | 16/9 | 51.2 (6.2–423.4) | |
| | | | > 20 | 9/2 | 275.6 (14.8–5106.5) | |
| Chen et al. (2002), Taichung, 1994–97 | 29 cases and 29 negative hospital controls from paraffin-embedded biopsies | Oral squamous-cell carcinoma [subsite not specified] | Betel-quid chewing | 19/5 | 17.1 (23–129.0) | Adjusted for gender, age, smoking, HPV6 and HPV11 |
| | | | HPV16 | 24/8 | 11.2 (1.2–103.2) | |
| | | | HPV18 | 20/3 | 6.6 (0.8–53.3) | |

CI, confidence interval; BQ, betel quid; D, alcohol drinking; S, cigarette smoking and 1992 (Lu *et al.*, 1996). Each case was matched to four neighbourhood non-cancer controls (136 men, 24 women) in Changhua County according to four criteria: sex, age, living in the same community residence as the case for at least 5 years and educational background. Information was gathered from a questionnaire administered by a social worker that covered demographic and socioeconomic factors, duration, type and daily amount of smoking, chewing and alcohol drinking. After adjustment for each individual risk factor, the authors showed that chewing betel quid without tobacco was highly associated with risk for oral cancer but that only a moderate non-significant association was noted for smoking and that no association was found for alcohol drinking. Adjusted odds ratios increased with duration of chewing and quantity of betel quid chewed per day, suggesting a trend for increasing duration and amount.

A case–control study on the association between human papillomavirus (HPV) infection, chewing betel quid without tobacco and cigarette smoking was conducted using biopsies from 29 cases of oral squamous-cell carcinoma and those from 29 controls that included normal or inflammatory mucosa obtained from a negative biopsy, teeth extraction or excision of a benign lesion (mucocele and haemangioma). Case and control biopsies were collected from the archives of the Medical and Dental University Hospital from 1994 to 1997. Betel-quid chewing remained the most significant factor, giving a 17-fold increase in risk after adjusting for HPV sequences 6, 11, 16 and 18, sex, age and smoking (Chen *et al.*, 2002).

### 2.1.3  *South-East Asia*

Epidemiological data from South-East Asia on the association between oral cancer and the habit of chewing betel quid are rare. However, age-standardized rates for oral cancer in men and women are available for some countries (Tables 45 and 46). Some descriptive studies on oral cancer without details on betel-quid chewing habits have been published from the South-East Asian region (Piyaratn, 1959; Lay *et al.*, 1982; Warnakulasuriya *et al.*, 1984; Kuek *et al.*, 1990; Ikeda *et al.*, 1995; Budhy *et al.*, 2001).

(*a*)  *Malaysia*

Ahluwalia and Duguid (1966) reported on the distribution of cancers in different ethnic groups of the Malay Peninsula (Malays, Chinese and Indians), using records from the Kuala Lumpur Institute for Medical Research. Of 4369 cases of cancer (1961–63), 476 (10.9%) were oral cancers in chewers of betel quid with and without tobacco. Of 912 cancers at all sites in Indians who are known to chew betel quid with tobacco, 306 (33.6%) were oral cancers. Of 776 cancers at all sites in Malays who are known to chew betel quid without tobacco, 74 (9.5%) had oral cancer.

Ramanathan and Lakshimi (1976) reported on racial variations of cancer in Indian, Malay and Chinese populations in Malaysia. Of a total of 898 cases of oral carcinoma, 31.1% occurred in Indian women, 29.1% in Indian men, 10.6% in Malay men, 11.1% in Malay women, 14.1% in Chinese men and 4% in Chinese women. Chewing and smoking

Table 45. Cancer of the oral cavity (men, all ages) in South-East Asia in 2000

| Country | Cases | Crude rate | ASR (W) | Deaths | Crude rate | ASR (W) |
|---|---|---|---|---|---|---|
| Cambodia | 113 | 2.1 | 4.6 | 66 | 1.2 | 2.8 |
| Indonesia | 1176 | 1.1 | 1.5 | 657 | 0.6 | 0.8 |
| Lao | 42 | 1.5 | 2.6 | 24 | 0.9 | 1.5 |
| Malaysia | 191 | 1.7 | 2.4 | 108 | 1.0 | 1.4 |
| Myanmar | 1387 | 6.1 | 8.6 | 805 | 3.5 | 5.1 |
| Philippines | 1304 | 3.4 | 5.8 | 755 | 2.0 | 3.4 |
| Singapore | 68 | 3.8 | 3.7 | 29 | 1.7 | 1.7 |
| Thailand | 1240 | 4.0 | 5.3 | 735 | 2.4 | 3.1 |
| Viet Nam | 920 | 2.3 | 3.7 | 520 | 1.3 | 2.1 |

From Ferlay et al. (2001)
ASR (W), age-standardized rates (world standard population)

Table 46. Cancer of the oral cavity (women, all ages) in South-East Asia in 2000

| Country | Cases | Crude rate | ASR (W) | Deaths | Crude rate | ASR (W) |
|---|---|---|---|---|---|---|
| Cambodia | 123 | 2.1 | 3.4 | 71 | 1.2 | 2.0 |
| Indonesia | 883 | 0.8 | 1.0 | 485 | 0.5 | 0.5 |
| Lao | 90 | 3.3 | 6.0 | 53 | 2.0 | 3.6 |
| Malaysia | 156 | 1.4 | 1.8 | 85 | 0.8 | 1.0 |
| Myanmar | 653 | 2.8 | 3.5 | 371 | 1.6 | 2.0 |
| Philippines | 1250 | 3.3 | 5.4 | 732 | 1.9 | 3.2 |
| Singapore | 38 | 2.1 | 1.9 | 16 | 0.9 | 0.8 |
| Thailand | 1139 | 3.7 | 4.0 | 673 | 2.2 | 2.4 |
| Viet Nam | 914 | 2.3 | 2.8 | 526 | 1.3 | 1.6 |

From Ferlay et al. (2001)
ASR (W), age-standardized rates (world standard population)

habits were not studied in particular. Ethnic differences in the pattern of oral carcinoma were evident and partly attributed to different oral habits such as betel-quid chewing, which is more prevalent in the Indian and Malay populations compared with the Chinese.

Ng et al. (1986) studied the betel-quid chewing and smoking habits, as well as alcohol consumption of 100 Indian, Chinese and Malay patients (39 men, 61 women) with histologically confirmed oral squamous-cell carcinoma. Betel-quid chewing was the most common single habit (85%), followed by alcohol consumption (55%) and smoking (29%). Seventy-one per cent of chewers used betel quid with tobacco. The location of the squamous-cell carcinoma in betel-quid chewers was associated with the site where the quid was retained in the mouth.

In one prevalence study of oral mucosal lesions in out-patients at two dental schools in Chiang-Mai, Thailand, and Kuala Lumpur, Malaysia, Axéll et al. (1990) found one case of oral carcinoma among 96 women from Kuala Lumpur (1.0%). This case was diagnosed in a 45-year-old Indian woman who had been chewing betel quid with tobacco daily for many years.

(b)  Myanmar

Sein et al. (1992) reported on 70 cases of oral cancer (35 men, 35 women) associated with smoking and betel-quid chewing (with or without tobacco) habits. Information was gathered from records of the Institute of Dental Medicine in Yangon (1985–88). The proportion of persons with oral cancer was 58.6% in regular betel-quid chewers, 12.8% in occasional users, 28.6% in non-chewers, 65.7% in regular smokers and 32.9% in non-smokers.

(c)  Thailand

A multivariate regression analysis was conducted in a case–control study in Thailand (Simarak et al., 1977). Over a period of 16 months (1971–72) at the University Hospital in Chiang Mai, patients with a confirmed diagnosis of cancer of the oral cavity and oropharynx (50 men, 38 women), of the larynx and hypopharynx (84 men, 12 women) or of the lung (60 men, 55 women) were selected as cases; 1113 controls (697 men, 416 women) were selected from among patients attending a radiology clinic, mainly with urogenital, respiratory or locomotor disorders; a small proportion of controls (7% of men, 15% of women) had cancers at sites other than those under study. Histological confirmation was obtained for about 50% of cases. A questionnaire administered by nurses provided information on personal habits and demographic factors. Variables that showed a significant relationship with cancer, after adjusting for age and residence, and that were included in the multivariate analysis comprised agricultural employment, rural residence and betel chewing for patients of each sex, lack of formal schooling, and cigarette and cigar smoking for men. After adjusting for the effects of covariables, the relative risk estimates for chewing betel were 2.3 ($p < 0.05$) for men and 3.2 ($p < 0.05$) for women for oral and oropharyngeal cancers and 2.4 ($p < 0.01$) for men for cancer of the larynx and hypopharynx. Among cancer cases who chewed betel, 25/26 added tobacco to the quid, whereas less than two-thirds of the control chewers used betel quid with tobacco.

In a case-only study in southern Thailand (1996–98), Kerdpon and Sriplung (2001) investigated the risk for developing advanced-stage oral squamous-cell carcinoma. Of 161 patients (117 men, 44 women) with early- or advanced-stage carcinoma of the oral cavity and lip (ICD-9 140–141, 143–145), 59/99 cases (59.6%) who presented the advanced stage were betel-quid chewers. [The composition of the betel quid (with or without tobacco) was not specified.] No significant association was observed between chewing and the development of advanced-stage cancer (crude odds ratio, 1.7; 95% CI, 0.9–3.2) at the time of diagnosis nor, upon further analysis, between dose or duration of chewing.

### 2.1.4  Papua New Guinea

In Papua New Guinea, the predominant habit is chewing betel quid with areca nut and slaked lime without tobacco, and oral cancer is generally the most common form of cancer. The earliest study (Eisen, 1946) concluded that betel-quid chewing does not appear to cause cancer of the buccal cavity. [The Working Group noted that this conclusion appeared to be based on the finding of no oral cancer in a cross-section of subjects.] In two reports by Farago (1963a,b), 99% and 98% of oral cancer patients were chewers of betel quid. Smoking was also reported to be common.

Two studies (Atkinson et al., 1964; Henderson & Aiken, 1979) were based on a cancer survey and a continuing cancer registration system. Atkinson et al. (1964) proposed that, since the occurrence of oral cancer correlated very well with the known distribution of the habit of betel-quid chewing, areca nut and slaked lime may have carcinogenic effects even when chewed without tobacco. [The Working Group noted that the authors did not take into consideration cigarette smoking, which was reported to be common.] Henderson and Aiken (1979) observed that the site distribution of their oral cancer cases was consistent with that reported of oral cancer among betel chewers from other parts of the world. Cooke (1969) observed that only 5% of all oral cancers occurred in people in the highlands [where 50% of the population lived, but where areca nut did not grow and betel-quid chewing was less popular (Henderson & Aiken, 1979)]. Cigarette smoking was reported to be common in both the highlands and lowlands.

In a study in 1971–78 from Papua New Guinea, the age-adjusted incidence rates of oral cancer were compared for different geographical areas (Atkinson et al., 1982). In the highlands, where very few people chew areca nut with slaked lime, the age-adjusted incidence of oral cancer per 100 000 compared with that in the lowlands, where a very high percentage of people practise this habit, was 1.01 versus 6.83 for men and 0.41 versus 3.03 for women. It was observed that, in a part of lowland western Papua, inhabited by a specific tribe among whom very few chew, the incidence of oral cancer was very low. The authors, while pointing out that the numbers were very small, noted that the finding had been consistent for 21 years.

In another study (Scrimgeour & Jolley, 1983), the changes in the incidence of oral cancer were compared with the changes in smoking and tobacco consumption during the periods 1965–69 and 1975–79. It was found that the incidence of oral cancer had increased among men as well as among women; the increase for men was not statistically significant, but that for women was ($p < 0.01$). During the same period, the proportion of adult women in a specific area of Papua who smoked commercial cigarettes had increased from 34 to 76%, although their betel-quid chewing habits had not changed greatly. Smoking habits among men had not changed significantly.

## 2.1.5 Migrant populations

Studies of migrant populations have proved of considerable interest to cancer epidemiologists in suggesting the extent to which environmental exposures are important in the etiology of specific cancers. Migrant studies on oral cancer risk have included several Asian groups who have migrated and settled in Britain.

### (a) South Africa

van Wyk et al. (1993) conducted a study among Indians in Natal, South Africa, during the period 1983–89, including 54 men and 89 women with oral and oropharyngeal cancer (ICD 140, 141, 143–146). Information on areca-nut chewing for the cases was obtained directly by patient interview ($n = 75$), from families or friends ($n = 42$) or was only available from hospital records ($n = 26$). Controls were of the same ethnicity, obtained from a random sample of households. The proportion of smokers among female cases was 7%, and 93% chewed areca nut with or without tobacco. Seventy per cent chewed areca nut without tobacco. The crude odds ratio in women (89 oral cancer cases, 735 controls) for chewing areca nut with or without tobacco was 47.4 (95% CI, 20.3–110.5) and that for chewing areca nut without tobacco was 43.9 (95% CI, 18.6–103.6). Of the male cases, 17% reported chewing betel quid with tobacco and 6% without tobacco. The proportion of smokers among male cases was 87%. [The percentage of female smokers was small, and it is known that drinking among these women is rare. This analysis is therefore close to a stratified analysis, but with no adjustment for age.]

### (b) United Kingdom

Marmot et al. (1984) reported on 15 oral cancer deaths in England and Wales between 1970 and 1972 among male Indian ethnic migrants. A higher than expected proportionate mortality ratio of 221 was observed in this ethnic group. Donaldson and Clayton (1984) reported a significant excess in the number of incident oral cancers during 1976–82 in Asian-named individuals in Leicestershire compared with what they referred to as non-Asians. From 1973 to 1985, Swerdlow et al. (1995) examined the risk of cancer mortality in persons born in the Indian subcontinent who migrated to England and Wales. Of the numerous cancers examined, highly significant risks in Indian ethnic migrants were noted for cancers of the mouth and pharynx (odds ratio, 5.5; 95% CI, 3.7–8.2). A later study in the Thames region, which has dense pockets of Asian ethnic communities, supported these observations (Warnakulasuriya et al., 1999). There was a significantly higher proportion of cancers of the oral cavity and pharynx among Asian ethnic migrant groups compared with other natives (for oral cancer in Asian versus other ethnicities, $\chi^2 = 13.6$; $p < 0.01$).

The incidence of oral cancer among migrant Asians is similar to that of Asians in the countries of birth; Asians also appear to retain their habit and their increased risk for oral cancer even several decades after migration (Swerdlow et al., 1995).

## 2.2 Some betel quid-associated lesions, and precancerous lesions and conditions

### 2.2.1 *Introduction*

Studies on the natural history of oral cancer suggest that several potentially malignant lesions and conditions precede the development of cancer of the oral cavity. Precancerous conditions include oral submucous fibrosis and oral lichen planus and oral precancerous lesions of relevance are leukoplakia and erythroplakia (Pindborg *et al.*, 1996; see Glossary B). There is no evidence to suggest that tobacco use (smoked or chewed) is associated with the development of oral submucous fibrosis (Murti *et al.*, 1995; Shah & Sharma, 1998).

The studies summarized here include those carried out in Asia and South Africa, with particular reference to the use of betel quid and areca nut with or without tobacco.

### 2.2.2 *Betel quid-associated oral lesions*

Besides oral precancerous lesions (oral leukoplakia and erythroplakia) and oral precancerous conditions (oral submucous fibrosis, oral lichen planus), some other betel quid-associated lesions of the oral mucosa may be observed. These include betel chewer's mucosa and oral lichenoid lesions, which are of some importance in differential diagnosis.

Areca-induced lichenoid lesions, mostly involving buccal mucosa or the tongue, have been reported at the sites of betel-quid retention (Daftary *et al.*, 1980). In areca-nut chewers, they are found at the site of quid placement and are unilateral in nature. The histology is suggestive of a lichenoid reaction and the lesion resolves following cessation of areca use.

Betel chewer's mucosa was first described by Mehta *et al.* (1971) and is characterized by a brownish-red discoloration of the oral mucosa. This discoloration is often accompanied by encrustation of the affected mucosa with quid particles, which are not easily removed, and a tendency for desquamation and peeling. The lesion is usually localized in and associated with the site of quid placement in the buccal cavity, and is strongly associated with the habit of betel-quid chewing, particularly in elderly women (Reichart *et al.*, 1996). Several epidemiological studies have shown that the prevalence of betel chewer's mucosa may vary between 0.2 and 60.8% in different South-East Asian populations (Table 47). At present, betel chewer's mucosa is not considered to be potentially malignant.

### 2.2.3 *Leukoplakia and erythroplakia*

The prevalence of oral leukoplakia among chewers of betel quid with or without tobacco in selected population samples in India, Malaysia and the Pacific area reported before 1984 is shown in Table 48.

**Table 47. Prevalence of betel chewer's mucosa in different populations**

| Country  | Year    | No.         | Prevalence (%) | Reference             |
|----------|---------|-------------|----------------|-----------------------|
| Cambodia | 1991    | 1319 (M + F)| < 1            | Ikeda et al. (1995)   |
|          | NG      | 102 (F)     | 60.8           | Reichart et al. (1996)|
|          | NG      | 48 (F)      | 85.4           | Reichart et al. (2002)|
| Malaysia | 1993/94 | NG          | 5.2            | Rahman et al. (1997)  |
|          | 1993/94 | 187 (M + F) | 1.6            | Zain et al. (1997)    |
| Thailand | 1979–84 | 1866 (M + F)| 13.1           | Reichart et al. (1987)|

M, men; F, women; NG, not given

(a) *India*

Gupta et al. (1995, 1997) reported on a cohort study conducted in Ernakulam district of Kerala state, India, that comprised 12 212 tobacco users, including betel-quid chewers and smokers, who were followed up for 10 years from 1977–78. All participated in a health education programme on cessation of tobacco use (chewing and smoking). The incidence of leukoplakia dropped significantly following cessation: the incidence among those who stopped chewing was 107 per 100 000 person–years compared with those who did not change their habit (265 per 100 000 person–years, men and women combined).

Gupta (1984) reported a dose–response relationship between the development of leukoplakia and chewing betel quid with or without tobacco. The age-adjusted prevalence of leukoplakia was higher among men than women and the prevalence increased with the number of quids chewed per day (Table 49).

Hashibe et al. (2000a) reported on a cross-sectional study in Kerala, India, that included 927 cases of oral leukoplakia (411 women, 516 men) and 47 773 population-based controls without oral disease (29 876 women, 17 897 men). A case–control study design was applied to the baseline data for a population screened by oral visual inspections and interviewed with structured questionnaires by health workers. Clinical diagnosis of oral precancers was confirmed by dentists and oncologists. Cases of leukoplakia who had other oral precancers or oral cancer were excluded. Elevated odds ratios for oral leukoplakia were observed for betel-quid chewing with tobacco, after adjustment for age, sex, education, body mass index, pack–years of smoking and years of alcohol drinking (Table 50). [The majority of chewers in this population chewed betel quid with tobacco.] The adjusted risk was higher for women than for men and higher for patients who swallowed the juice while chewing, or kept the quid in their mouth overnight. Dose–response relationships were observed for both the frequency (times per day, $p$-value for trend = 0.0001) and duration (years; $p$-value for trend = 0.0001) of betel-quid chewing and the risk for oral leukoplakia.

Within the same study population, 100 cases of erythroplakia (49 women, 51 men) were identified and included in a case–control study with the same 47 773 controls

## Table 48. Prevalence of oral leukoplakia among chewers in selected studies in Asia and the Pacific

| Reference | Location | Chewing habit | Size of sample | Prevalence No. | % |
|---|---|---|---|---|---|
| Gerry et al. (1952) | Guam | Betel quid | 822 | 4 | 0.5 |
| Mehta et al. (1961) | Mumbai, India (police) | Betel quid with tobacco | 1898 | 80 | 4.2 |
| | | Betel quid and smoking | 595 | 42 | 7.1 |
| | | No habit | 1112 | 1 | 0.001 |
| Forlen et al. (1965) | Papua New Guinea | Areca nut and smoking | 610 | – | 9.7–36.3 |
| Pindborg et al. (1967) | Lucknow, India (out-patient clinic) | Tobacco alone | 206 | 15 | 7.3 |
| | | Betel quid with tobacco | 672 | 30 | 4.5 |
| | | Betel quid without tobacco | 181 | 6 | 3.3 |
| | | No habit | 6699 | 2 | 0.03 |
| Pindborg et al. (1968) | Papua New Guinea | Areca nut | 162 | 2 | 1.2 |
| | | Areca nut and smoking | 767 | 29 | 3.8 |
| | | No habit | 165 | – | – |
| Chin & Lee (1970) | Perak, West Malaysia | Betel quid with tobacco | 167 | 67 | 40.1 |
| | | Betel quid without tobacco | 45 | 9 | 20.0 |
| | | Betel quid with *gambir* | 45 | 5 | 11.1 |
| Mehta et al. (1971) | Ernakulam (Kerala), India | Betel quid with tobacco | 2661 | 47 | 1.8 |
| | | Betel quid without tobacco | 38 | – | – |
| | | Chewing and smoking | 1106 | 67 | 6.1 |
| | | No habit | 4210 | 8 | 0.2 |
| | Srikakulam (Andhra Pradesh), India | Betel quid with tobacco | 281 | – | – |
| | | Betel quid without tobacco | 56 | – | – |
| | | Chewing and smoking | 803 | 23 | 2.9 |
| | | No habit | 2620 | 3 | 0.1 |
| | Bhavnagar (Gujarat), India | Betel quid with tobacco | 299 | 3 | 1.0 |
| | | Betel quid without tobacco | 157 | 1 | 0.6 |
| | | Mishri | 714 | 2 | 0.3 |
| | | Chewing and smoking | 320 | 19 | 5.9 |
| | | No habit | 5647 | – | – |
| | Darbhanga (Bihar), India | Betel quid with tobacco | 1572 | 6 | 0.4 |
| | | Betel quid without tobacco | 138 | 2 | 1.4 |
| | | Chewing and smoking | 1485 | 6 | 0.4 |
| | | No habit | 3719 | – | – |
| | Singhbhum (Bihar), India | Betel quid with tobacco | 1293 | 5 | 0.4 |
| | | Betel quid without tobacco | 41 | – | – |
| | | *Gudakhu* | 832 | – | – |
| | | Chewing and smoking | 730 | 2 | 0.3 |
| | | No habit | 4454 | 1 | 0.02 |

**Table 48 (contd)**

| Reference | Location | Chewing habit | Size of sample | Prevalence No. | % |
|---|---|---|---|---|---|
| Smith et al. (1975) | Ahmedabad (Gujarat), India (mainly textile-mill workers) | Tobacco chewing | 1515 | 193 | 12.7 |
| | | Smoking and tobacco chewing | 2319 | 300 | 12.9 |
| | | Betel quid/areca nut without tobacco | 2687 | 144 | 5.4 |
| | | Smoking and betel quid | 12 907 | 2264 | 17.5 |
| | | No habit | 8710 | 112 | 1.3 |
| Lin et al. (1983) (cited in Pindborg et al., 1984a) | Hainan Island, China | Betel quid | 954 | – | 2.5 |

**Table 49. Age-adjusted prevalence of leukoplakia in India by number of quids chewed per day**

| Gender | 1–10 quids per day | | | > 10 quids per day | | |
|---|---|---|---|---|---|---|
| | No. in study | No. of leukoplakias | Age-adjusted prevalence/1000 | No. in study | No. of leukoplakias | Age-adjusted prevalence/1000 |
| Men | 1059 | 34 | 26.6 | 195 | 12 | 49.1 |
| Women | 3099 | 35 | 8.4 | 261 | 5 | 14.6 |

From Gupta (1984)

(Hashibe et al., 2000b). An association was observed between chewing betel quid with tobacco and the risk for erythroplakia, after adjustment for age, sex, education, body mass index, pack–years of smoking and years of alcohol drinking (Table 50). [The majority of chewers in this population chewed betel quid with tobacco.] An increase in the risk for erythroplakia was observed with an increase in the frequency and duration of betel-quid chewing, as well as for swallowing the juice and keeping the quid in mouth overnight. [Cases of erythroplakia were clinically diagnosed by dentists and oncologists without histopathological exclusion of other possible oral erythematous lesions. This may contribute to non-specific oral lesions being included in this clinical category.]

(b)  Taiwan, China

Three recent studies addressed the association between chewing betel quid and the occurrence of oral leukoplakia. The details of design, method and results are summarized in Table 51.

Table 50. Epidemiological studies of the association between chewing betel quid and oral precancerous lesions in India

| Reference, place | Methods | Precancerous lesion | Exposure measurement | Odds ratio (95% CI) | Comments |
|---|---|---|---|---|---|
| Hashibe et al. (2000a) Kerala | Cross-sectional study within large intervention study on oral cancer screening. Case–control design with 927 cases (411 women, 516 men) and 47 773 controls (29 876 women, 17 897 men) from intervention cohort | Oral leukoplakia | Non-chewers<br>Ever chewers<br><br><br><br><br>Current chewers<br>Former chewers<br>Occasional chewers<br>Swallowed chewed tobacco fluid<br>No<br>Yes<br>Kept quid in mouth overnight<br>No<br>Yes | 1.0<br>Men + women<br>7.0 (5.9–8.3)<br>Women<br>37.7 (24.2–58.7)<br>Men<br>3.4 (2.8–4.1)<br>9.4 (8.0–11.2)<br>3.9 (2.8–5.6)<br>2.4 (1.7–3.3)<br><br><br>7.5 (6.4–8.8)<br>13.3 (9.0–16.9)<br><br><br>7.6 (6.5–8.9)<br>13.8 (9.3–20.3) | Adjusted for age, sex, education, body mass index, smoking and drinking |

**Table 50 (contd)**

| Reference, place | Methods | Precancerous lesion | Exposure measurement | Odds ratio (95% CI) | Comments |
|---|---|---|---|---|---|
| Hashibe et al. (2000b) Kerala | Same study base as Hashibe et al. (2000a) 100 cases (49 women, 51 men) and 47 773 controls | Oral erythroplakia | Non-chewers<br>Ever chewers<br>Current chewers<br>Former chewers<br>Occasional chewers<br>Frequency of chewing (times per day)<br>  Continuous<br>  1–10<br>  11–20<br>  > 20<br>  $p$ for trend<br>Duration of chewing (years)<br>  Continuous<br>  1–20<br>  21–40<br>  > 40<br>  $p$ for trend<br>Swallowed chewed tobacco fluid<br>  No<br>  Yes<br>Kept quid in mouth overnight<br>  No<br>  Yes | 1.0<br>19.8 (9.8–40.0)<br>27.6 (10.8–70.4)<br>25.8 (12.6–52.8)<br>2.3 (0.5–10.9)<br><br>1.04 (1.02–1.06)<br>28.6 (14.0–58.7)<br>49.8 (22.0–113.1)<br>130.8 (52.5–326.3)<br>0.0001<br><br>1.01 (0.99–1.03)<br>29.3 (14.2–60.8)<br>53.3 (24.7–114.8)<br>52.8 (18.3–152.6)<br>0.0001<br><br>20.8 (9.8–44.4)<br>50.6 (17.9–143.4)<br><br>21.2 (10.0–45.2)<br>36.3 (11.9–111.6) | Adjusted for age, sex, education, body mass index, smoking and drinking<br><br><br><br><br><br><br><br><br><br><br><br><br><br><br><br><br>Also adjusted for tobacco chewing (years and times per day) |

CI, confidence interval

Table 51. Epidemiological studies of the association between chewing betel quid and oral precancerous lesions and conditions in Taiwan, China

| Reference, place, period | Characteristics of cases and controls | Precancerous lesion and condition | Exposure measurement | Odds ratio (95% CI) | | | Comments |
|---|---|---|---|---|---|---|---|
| Shiu et al. (2000), Taipei, 1988–98 | Nested case–control study; 100 cases selected among cohort of 435 leukoplakia patients, and 100 hospital controls matched on age, gender and date of diagnosis, selected among 25 882 patients with periodontal disease | Leukoplakia | No habit<br>Former chewer<br>Current chewer<br>Former smoker<br>Current smoker<br>Former drinker<br>Current drinker<br>*Level of habit*<br>Chewing   Low<br>              High<br>Smoking  Low<br>              High | 1.0<br>2.4 (0.3–16.8)<br>17.4 (1.9–156.3)<br>1.04 (0.2–4.6)<br>3.2 (1.06–9.8)<br>0.3 (0.03–2.6)<br>3.0 (0.3–33.5)<br><br>9.06 (1.0–81.6)<br>22.5 (1.4–351.0)<br>1.7 (0.5–6.3)<br>3.1 (0.9–10.3) | | | Multivariate analysis adjusted for the effects of the three factors on each other |
| Yang et al. (2001), Pingtung, 1997 | Prevalence study including 312 participants (119 men, 193 women) out of a source population of 3623 in Mutan country (aboriginal community) | Oral submucous fibrosis (OSF) and oral leukoplakia (OL) | *Duration of chewing (years)*<br>0–10<br>11–20<br>21–30<br>≥ 31<br>*No. of quids/day*<br>1–10<br>11–20<br>≥ 21<br>*Multivariate analysis*<br>Areca/betel-quid chewing<br>Smoking<br>Drinking<br>Smoking/drinking | OSF<br>1.0<br>1.8 (0.7–4.8)<br>2.4 (1.01–5.6)<br>2.4 (1.1–5.0)<br><br>1.0<br>1.2 (0.7–2.04)<br>1.3 (0.7–2.2) | OL<br>1.0<br>1.9 (0.9–4.1)<br>1.9 (0.9–3.9)<br>2.03 (1.1–3.7)<br><br>1.0<br>1.03 (0.6–1.7)<br>1.5 (0.9–2.2) | OL or OSF<br>1.0<br>1.7 (0.9–3.1)<br>1.9 (1.09–3.3)<br>2.09 (1.3–3.4)<br><br>1.0<br>1.2 (0.8–1.8)<br>1.5 (1.04–2.08)<br><br>8.2 (1.8–37.5)<br><br>1.05 (0.5–2.2)<br>1.8 (0.9–3.7)<br>1.4 (0.6–3.1) | [Relative risks calculated by the Working Group]<br><br>Adjusted for each other, age and gender |

## Table 51 (contd)

| Reference, place, period | Characteristics of cases and controls | Precancerous lesion and condition | Exposure measurement | Odds ratio (95% CI) | | Comments |
|---|---|---|---|---|---|---|
| | | | | OL | OSF | |
| Lee et al. (2003), Kaohsiung, 1994–95 | 125 histologically confirmed cases of OL (118 men, 7 women) and 94 cases of OSF (93 men, 1 woman); 876 population controls (844 men, 32 women) matched on age and sex | Oral leukoplakia (OL) and oral submucous fibrosis (OSF) | *Betel-quid chewing*<br>Never chewed<br>Former chewer<br>Current chewer<br>Dose-response | 1.0<br>7.1 (2.3–21.5)<br>22.3 (11.3–43.8)<br>4.6 (3.3–6.4) | 12.1 (2.8–51.9)<br>40.7 (16.0–103.7)<br>6.2 (3.9–9.7) | Adjusted for education and occupation |
| | | | *Age started chewing (years)*<br>≥ 26<br>< 26<br>Dose-response | 20.6 (9.9–42.7)<br>19.5 (9.3–41.0)<br>4.3 (3.1–6.0) | 32.3 (12.1–86.6)<br>39.4 (14.8–105.3)<br>5.8 (3.8–8.8) | |
| | | | *Duration of chewing (years)*<br>1–10<br>11–20<br>≥ 21<br>Dose-response | 15.9 (7.1–35.6)<br>20.7 (8.9–48.2)<br>24.0 (10.8–53.4)<br>3.0 (2.3–3.9) | 30.9 (11.3–84.7)<br>41.9 (14.1–124.9)<br>39.3 (11.7–131.7)<br>4.2 (3.0–6.1) | |
| | | | *No. of quids chewed per day*<br>1–10<br>11–20<br>≥ 21<br>Dose-response | 16.6 (8.2–33.8)<br>21.0 (8.9–49.7)<br>38.5 (14.1–105.1)<br>3.8 (2.8–5.1) | 31.4 (11.9–82.5)<br>37.4 (12.6–110.4)<br>53.5 (16.4–174.8)<br>4.1 (2.9–5.8) | |
| | | | *Cumulative quid–years*<br>1–10<br>11–20<br>≥ 21<br>Dose-response | 12.0 (5.6–25.7)<br>23.7 (9.1–61.7)<br>31.4 (14.2–69.2)<br>3.1 (2.4–3.9) | 26.5 (10.0–70.3)<br>47.0 (15.8–139.8)<br>51.4 (16.5–159.7)<br>4.1 (2.9–5.8) | |
| | | | *Type of material*<br>Lao-hwa<br>Betel quid<br>Mixed (betel quid + lao-hwa) | 24.5 (11.8–50.7)<br>11.5 (4.2–32.0)<br>17.4 (7.6–39.8) | 38.7 (14.7–101.9)<br>18.7 (5.3–66.1)<br>37.4 (13.1–107.2) | |

## Table 51 (contd)

| Reference, place, period | Characteristics of cases and controls | Precancerous lesion and condition | Exposure measurement | Odds ratio (95% CI) | | Comments |
|---|---|---|---|---|---|---|
| | | | | OL | OSF | |
| Lee et al. (2003) (contd) | | | **Synergistic effects** | | | Adjusted for education, occupation and alcohol drinking |
| | | | *Betel chewing/smoking* | | | |
| | | | No habit | 1.0 | | |
| | | | Smoking only | 2.4 (1.0–5.5) | 2.3 (0.6–9.1) | |
| | | | Chewing only | 10.0 (3.1–32.7) | 39.3 (7.5–206.9) | |
| | | | Chewing + smoking | 40.2 (16.3–99.2) | 57.9 (16.0–209.6) | |
| | | | Synergy index | 3.8 (1.4–10.5) | 1.4 (0.4–4.7) | |
| | | | *Betel chewing/alcohol drinking* | | | Adjusted for education, occupation and cigarette smoking. Synergy index estimated by an additive interaction model |
| | | | No habit | 1.0 | 1.0 | |
| | | | Drinking only | 1.0 (0.4–2.6) | 0.7 (0.1–3.4) | |
| | | | Chewing only | 15.6 (7.1–34.3) | 26.5 (9.5–74.1) | |
| | | | Chewing + drinking | 16.8 (7.2–39.5) | 31.7 (10.1–99.3) | |
| | | | Synergy index | 1.1 (0.6–2.1) | 1.2 (0.6–2.5) | |

CI, confidence interval

Shiu et al. (2000) used a retrospective leukoplakia cohort that included 435 hospital patients diagnosed according to WHO criteria between June 1988 and February 1998 to study the effects of betel chewing, smoking and drinking on the occurrence of leukoplakia and malignant transformation to oral cancer. To investigate the association between betel quid and risk for oral leukoplakia, a nested case–control study was conducted with 100 cases randomly selected from among the leukoplakia cohort and 100 controls selected from patients with periodontal disease in the same hospital and period as the cases, and matched by age, sex and date of diagnosis. Information on betel-quid chewing (without tobacco), tobacco smoking and alcohol drinking was collected from medical charts and telephone interviews. Duration and frequency of the three habits was also ascertained. Level of chewing (frequency × duration) was classified as high or low according to the distribution of median values. After adjusting for tobacco smoking and alcohol drinking using conditional logistic regression, a 17-fold significant risk was observed among current betel-quid chewers, whereas the risk for former chewers was only twofold and was non-significant. The risk for oral leukoplakia also increased with the level of intensity, suggesting a dose–response relationship between areca-nut chewing and oral leukoplakia.

A population-based survey, using 312 samples obtained by stratified random sampling with a 62.3% response rate, selected from 2059 residents composed mainly of one aboriginal tribe (Paiwan) in southern Taiwan, China, found the prevalences of oral submucous fibrosis and leukoplakia to be 17.6 and 24.4%, respectively (Yang et al., 2001). The prevalence of chewing areca/betel quid was 69.5% and more women (78.7%) than men (60.6%) chewed. Dose–response relationships between duration and frequency of chewing betel quid and precancerous lesions and conditions were also demonstrated [see Table 51; relative risks calculated by the Working Group]. In a multiple logistic regression analysis, the adjusted odds ratio for chewing areca/betel quid was 8.2 (95% CI, 1.8–37.5) for either oral leukoplakia or oral submucous fibrosis.

Lee et al. (2003) designed a case–control study to elucidate the relationships of betel-quid chewing, tobacco and alcohol with oral leukoplakia and oral submucous fibrosis. Cases were selected during 1994–95 among patients of the Kaohsiung Hospital dentistry department and were histologically confirmed. Patients with both oral leukoplakia and oral submucous fibrosis were excluded. There were 125 cases of oral leukoplakia (118 men, seven women) and 94 cases of oral submucous fibrosis (93 men, one woman). Population controls were recruited randomly in the greater Kaohsiung area, and matched to cases by age and sex. A total of 876 controls (844 men, 32 women) participated in the study. All subjects were interviewed by research workers. The major finding was that betel quid conferred a significantly increased risk not only for oral leukoplakia (adjusted odds ratio for current chewers, 22.3; 95% CI, 11.3–43.8), but also for oral submucous fibrosis (adjusted odds ratio for current chewers, 40.7; 95% CI, 16.0–103.7). Chewers of *lao-hwa* quid had the highest risk for oral leukoplakia (adjusted odds ratio, 24.5; 95% CI, 11.8–50.7) and oral submucous fibrosis (adjusted odds ratio, 38.7; 95% CI, 14.7–101.9). Significant dose–response relationships were also demonstrated with respect to duration and frequency of betel-quid chewing. Using an additive interaction model, the synergistic effects in terms of the interaction between betel quid chewing and cigarette smoking were statistically significant for oral leukoplakia but not for oral submucous fibrosis. No synergistic effect between betel quid chewing and drinking was found for oral leukoplakia or oral submucous fibrosis. The proportion of betel-quid chewing contributing to precancerous lesions and conditions in the underlying population (population attributable proportion) was quantified as 73.2% for oral leukoplakia and 85.4% for oral submucous fibrosis.

(c) *South-East Asia*

(i) *Cambodia*

Among 953 Cambodian women, of whom 311 (32.6%) chewed betel quid [with or without tobacco not specified], oral leukoplakia was recorded in six (1.9%) (Ikeda *et al.*, 1995).

In a study of 102 rural Cambodian women who chewed betel quid with tobacco, three (2.9%) showed homogeneous leukoplakia (Reichart *et al.*, 1996). In another study in Cambodia that included 48 women who chewed betel quid with tobacco, four (8.3%) had oral leukoplakia (Reichart *et al.*, 2002).

(ii) *Thailand*

In a field study, Reichart *et al.* (1987) investigated oral mucosal lesions in relation to smoking and chewing habits including betel quid with tobacco in northern Thai tribes. Among betel-quid chewers, oral leukoplakia was recorded in 1.5% of Lahu men, 2.3% of Karen men, 2.6% of Karen women and 3.1% of Lisu men.

(d) *Migrants*

Pearson (1994) reported areca-nut habits of Bangladeshi adults in London, United Kingdom, in a sample of 158 individuals attending general practices. Seventy-eight per cent chewed *paan* with or without tobacco, and the most common lesion was leukoplakia (22%). In a subsequent study on *paan* chewing and smoking habits among the same subjects, the prevalence of leukoplakia had increased to 24.8% (Pearson *et al.*, 2001).

2.2.4 *Oral submucous fibrosis*

(a) *India and Pakistan*

In a survey of over 10 000 villagers in five areas of India, Mehta *et al.* (1971) found submucous fibrosis in people with various chewing and smoking habits. The prevalences are shown in Table 52.

In a 2-year follow-up study of 43 654 industrial workers in Gujarat, India (1969–71), Bhargava *et al.* (1975) found seven new cases of submucous fibrosis among 2105 (0.3%) people who chewed betel quid with areca nut, six new cases among 9506 (< 0.1%) who both chewed and smoked, three new cases among 1161 (0.3%) who chewed tobacco alone and 10 new cases among 7065 (0.1%) with no such habit.

**Table 52. Prevalence of submucous fibrosis and lichen planus in five areas of India**

| Area | Chewing habit | No. | Prevalence of submucous fibrosis | | Prevalence of lichen planus | |
|---|---|---|---|---|---|---|
| | | | No. | % | No. | % |
| Ernakulam (Kerala) | Betel quid with tobacco | 2661 | 29 | 1.1 | 50 | 1.9 |
| | Betel quid without tobacco | 38 | – | – | – | – |
| | Chewing and smoking | 1106 | 5 | 0.4 | 41 | 3.7 |
| | No habit | 4210 | 2 | 0.05 | 3 | 0.07 |
| Srikakulam (Andhra Pradesh) | Betel quid with tobacco | 281 | 1 | 0.4 | 1 | 0.4 |
| | Betel quid without tobacco | 56 | – | – | – | – |
| | Chewing and smoking | 803 | – | – | 7 | 0.9 |
| | No habit | 2620 | – | – | 1 | 0.04 |
| Bhavnagar (Gujarat) | Betel quid with tobacco | 299 | – | – | 1 | 0.3 |
| | Betel quid without tobacco | 157 | – | – | – | – |
| | *Mishri* | 714 | – | – | – | – |
| | Chewing and smoking | 320 | – | – | 1 | 0.3 |
| | No habit | 5647 | 16 | 0.3 | – | – |
| Darbhanga (Bihar) | Betel quid with tobacco | 1572 | – | – | 5 | 0.3 |
| | Betel quid without tobacco | 138 | 2 | 1.4 | – | – |
| | Chewing and smoking | 1485 | 3 | 0.2 | 3 | 0.2 |
| | No habit | 3719 | – | – | – | – |
| Singhbhum (Bihar) | Betel quid with tobacco | 1293 | – | – | 4 | 0.3 |
| | Betel quid without tobacco | 41 | – | – | – | – |
| | *Gudakhu* | 832 | – | – | – | – |
| | Chewing and smoking | 730 | – | – | – | – |
| | No habit | 4454 | – | – | 2 | 0.04 |

From Mehta *et al.* (1971)

In the 10-year follow-up survey of Gupta *et al.* (1980), the age-adjusted incidences per 100 000 for submucous fibrosis were 7.0 for men and 17.0 for women in Ernakulam. The annual incidences per 100 000 were 2.6 for men and 8.5 for women in Bhavnagar; of the four new cases seen in 38 818 persons, two had no tobacco habit, one chewed and one smoked. In Ernakulam, all 11 new cases (out of 39 828 person–years) occurred among chewers of tobacco or of tobacco and betel quid or those with a mixed habit (including smoking).

Murti *et al.* (1990) calculated the incidence of oral submucous fibrosis from a 10-year prospective intervention study of 12 212 individuals in an intervention cohort and 10 287 in a non-intervention cohort. The intervention consisted in a health education programme on cessation of tobacco habits (smoking and chewing) and betel-quid chewing. The intervention cohort consisted of tobacco chewers or smokers selected from a baseline survey undertaken in 1977–78 on 48 000 individuals from 23 villages. Controls were provided by an earlier random sample in Ernakulam district, followed up from 1966–67 but without health education. Two new cases occurred among men and nine among women in the intervention group and three new cases in men and eight in women among the non-intervention group. The annual incidence was 8.0 per 100 000 among men and 29.0 per 100 000 among women in the intervention cohort and 21.3 per 100 000 among men and 45.7 per 100 000 among women in the non-intervention cohort. However, there was only a small number of oral submucous fibrosis patients and the decrease in incidence in the intervention group was not statistically significant.

A case–control study was conducted at a dental clinic in Bhavnagar, Gujarat, and comprised 60 oral submucous fibrosis patients and an equal number of hospital controls matched on age, sex, religion and socioeconomic status. Relative risks were 78 for chewing areca nut without tobacco ($p < 0.01$), 106 for chewing *mawa* ($p < 0.01$) and 30 for chewing areca nut without *mawa* but with tobacco ($p < 0.01$) were observed. The relative risk increased with increasing frequency and duration of chewing (Sinor et al., 1990).

Another case–control study was conducted in Karachi in 1989–90 comprising 157 histologically confirmed cases and 157 hospital-based controls matched on age, sex and ethnicity. Odds ratios for developing oral submucous fibrosis were similar in men and women, although women were predominant (ratio of men:women, 1:2.3). The risk associated with chewing areca nut alone was 154 (95% CI, 34–693) and that associated with chewing areca nut with tobacco was 64 (95% CI, 15–274). The risk increased with frequency of quids chewed, up to 10 per day, and duration of the habit, up to 10 years (Maher et al., 1994).

Babu et al. (1996) reported on a clinico-pathological study of oral submucous fibrosis in Hyderabad. The study included 90 subjects consisting of 50 chewers of betel quid with tobacco and *pan masala* (alone or in combination) who had oral submucous fibrosis (cases) and 40 non-chewers without oral submucous fibrosis (randomly selected hospital controls). Smokers were excluded from the study. *Pan masala/gutka* chewers developed oral submucous fibrosis after 2.7 ± 0.6 years of use, whereas betel-quid chewers developed oral submucous fibrosis after 8.6 ± 2.3 years of use.

Gupta et al. (1998) found the highest prevalence of oral submucous fibrosis among users of *mawa* (10.9%) and the lowest among those who did not use areca nut, in a house-to-house survey conducted in 20 villages in Bhavnagar, Gujarat, that included 11 262 men and 10 590 women. This study also showed that the highest relative risk (age-adjusted) for developing oral submucous fibrosis was among users of *mawa* (75.6) followed by users of any kind of areca nut (60.6), including chewing *mawa*, smoking tobacco and chewing tobacco, compared with non-users of areca nut (Table 53).

Shah and Sharma (1998) reported a case–control study conducted in New Dehli on 236 cases of oral submucous fibrosis (188 men, 88 women) and 221 hospital controls (120 men, 101 women) without oral submucous fibrosis matched on age, sex and socio-

**Table 53. Survey of areca-nut and tobacco use and oral submucous fibrosis, Gujarat, India**

| Areca nut habits | No. of users | No. of cases | Prevalence (%) (age-adjusted) | Relative risk (age-adjusted) |
|---|---|---|---|---|
| No areca nut use | 3 232 | 4 | 0.12 (0.16) | 1.0 |
| Areca nut use | 11 786 | 160 | 9.0 (9.7) | 60.6 |
| *Mawa* | 1 326 | 144 | 10.9 (12.1) | 75.6 |
| With tobacco | 136 | 2 | 1.5 (1.5) | 9.4 |
| With smoking | 324 | 14 | 4.3 (5.0) | 31.3 |
| Total | 15 018 | 164 | 3.2 (3.3) | – |

From Gupta *et al.* (1998)

economic status. No case was found who did not practise any form of areca-nut chewing, whereas in the control group, 165 subjects (74.7%) had no chewing habit. Among cases, 34.7% chewed betel quid without tobacco, 46.2% chewed betel quid with tobacco and none of them smoked tobacco only. Among controls, 7.3% chewed betel quid without tobacco, 4.5% chewed betel quid with tobacco and 11% were tobacco smokers only. Oral submucous fibrotic changes occurred earlier in people who chewed *pan masala* (41.4 months) compared with those who chewed betel quid (77.9 months) [with or without tobacco not specified].

Hazare *et al.* (1998) reported the results of a case–control study conducted for 1 year (June 1996–May 1997) on 200 cases of oral submucous fibrosis (168 men, 32 women) and 197 age-matched hospital controls (122 men, 75 women) in Nagpur, Maharashtra, India. A statistically significant increase in risk was observed with an increase in the frequency of areca-nut use in the form of betel quid that almost always contained tobacco (Table 54).

**Table 54. Dose–response relationship between frequency of areca-nut use and oral submucous fibrosis in India**

| Frequency/day | Cases | Controls | Relative risk |
|---|---|---|---|
| Non-users | 5 | 110 | 1.0 |
| 1 | 11 | 24 | 10.1 |
| 2–3 | 65 | 42 | 34.0 |
| 4–5 | 61 | 16 | 83.9 |
| > 5 | 58 | 5 | 255.2 |
| Total | 200 | 197 | $p$ for trend < 0.01 |

From Hazare *et al.* (1998)

From the study population described in Section 2.2.3 on oral leukoplakia and erythroplakia (Hashibe et al., 2000a,b; Thomas et al., 2003), a case–control study was conducted in Kerala on 170 cases of oral submucous fibrosis (139 women, 31 men) and 47 773 controls (Hashibe et al., 2002). Only nine cases of oral submucous fibrosis reported not to be occasional, past or current chewers of betel quid with or without tobacco. Betel-quid chewing (with and without tobacco) was associated with an increased risk for oral submucous fibrosis adjusted for age, sex, education, occupation, body mass index, pack–years of smoking, years of alcohol drinking and fruit and vegetable intake (Table 55). [The majority of chewers in this population chewed betel quid with tobacco.] Dose–response trends were apparent for the frequency and duration of betel-quid chewing.

Table 55. Association between chewing betel quid with and without tobacco and oral submucous fibrosis in India

| Chewing habit | No. of cases/controls (women and men) | Odds ratio[a] (95% CI) |
|---|---|---|
| Non-chewer | 9/34 373 | 1.0 (reference) |
| Ever chewer | 161/13 400 | 44.1 (22.0–88.2) |
|   Former chewer | 29/1276 | 125.2 (56.7–276.3) |
|   Occasional chewer | 7/2625 | 12.7 (4.7–34.4) |
|   Current chewer | 125/9499 | 49.2 (24.3–99.6) |
| Frequency of chewing (times/day) | | |
|   1–20 | 114/8991 | 28.9 (16.5–50.5) |
|   21–40 | 30/1443 | 46.8 (24.3–90.2) |
|   > 40 | 8/271 | 84.3 (32.8–216.8) |
|   $p$ for trend | | < 0.0001 |
| Duration of chewing (years) | | |
|   1–20 | 88/5971 | 30.8 (17.6–53.8) |
|   21–40 | 54/3470 | 34.7 (18.6–64.5) |
|   > 40 | 9/1217 | 22.7 (9.0–57.5) |
|   $p$ for trend | | < 0.0001 |

From Hashibe et al. (2002)
[a] Adjusted for age, sex, education, occupation, body mass index, drinking (years), smoking (pack-years), vegetable intake and fruit intake
CI, confidence interval

*(b) People's Republic of China*

In a population-based survey of 11 406 people in Xiangtan in 1986, using a method of cluster sampling, 3907 (35.4%) users of betel quid were found. All chewers used areca nut without tobacco. Among betel-quid chewers, a total of 335 cases of oral submucous fibrosis were diagnosed, indicating a prevalence of 3%. No case of oral submucous fibrosis was found among those who did not chew betel quid. The development of oral submucous fibrosis was related to the duration and frequency of chewing (Tang *et al.*, 1997).

On Hainan Island, no oral submucous fibrosis was found among 100 persons (44 men, 56 women) examined within a pilot survey of oral mucosa in betel-nut chewers [with or without tobacco not specified]. However, two cases were suggestive of an early-stage precancerous lesion resembling leukoplakia (Pindborg *et al.*, 1984a).

(c)  *Taiwan, China*

Two studies reporting on oral submucous fibrosis in Taiwan have been reported in Section 2.2.3 (Table 51).

(d)  *South-East Asia*

(i)  *Cambodia*

In a prevalence study of oral mucosal lesions, submucous fibrosis was diagnosed in two of 1319 individuals (0.2%), one man without any distinctive oral habit and one woman who reported betel chewing and tobacco smoking (Ikeda *et al.*, 1995).

(ii)  *Thailand*

Reichart *et al.* (1984) observed one case of submucous fibrosis among the Lisu hill tribe ($n = 139$) who chewed betel quid with tobacco.

(e)  *Migrants*

(i)  *South Africa*

In a survey of 1000 consecutive, unselected Indians from the municipal areas of Johannesburg and Pretoria, all five cases of oral submucous fibrosis detected were in women who chewed areca nut, giving an incidence of 0.5% (Shear *et al.*, 1967). In a further series, five cases of oral submucous fibrosis detected in hospitals by the same authors were also areca-nut chewers. The most frequent habit was chewing betel nut with tobacco in the form of *pan*.

In a stratified survey of 2058 randomly selected Indians in the Durban area in 1981–83, 5% were areca-nut chewers [with or without tobacco not specified]; 71 cases (70 women, one man) of oral submucous fibrosis were detected, all of whom chewed areca nut. Of the cases, 46% had established fibrous bands and 54% were early cases (Seedat & van Wyck, 1988). [The Working Group noted that the criteria for detection of oral submucous fibrosis included very early forms.]

(ii)  *United Kingdom*

Canniff *et al.* (1986) described a large case series of 44 Asian patients (eight men, 36 women) treated at a London hospital (22 Indians, 17 Indians who arrived via East Africa and five non-residents including one Pakistani) for oral submucous fibrosis. All had chewed areca nut either alone or with additives of *pan*. The nature of their chewing habits is shown in Table 56. The case series predominantly consisted of chewers of areca nut only (77%); tobacco was used by only a few, although some added other substances to the nut.

**Table 56. Details of chewing habits in a case series of oral submucous fibrosis patients among migrants, United Kingdom**

| Material chewed | No. of patients (%) |
|---|---|
| Roasted areca nut | 28 (64) |
| Raw areca nut | 6 (14) |
| Roasted nut/slaked lime/betel leaf | 4 (9) |
| Roasted nut/slaked lime/betel leaf/tobacco | 2 (5) |
| Roasted nut/slaked lime/betel leaf/aniseed | 1 (2) |
| Pan parag[a] | 3 (6) |

From Canniff et al. (1986)
[a] Preparation consisting in small pieces of roasted areca nut dusted with a powder of slaked lime and undisclosed flavouring agents

McGurk and Craig (1984) described three cases (two Indians and one Pakistani) of oral submucous fibrosis, two of whom had concomitant oral carcinoma, but whose chewing habits were not accurately recorded. Several other single case studies of oral submucous fibrosis have been reported in Asian migrants to Australia (Oliver & Radden, 1992), Canada (Hayes, 1985) and Great Britain (Zafarulla, 1985; Shah et al., 2001). Some of these cases were in young children who had never been exposed to tobacco or alcohol before and had consumption of areca nut only as a sole risk factor.

### 2.2.5 Oral lichen planus

(a) India

The prevalence of lichen planus in five areas of India (Mehta et al., 1971) is given in Table 52.

In a house-to-house survey in Ernakulam (Kerala) of 7639 villagers, oral lichen planus was found in 1.5% of men and 1.6% of women. The prevalence in various habit groups is given in Table 57. The highest prevalence was found in chewers of betel quid with tobacco (Pindborg et al., 1972).

In the 10-year follow-up survey of Gupta et al. (1997), age-adjusted incidences of lichen planus per 100 000 per year in Ernakulam were 251 for men with mixed habits (including smoking), 329 for men who chewed tobacco or betel quid plus tobacco, 146 for women with mixed habits and 385 for women who chewed betel quid with tobacco.

**Table 57. Prevalence of lichen planus in subjects with various habits in Kerala, India**

| Habit | No. in study | Lichen planus | |
|---|---|---|---|
| | | No. | % |
| Chewing | | | |
|   Tobacco and lime | 212 | 3 | 1.4 |
|   Betel quid without tobacco | 24 | – | – |
|   Betel quid with tobacco | 1925 | 61 | 3.2 |
| Smoking | | | |
|   Bidi | 1334 | 10 | 0.7 |
|   Other | 386 | 3 | 0.8 |
| Chewing and smoking | 845 | 31 | 3.7 |
| None | 2911 | 10 | 0.3 |

From Pindborg et al. (1972)

*(b)  South-East Asia*

Among 953 Cambodian women studied for oral mucosal lesions, 365 chewed betel quid only or in combination with smoking. Oral lichen planus was recorded in 20 of these women (5.5%); 19 of the 20 women used betel quid with tobacco (Ikeda et al., 1995).

2.2.6   *Multiple and mixed lesions*

A case–control design was applied to analyse data collected from a screening programme conducted in Sri Lanka. Three hundred and fifty-nine precancer cases (316 men, 43 women, with leukoplakia and submucous fibrosis), age- and sex-matched to population controls from the same villages as the cases, were included in the study. Controls were disease-free following oral examination. The relative risk for chewing betel quid without tobacco among nonsmokers was 5.3 in men and 5.0 in women; both were statistically non-significant. The relative risk for chewing betel quid with tobacco among nonsmoking men was 15.0 ($p < 0.005$) and that among nonsmoking women was 33.0 ($p < 0.001$) (Warnakulasuriya, 1990). Chewers were at higher risk than smokers.

An additional 115 subjects with multiple premalignant oral lesions and conditions (defined as having one or more of the following: oral leukoplakia, erythroplakia, oral submucous fibrosis; 73 women, 42 men) from the Kerala, India, study population with the 47 773 controls described in Section 2.2.3 (Hashibe et al., 2000a,b) were included in another case–control study (Thomas et al., 2003). The odds ratios were 52.8 (95% CI, 22.4–124.4) for chewing betel quid with tobacco and 22.2 (95% CI, 6.6–74.0) for chewing betel quid without tobacco, after adjustment for age, sex, education, body mass index, pack–years of smoking, years of alcohol drinking and fruit and vegetable intake. Dose–response trends were observed for the frequency (times per day; *p*-value for trend < 0.0001) and duration (years; *p*-value for trend < 0.0001) of chewing betel quid (with and without tobacco) and the risk for multiple premalignant oral lesions and conditions.

2.2.7   *Malignant transformation*

(*a*)   *India and Pakistan*

In many of the earlier histological studies of oral cancer, e.g. Paymaster (1956), leukoplakia was seen concomitantly with the cancer.

In the 10-year follow-up study of Mumbai policemen (Mehta *et al.*, 1961, 1969, 1972a), one oral cancer developed among 117 cases of leukoplakia in an individual who chewed betel quid (presumably with tobacco) and who also smoked bidis.

In the follow-up of Bhargava *et al.* (1975) in Gujarat, India, 22 histologically confirmed cases of oral cancer were seen among 43 654 persons re-examined after 2 years. The authors stated that seven (0.13%) of the cases had developed from leukoplakia.

Of the 4762 persons with leukoplakia who were re-examined after 2 years by Silverman *et al.* (1976), six had developed oral carcinoma, giving an annual incidence of malignant transformation of leukoplakia of 63 per 100 000. One man chewed tobacco plus betel quid only, two both chewed (one tobacco, the other tobacco plus betel quid) and smoked bidis, two smoked bidis only and the one woman took nasal snuff only.

In a 10-year follow-up in Ernakulam (Kerala), South India, of 410 leukoplakia patients, all of whom were chewers of betel quid with tobacco, nine (six men, three women) developed oral carcinoma (Gupta *et al.*, 1980). The crude annual rate of malignant transformation was 3.9 per 1000 in men and 6.0 per 1000 in women. Four other oral cancers were observed: two in patients who had been diagnosed with early leukoplakic changes (preleukoplakia), one in a patient with submucous fibrosis and the other in a case of lichen planus. No oral cancer was seen in subjects who had had normal mucosa at the previous examination.

In an 8-year follow-up of 12 212 tobacco users that started in 1977, the relative risk for developing oral cancer from nodular leukoplakia was 3243 (6 new cases of oral cancer among 13 cases), that from homogeneous leukoplakia was 25.6 (three new cases of oral cancer among 489 cases) and that from lichen planus was 15.8 (one among 344 cases). The relative risk for malignant transformation among individuals with oral submucous fibrosis was 397, based on three new cases of oral cancer among 25 cases of oral submucous fibrosis versus four new cases of oral cancer among 10 145 persons with no precancerous condition (Gupta *et al.*, 1989). The risk for malignant transformation was significant for all lesions except lichen planus.

Gupta *et al.* (1980) also reported malignant transformation in one of 44 cases of oral submucous fibrosis in Ernakulam (Kerala); none were found among five cases in Srikakulam.

A follow-up study over 4–15 years of 66 patients with submucous fibrosis was carried out in Ernakulam. Malignant transformation was observed in three patients 3, 4 and 7 years after initial examination, giving an overall transformation rate of 4.5% (Pindborg et al., 1984b).

In a population sample of 27 600 individuals in Ernakulam district, Kerala, 66 had oral submucous fibrosis and were followed up for 17 years. Five developed oral cancer, giving a malignant transformation rate of 7.6% (Murti et al., 1985).

A study conducted in Karachi, Pakistan (1996–98), on 79 cases of oral squamous-cell carcinoma and 149 hospital controls showed that the risk for developing oral cancer was 19 times higher (95% CI, 4.2–87.7) among cases of oral submucous fibrosis than among subjects with no precancerous condition (Merchant et al., 2000).

Gupta et al. (1980) observed one oral cancer case among 332 individuals seen with lichen planus.

(b) *Taiwan, China*

In the study by Shiu et al. (2000), 60 cases of oral and pharyngeal cancer (including lip, tongue, gum, mouth floor, buccal palate, oropharynx and hypopharynx) were ascertained by linking a retrospective leukoplakia cohort consisting of 435 patients recruited from hospital between 1988 and 1998 to a population cancer registry. The risk for malignant transformation increased with time, particularly for areca-nut chewers. Using a Weibull survival model, the adjusted hazard ratio for chewing areca nut without tobacco was 4.6 (95% CI, 1.3–16.9) after adjusting for age and sex.

(c) *Migrants*

McGurk and Craig (1984) reported malignant transformation of submucous fibrosis in two Indian women living in the United Kingdom. Only one of the women had chewed areca nut and both had latent iron deficiency.

## 2.3 Other upper aerodigestive cancer

### 2.3.1 *India*

The study by Hirayama (1966) described in Section 2.1.1(c) reported a statistically significant six-fold increase in risk for oropharyngeal cancer among nonsmokers chewing betel quid with tobacco.

A comprehensive evaluation of cancer risk among betel-quid chewers and smokers was reported by Jussawalla and Deshpande (1971) in a case–control study in Mumbai. They selected 2005 histologically confirmed cancer patients with cancers of the oral cavity, pharynx, larynx and oesophagus. Equal numbers of controls were selected from the population using electoral roll and were matched to cases for age, sex and religion. Information was collected by interviewing patients and controls. Table 58 shows the assessment of risk for cancer at each site in chewers and non-chewers. The relative risks were highly significant for all studied cancers combined, oral cavity as a whole, and for cancers of the tongue, alveolus, buccal mucosa, hard palate, tonsils, oropharynx, hypopharynx, larynx

Table 58. Relative risks for oral cancer and other cancers of the upper aerodigestive tract among betel-quid chewers, assuming the risk among non-chewers to be unity

| Group | Habit | | Relative risk |
|---|---|---|---|
| | None (no.) | Chewing (no.) | |
| Controls | 1340 | 665 | |
| Cancer patients | 853 | 1152 | 2.7*** |
| Oral cavity | 129 | 282 | 4.4*** |
| Base of tongue | 175 | 187 | 2.2*** |
| Soft palate | 35 | 18 | 1.0 NS |
| Tonsils | 99 | 128 | 2.6*** |
| Lip | 8 | 6 | 1.5 NS |
| Anterior two-thirds of tongue | 36 | 54 | 3.0*** |
| Floor of mouth | 10 | 4 | 0.8 NS |
| Alveolus | 26 | 44 | 3.4*** |
| Buccal mucosa | 42 | 160 | 7.7*** |
| Hard palate | 7 | 14 | 4.0** |
| Oropharynx | 309 | 333 | 2.2*** |
| Nasopharynx | 10 | 7 | 1.4 NS |
| Hypopharynx | 21 | 49 | 4.7*** |
| Larynx | 246 | 314 | 2.6*** |
| Oesophagus | 138 | 167 | 2.4*** |

From Jussawalla & Deshpande (1971)
**, $p < 0.01$; ***, $p < 0.001$; NS, $p > 0.05$

and oesophagus. Table 59 shows the relative risks for cancers at different sites for chewers only, chewers and smokers and smokers only. The relative risks were highly significant for all cancers, except cancer of the nasopharynx, in all habit groups.

A summary of the case–control studies of other upper aerodigestive cancers in India published since 1984 is given in Table 60.

Sankaranarayanan et al. (1991) reported a case–control study of cancer of the oesophagus conducted in Kerala, India, in 1983–84, that included 267 cases (207 men, 60 women) and 895 controls comprised of 271 non-cancer cases from the cancer center and 624 patients diagnosed with acute respiratory, gastrointestinal or genitourinary infection. Sixty-seven per cent of cases were histologically confirmed (33% by radiology only). Only four men (controls) and six women (three cases, three controls) chewed betel quid without tobacco. Among men, an elevated risk was suggested for chewing betel quid with tobacco for the age group 31–40 years (odds ratio, 1.2; 95% CI, 0.6–2.1) and a significant risk for chewing betel quid with tobacco was observed for subjects over 40 years of age (odds ratio, 2.0; 95% CI, 1.03–3.9). Among women, risks were elevated for chewing betel quid with tobacco for the age group 30–40 years (odds ratio, 1.4; 95% CI, 0.5–4.3) and

**Table 59. Relative risks for oral and other cancers by habit, assuming the risk among persons with no habit to be unity**

| Group | No habit (no.) | Chewing only (no.) | Relative risk | Chewing and smoking (no.) | Relative risk | Smoking only (no.) | Relative risk |
|---|---|---|---|---|---|---|---|
| Controls | 925 | 521 | | 144 | | 415 | |
| Cancer patients | 243 | 557 | 4.1*** | 595 | 15.7*** | 610 | 5.6*** |
|   Oral cavity | 57 | 192 | 6.0*** | 90 | 10.1*** | 72 | 2.8*** |
|   Oropharynx | 49 | 91 | 3.3*** | 242 | 31.7*** | 260 | 11.8*** |
|   Nasopharynx | 4 | 4 | 1.8 NS | 3 | 4.8 NS | 6 | 3.3 NS |
|   Hypopharynx | 8 | 28 | 6.2*** | 21 | 16.9*** | 13 | 3.6** |
|   Larynx | 55 | 142 | 4.6*** | 172 | 20.1*** | 191 | 7.7*** |
|   Oesophagus | 70 | 100 | 2.5*** | 67 | 6.2*** | 68 | 2.2*** |

From Jussawalla & Deshpande (1971)
**, $p < 0.01$; ***, $p < 0.001$; NS, $p > 0.05$

for subjects over 40 years of age (odds ratio, 2.2; 95% CI, 0.6–8.1). [The Working Group noted that, among men, risk estimates were potentially confounded by bidi smoking.]

From 1997 to 1998, a hospital-based case–control study on oesophageal cancer in Assam, India, included 502 cases (358 men, 144 women) and 994 controls (706 men, 288 women) who were attendants to cancer patients. Controls were matched on sex and age. The risk for chewing betel quid (with or without tobacco), adjusted for smoking and alcohol consumption, was 2.6 (95% CI, 1.3–7.4) for men and 1.9 (95% CI, 0.02–7.8) for women. The risk increased with increasing frequency of chewing betel quid with or without tobacco and increased substantially when the chewing habit had lasted 20 years or more. A dose–response relationship was also observed for age at starting the habit, with a higher risk for starting at a younger age (Phukan et al., 2001).

Znaor et al. (2003) reported a study conducted in men in two centres in South India, Chennai and Trivandrum, in 1993–99 that included 636 cases of pharyngeal cancer (except nasopharynx) and 566 cases of oesophageal cancer, who were compared with 1711 cancer controls and 1927 healthy hospital visitor controls. For oesophageal cancer, significantly elevated risks were found for chewing betel quid without tobacco (odds ratio,1.6; 95% CI, 1.1–2.5) and for chewing betel quid with tobacco (odds ratio, 2.1; 95% CI, 1.6–2.6). For pharyngeal cancer, the odds ratios (adjusted for age, educational level, smoking, alcohol consumption and centre) were 1.4 (95% CI, 0.9–2.1) for chewing betel quid without tobacco and 1.8 (95% CI, 1.4–2.3) for chewing betel quid with tobacco. Significant dose–response relationships were observed for duration of chewing with or without tobacco, number of quids consumed per day and cumulative years of chewing for both oesophageal and pharyngeal cancers (Table 61). A non-significant substantial decrease in risk was seen 10 years after quitting the chewing habit. Likelihood ratio tests

Table 60. Case–control studies of upper aerodigestive cancers other than oral cancers and risk associated with chewing betel quid in India (1985–2003)

| Location (years) | Cancer site | ICD code | No. of cases | Habit | No. of controls | Habit | Relative risk (95% CI) | Reference | Comments |
|---|---|---|---|---|---|---|---|---|---|
| Kerala, South India (1983–84) | Oesophagus | 150 | 207 (M) 60 (F) | BQ + T, 35.4% BQ + T, 45.5% | 546 (M) 349 (F) | BQ + T, 33.5% BQ + T, 51.3% | BQ + T, 1.09 (0.8–1.5) BQ + T, 0.8 (0.4–1.4) | Sankaranarayanan et al. (1991) | Crude relative risk |
| Assam (1997–98) | Oesophagus | 150 | 358 (M) 144 (F) | Q, 92% Q, 76% | 706 (M) 288 (F) | Q, 65% Q, 47% | Q, 3.4 (1.2–9.5) Q, 3.5 (1.4–10.3) | Phukan et al. (2001) | Crude relative risk |
| Chennai & Trivandrum (1993–99), South India | Pharynx Oropharynx Hypopharynx Pharynx, unspecified | 146 148 149 | 636 (M) | BQ, 5% BQ + T, 28% S, 86% | 3638 (M) | BQ, 5% BQ + T, 10% S, 51% | BQ, 1.4 (0.9–2.1) BQ + T, 1.8 (1.4–2.3) | Znaor et al. (2003) | Adjusted for age, center, education, drinking and smoking |
| | Oesophagus | 150 | 566 (M) | BQ, 5% BQ + T, 25% S, 72% | | | BQ, 1.6 (1.1–2.5) BQ + T, 2.1 (1.6–2.6) | | |
| Bhopal, Central India (1986–92) | Oropharynx | 146 | 247 (M) | BQ, 1.6% BQ + T, 42.1% S + T, 32.8% | 260 (M) | BQ, 4.6% BQ + T, 41.5% S + T, 16.5% | BQ + T, 1.2 (0.8–1.8) | Dikshit & Kanhere (2000) | Adjusted for age and smoking |
| Kerala, South India (1983–84) | Larynx | 161 | 171 (M) | BQ + T, 29% | 541 (M) | BQ + T, 33% | BQ + T, 0.8 (0.6–1.2) | Sankaranarayanan et al. (1990b) | Crude relative risk |

CI, confidence interval; M, men; F, women; BQ, betel quid without tobacco; T, tobacco S, smoking only; Q, betel quid with or without tobacco

**Table 61. Odds ratio for pharyngeal and oesophageal cancer by duration, level and cumulative chewing, South India**

| Site | Pharynx | | | | Oesophagus | | |
|---|---|---|---|---|---|---|---|
| | Controls | Cases | Odds ratio [a] | 95% CI | Cases | Odds ratio [a] | 95% CI |
| Never chewed | 3079 | 424 | 1.0 | – | 371 | 1.0 | – |
| *Duration of chewing (years)* | | | | | | | |
| 0–19 | 286 | 67 | 1.2 | 0.9–1.7 | 71 | 1.8 | 1.3–2.5 |
| 20–39 | 209 | 101 | 1.97 | 1.5–2.7 | 84 | 2.05 | 1.5–2.8 |
| ≥ 40 | 64 | 44 | 2.6 | 1.6–4.2 | 40 | 2.3 | 1.4–3.6 |
| $p$ for trend | | | | < 0.001 | | | < 0.001 |
| *Average daily amount (no. of quids)* | | | | | | | |
| 1–3 | 343 | 101 | 1.2 | 0.9–1.6 | 81 | 1.2 | 0.9–1.6 |
| 4–5 | 135 | 55 | 1.9 | 1.3–2.8 | 51 | 2.2 | 1.5–3.2 |
| > 5 | 800 | 56 | 4.2 | 2.7–6.6 | 63 | 6.1 | 4.0–9.1 |
| $p$ for trend | | | | < 0.001 | | | < 0.001 |
| *Cumulative exposure to chewing* | | | | | | | |
| < 1000 | 158 | 101 | 1.4 | 0.97–1.9 | 69 | 0.9 | 0.7–1.3 |
| > 1000 | 26 | 31 | 1.97 | 1.05–3.7 | 23 | 1.7 | 0.9–3.3 |
| $p$ for trend | | | | = 0.03 | | | = 0.029 |
| *Time since quitting chewing (years)* | | | | | | | |
| Current chewers | 460 | 171 | 1.0 | – | 160 | 1.0 | – |
| 2–4 | 41 | 15 | 0.8 | 0.4–1.7 | 12 | 0.5 | 0.2–1.1 |
| 5–9 | 20 | 10 | 1.2 | 0.5–3.0 | 8 | 0.9 | 0.4–2.3 |
| 10–14 | 19 | 6 | 0.5 | 0.2–1.3 | 8 | 0.6 | 0.2–1.6 |
| ≥ 15 | 19 | 10 | 0.6 | 0.2–1.4 | 7 | 0.4 | 0.2–1.1 |
| $p$ for trend | | | | = 0.62 | | | = 0.586 |

From Znaor *et al.* (2003)
[a] Adjusted for age, centre, level of education, alcohol consumption and smoking
CI, confidence interval

were statistically significant ($p < 0.05$) for (a) the combination of the three habits of chewing, smoking and drinking for oesophageal and pharyngeal cancers; (b) for chewing and drinking, and chewing and smoking, for oesophageal cancer and (c) for the interaction between drinking and smoking, and chewing and smoking, for pharyngeal cancer. Interaction was not tested separately for chewing betel quid without tobacco because only 33 oesophageal and 34 pharyngeal cancer cases had chewed betel quid without tobacco.

A case–control study conducted in 1986–92 on 247 cases of oropharyngeal cancer (all men) registered in the population-based Bhopal Cancer Registry and 260 population controls showed a non-significant risk for oropharyngeal cancer associated with chewing betel quid with tobacco. Those who chewed more than 10 quids with tobacco per day (odds ratio, 3.6; 95% CI, 1.7–7.4) and those who had chewed quid with tobacco for more than 30 years (odds ratio, 3.1; 95% CI, 1.6–5.7) had statistically significant risks (Dikshit & Kanhere, 2000).

A case–control study was conducted in Kerala in 1983–84 on 191 men with histologically confirmed laryngeal cancer and 549 hospital controls; after excluding occasional chewers, the number of cases and controls (hospital patients without cancer) were 171 and 541, respectively. The risk associated with chewing betel quid with tobacco was not increased (Sankaranarayanan et al., 1990b).

### 2.3.2　Taiwan, China

One case–control study in Taiwan, China, in 1996–2000, included 104 cases of histologically confirmed oesophageal squamous-cell carcinoma (94 men, 10 women) and 277 age- and sex-matched controls (256 men, 21 women) without malignant disease from the same hospital. The results showed that subjects who chewed moderate amounts of betel quid without tobacco (lifetime consumption, 1–495 quid–years) had a 3.6-fold (95% CI, 1.3–10.1) risk and those who chewed greater amounts (lifetime consumption, ≥ 495 quid–years) had a 9.2-fold (95% CI, 1.8–46.7) risk for oesophageal cancer after controlling for cigarette smoking and alcohol consumption (Wu et al., 2001).

## 2.4　Other cancers

The studies from India on cancers of the stomach, lung or cervix are summarized in Table 62.

### 2.4.1　Stomach cancer

A case–control study of stomach cancer conducted in Chennai, India, in 1988–90 included 388 incident cases of stomach cancer (287 men, 101 women; 75% histologically confirmed) and an equal number of cancer controls matched on age, sex, religion and native language, showed a non-significantly increased risk, when adjusted for income group, level of education and area of residence, for current chewing of betel quid with or without tobacco (relative risk, 1.4; 95% CI, 0.96–1.93). This risk disappeared when further adjustment was made for smoking, alcohol drinking and dietary items (relative risk, 0.8; 95% CI, 0.5–1.4) (Gajalakshmi & Shanta, 1996).

### 2.4.2　Lung cancer

A case–control study conducted on 163 male lung cancer cases registered at the population-based Bhopal (India) Cancer Registry and 260 population controls showed no association between chewing betel quid with tobacco and lung cancer (Dikshit & Kanhere, 2000).

Table 62. Case–control studies of chewing betel quid and cancers of the stomach, lung and cervix, India

| Location (years) | Cancer site | No. of cases | Habit | No. of controls | Habit | Relative risk (95% CI) | Reference | Comments |
|---|---|---|---|---|---|---|---|---|
| Chennai, South India (1988–90) | Stomach | 287 (M) 101 (F) | Q, 38.9% | 287 (M) 101 (F) | Q, 33.7% | Q, 1.3 (0.95–1.8) BQ, 1.3 (0.8–2.1) BQ + T, 1.3 (0.9–1.98) | Gajalakshmi & Shanta (1996) | Adjusted for income, education and residence |
| Bhopal, Central India (1986–92) | Lung | 163 | BQ, 2.5% BQ + T, 31.9% S + T, 27.6% | 260 (M) | BQ, 4.6% BQ + T, 41.5% S + T, 16.5% | BQ + T, 0.7 (0.4–1.2) | Dikshit & Kanhere (2000) | Adjusted for age and smoking |
| Chennai and Trivandrum, South India (1993–99) | Lung | 778 (M) | NS | 3430 (M) | NG | Q, 0.8 (0.6–1.02) | Gajalakshmi et al. (2003) | Adjusted for age, education, centre and smoking |
| Chennai, South India (1998–99) | Cervix | 205 (F) | BQ, 4.9% BQ + T, 13.7% | 213 (F) | BQ, 2.8% BQ + T, 4.2% | BQ, 2.6 (0.7–9.8) BQ + T, 2.1 (0.8–5.9) | Rajkumar et al. (2003c) | |

CI, confidence interval; M, men; F, women; Q, betel quid with or without tobacco; BQ, betel quid without tobacco; T, tobacco; S, smoking only; NG, not given

In a case–control study conducted in men in Chennai and Trivandrum, India, in 1993–99 comprising 778 lung cancer patients, 1711 cancer (non-tobacco related) controls and 1927 healthy controls, no significant association was found between chewing betel quid with or without tobacco and risk for lung cancer, nor was there evidence for increasing trend with prolonged duration of chewing (Gajalakshmi et al., 2003).

### 2.4.3 Cervical cancer

A case–control study of 205 cases of invasive cervical cancer and 213 age-matched hospital controls was conducted in Chennai, India, in 1998–99. A twofold non-significantly elevated risk was noted for chewing betel quid with and without tobacco. A statistically significant association was seen among those who chewed more than five quids with or without tobacco per day and the dose–response relationship was also significant ($p = 0.02$). [The Working Group noted that the number of subjects analysed for the dose–response relationship was small.] (Table 63) (Rajkumar et al., 2003).

**Table 63. Dose–response relationship: cervical cancer study in Chennai**

| Average daily amount (no. of quids) | Cases | Controls | Odds ratio[a] | 95% CI |
|---|---|---|---|---|
| Never chewed | 167 | 198 | 1.0 | |
| < 5 | 16 | 9 | 1.4 | 0.5–4.1 |
| ≥ 5 | 22 | 6 | 4.0 | 1.2–13.3 |
| Trend test, $p = 0.02$ | | | | |

From Rajkumar et al. (2003)
[a] Adjusted for age, area of residence, education, occupation, marital status, age at first marriage, number of pregnancies and husband's extramarital affairs

### 2.4.4 Liver cancer

(a) Taiwan, China

An association was seen in one case report (Liu et al., 2000) of a histologically confirmed hepatocellular carcinoma in a 54-year-old Taiwanese man who had chewed betel quid without tobacco for at least 32 years. He also had an oral squamous-cell carcinoma. He had smoked 1.5 packs of cigarettes daily and consumed alcohol occasionally and in moderate amounts; he was not infected by hepatitis viruses. High concentrations of safrole (a product of the inflorescence of *Piper betle*)-like DNA adducts were detected in oral and liver cells. [The specificity of the DNA adducts was questioned by the Working Group.]

In a prospective study in Taiwan, China, Sun et al. (2003) followed a total of 12 008 men aged 30–64 years with no history of hepatocellular carcinoma at baseline from 1990 to 2001. At baseline, information on betel-quid chewing was available for 11 989 subjects; of these, 1463 (12.2%) had a history of chewing. Among the 1463 chewers and 10 526 non-chewers, 10 and 102 cases of hepatocellular carcinoma were ascertained, respectively, to give incidence rates of 74.8 per 100 000 person–years for chewers and 105.7 per 100 000 person–years for non-chewers, and a crude relative risk of 0.7 (95% CI, 0.4–1.3). In a multiple regression model with adjustment for age, smoking, hepatitis B virus surface antigen (HBsAg) status, and family history of liver cirrhosis and/or liver cancer, the relative risks for the combination of hepatitis C virus (HCV) infection and betel-quid chewing were 0.8 (95% CI, 0.4–1.6) for chewers without HCV infection, 2.6 (95% CI, 1.5–4.6) for non-chewers with HCV infection and 6.8 (95% CI, 1.7–28.2) for chewers with HCV infection, compared with non-chewers without HCV infection. The corresponding synergy factor was 4.2 (95% CI, 0.6–30.7), suggesting that the effect of HCV infection on the risk for hepatocellular carcinoma may be modified by betel-quid chewing.

Another case–control study in Kaohsiung in 1996–97 included 263 cases of hepatocellular carcinoma (205 men, 58 women), matched with 263 controls selected from community residents who received a health check-up in the same hospital and had normal serum aminotransferase levels and no space-occupying lesion in the liver (Tsai et al., 2001). Chewing betel quid (without tobacco) was associated with the risk for hepatocellular carcinoma (odds ratio, 3.5; 95% CI, 1.7–7.0) after controlling for sex, age, alcohol drinking, smoking, HBsAg, anti-HCV and education, using a conditional logistic regression model. The risk for hepatocellular carcinoma increased with increasing duration of areca-nut chewing and with frequency of chewing (Table 64). The risk increased in subjects with HCV infection and an interaction between HCV infection and chewing was demonstrated. The risk was also strongly associated with the presence of HBsAg and chewing betel quid (Table 65). Both interactions, in terms of synergism index, were greater than 1, with 5.37 for HBV–areca-nut chewing and 1.66 for HCV–areca-nut chewing. [This finding suggests that the effect of areca-nut chewing on hepatocellular carcinoma may confer an increased risk among subjects who have HBV or HCV infections.]

*(b)   Thailand*

A case–control study conducted in 1987–88 (Parkin et al., 1991) included 103 cases (71 men, 32 women) of cholangiocarcinoma admitted to three hospitals in North-East Thailand and 103 hospital controls matched by age, sex and residence. The criteria for definition of cases included histology, typical findings on ultrasound examination or percutaneous cholangiography. Controls were selected from individuals visiting various clinics in the same hospital or from a variety of non-malignant diseases considered to be unrelated to tobacco or alcohol consumption. Interviews were conducted using a structured questionnaire, including information on family history, smoking, betel chewing, dietary habits and alcohol use. Blood specimens were examined for HBV serology, antibodies to *Opisthorchis viverrini* and aflatoxin–albumin adducts. The final conditional logistic regression model included anti-

Table 64. Dose–response relationship between duration and frequency of chewing and risk for hepatocellular carcinoma in Taiwan, China

| Chewing habits | No. of cases/controls | Odds ratio (95% CI) |
| --- | --- | --- |
| Non-chewer | 192/241 | 1.0 |
| Duration of chewing (years) | | |
| < 20 | 8/14 | 0.7 (0.3–1.9) |
| 20–30 | 27/5 | 6.8 (2.4–20.5) |
| > 30 | 36/3 | 15.1 (4.4–39.1) |
| $p$ for trend | | < 0.0001 |
| Total amount consumed (quids × 1000) | | |
| < 100 | 11/10 | 1.4 (0.5–3.6) |
| 100–199 | 31/7 | 5.6 (2.3–14.2) |
| 200–299 | 15/3 | 6.3 (1.7–20.7) |
| > 299 | 14/2 | 8.8 (1.9–34.0) |

From Tsai et al. (2001)
CI, confidence interval

Table 65. Interactions between betel-quid chewing and anti-HCV, and betel-quid chewing and HBsAg, and risk for hepatocellular carcinoma in Taiwan, China

| Betel-quid chewer | Anti-HCV | HBsAg | No. of cases/ controls | Odds ratio (95% CI) | Synergy index |
| --- | --- | --- | --- | --- | --- |
| − | − | | 121/230 | 1.0 | |
| − | + | | 71/11 | 12.3 (6.0–25.5) | |
| + | − | | 57/21 | 5.2 (2.9–9.3) | |
| + | + | | 14/1 | 26.6 (3.6–116.6) | 1.66 |
| − | | − | 74/187 | 1.0 | |
| − | | + | 118/54 | 5.5 (3.6–8.6) | |
| + | | − | 18/18 | 2.5 (1.2–5.4) | |
| + | | + | 53/4 | 33.5 (11.1–72.7) | 5.37 |

From Tsai et al. (2001)
Anti-HCV, antibodies to hepatitis C virus; HBsAg, hepatitis B surface antigen; CI, confidence interval

*O. viverrini* status, rice consumption and betel-quid chewing with or without tobacco. The odds ratio for betel-quid chewing, comparing weekly to less than monthly use, was 6.4 (90% CI, 1.1–39.3).

A case–control study conducted within the same investigation of liver cancer in Thailand (Parkin *et al.*, 1991) included 65 cases (47 men, 18 women) of hepatocellular carcinoma admitted to the same three hospitals in North-East Thailand and 65 controls matched by age, sex and residence (Srivatanakul *et al.*, 1991). The criteria for definition of cases included cytology, typical findings on ultrasound, or radiological examination. Controls were selected from the same source as in Parkin *et al.* (1991) and interviews were conducted similarly. Blood specimens were examined for HBV and HCV serology, antibodies to *O. viverrini* and aflatoxin–albumin adducts. The final conditional logistic regression model included HBsAg status, alcohol consumption, some dietary items and betel-quid chewing with or without tobacco. The odds ratio for betel-quid chewing, comparing weekly to less than monthly use, was 11.0 (90% CI, 1.0–115.8; $p < 0.05$).

## 3. Studies of Cancer in Experimental Animals

### 3.1 Oral administration

#### 3.1.1 *Mouse*

Groups of 15–21 male Swiss mice, 8–10 weeks of age, were administered by gavage 0.1 mL of aqueous extracts of areca nut (containing 1.5 mg arecoline and 1.9 mg polyphenol) or betel leaf or a polyphenol fraction of areca nut (containing 1.9 mg tannic acid) on 5 days a week for life. A group of 30 male C17 mice received 0.1 mL of an aqueous extract of areca nut by gavage. Groups of 20 male Swiss and 20 male C17 mice served as untreated controls. Of the animals treated with aqueous areca-nut extract, 12/21 Swiss mice developed tumours (five hepatocellular carcinomas, two haemangiomas of the liver, two adenocarcinomas of the lung, one adenocarcinoma and one squamous-cell carcinoma of the stomach, and one leukaemia) and 8/30 C17 mice developed tumours (three squamous-cell carcinomas and two adenocarcinomas of the stomach, two leukaemias and one adenocarcinoma of the lung). In Swiss mice fed the areca-nut polyphenol fraction, two developed tumours of the salivary gland and one a haemangioma of the liver. No tumour was observed in either of the control groups or in the mice fed aqueous betel-leaf extract (Bhide *et al.*, 1979). [The Working Group noted the absence of survival data and indication of duration of the experiment for the treated and control mice.]

A group of 14 male and 18 female C17 mice, 10–12 weeks of age, was fed a diet containing 10% (w/w) areca nut coated with saccharin [concentration not specified] for 40 weeks, and the animals were followed for life. Another group of 12 males and 22 females served as untreated controls. In the group fed areca nut, two males developed squamous-cell carcinomas of the forestomach and three females developed uterine malignancies (reticular-cell neoplasm type A). Two similar uterine tumours were observed in the untreated controls. No statistically significant increase in tumour incidence was observed in animals treated with areca nut compared with controls (Pai et al., 1981).

Groups of 20 male Swiss mice, 8–10 weeks of age, were administered by gavage 0.1 mL of aqueous extracts of betel quid, betel quid and tobacco, areca nut, betel leaf, or areca nut and betel leaf five times per week for life or served as untreated controls. Animals were killed when moribund. All lesions reported were lung adenocarcinomas [histological details not given]; the incidences are given in Table 66 (Shirname et al., 1983). [The Working Group noted that the reason for the difference between the initial number of animals and the number of animals assessed for the presence of tumours is unknown.]

Table 66. Design and results of experiments in Swiss mice given aqueous extracts of betel quid and its components by gavage

| Group | No. at start | No. of mice alive between 10 and 24 months | No. of mice with lung tumours (%) |
|---|---|---|---|
| Control | 20 | 20 | 1 (5) |
| Betel quid | 20 | 15 | 4 (26) |
| Betel quid and tobacco | 20 | 18 | 4 (22) |
| Areca nut | 20 | 19 | 9 (47)* |
| Betel leaf | 20 | 14 | 1 (7) |
| Areca nut and betel leaf | 20 | 16 | 6 (38)* |

From Shirname et al. (1983)
*Statistically significant compared with controls ($p < 0.05$)

Groups of 8–20 female and 16–35 male Swiss mice, 6 weeks of age, were given 1 mg arecoline hydrochloride (in 0.1 mL distilled water) daily by gavage on 5 days a week, either alone or in combination with potassium nitrate ($KNO_3$) (1 mg daily), or $KNO_3$ with slaked lime (1 mg daily); controls were either untreated or received $KNO_3$ and lime. Treatment was continued for up to 25 months. A total of 15/35 (43%) males given arecoline alone developed tumours (8/18 between 12 and 18 months and 7/17 between 19 and 25 months) compared with 1/20 untreated males. Of the 15 tumours in the arecoline group, eight were liver haemangiomas, four were lung adenocarcinomas and three were squamous-cell carcinomas of the stomach. No tumour was reported in any of the 18 arecoline-treated or 20 control females. The incidence of tumours in male mice given arecoline in combination with either $KNO_3$ (3/19) or $KNO_3$ + lime (1/16) did not differ from that in corresponding control males given $KNO_3$ + lime (2/17). No tumour was found in females treated similarly (Bhide et al., 1984). [The Working Group noted the lack of information on the time of appearance of specific neoplasms and the inadequate reporting of the pathological findings. The lack of tumours in females was not explained.]

Groups of 18 male and 18 female Swiss mice, 10–12 weeks of age, were administered by gavage a daily ration of 0.1 mL of a fraction of areca nut containing ~1.9 mg tannin for life. Two animals developed tumours of the parotid gland, which were diagnosed as adenocystic carcinomas. One of the tumours was transplantable and was maintained as a model system by serial transplantation in Swiss mice (Gothoskar & Pai, 1986). [This study was only aimed at describing the derivation of a transplantable tumour model and did not yield any data on concentration or constituents of the areca-nut component used. The Working Group deemed it to be inadequate for evaluation.]

A total of 690 inbred Swiss mice, 6–7 weeks of age, divided into groups of 20–25 males and 20–25 females, were fed diets containing the following areca-nut products: (a) ripe, unprocessed, sun-dried areca nut (R-UP-SD), (b) ripe, processed, sun-dried areca nut (R-P-SD), (c) unripe, processed, sun-dried areca nut (UR-P-SD), (d) ripe, unprocessed, sun-dried, water-soaked areca nut (R-UP-SD-WS) or (e) ripe, unprocessed, sun-dried, water-soaked areca nut (R-UP-UD-WS) for 12 months. Diet was prepared using different types of areca nut from the market. The preparations were dehydrated, powdered and added wt/wt to pulverized feed to obtain diets containing 0.25, 0.5 and 1% areca nut. Control mice were maintained on normal diet for 12 months. In a second experiment, areca-nut paste was applied to the oral cavity of groups of 20–25 male and 20–25 female mice using a dispenser at dose levels of 0.25, 0.5 or 1.0 g/kg bw twice a day on 5 days per week for 12 months. The paste was prepared by grinding 10 g powdered areca-nut preparation of each type (as in experiment 1) with 25–30 mL drinking-water to obtain a smooth paste. Drinking-water was not provided to animals for 1 h following administration of the paste to facilitate intimate contact of the paste with the oral, pharyngeal and oesophageal epithelium. Control mice received oral applications of 0.05 mL water. In both experiments, animals were killed at the end of 12 months, internal organs were screened for tumour development and oral, pharyngeal, oesophageal, gastric and liver tissues were processed for histology. Cellular atypia (in three males and two females) and papilloma and carcinoma (in two males and one female) were observed in the oesophagus of animals treated with R-UP-SD at the highest dose (1% in diet). Two of 23 males receiving 1% R-UP-SD-WS developed papillomas in the oesophagus; 2/23 males and 1/21 females receiving 1% R-UP-UD-WS developed oesophageal papillomas and carcinomas. Following oral application of areca-nut paste, animals exposed to 1 g/kg bw R-UP-SD paste developed oesophageal papillomas and carcinomas (2/23 males and 2/24 females). One male and one female mouse receiving 1 g/kg bw R-UP-SD-WS developed papilloma and carcinoma of the oesophagus. In the R-UP-UD-WS-treated group, 2/23 males and 1/21 females developed oesophageal papilloma and carcinoma. In both experiments, oesophageal tumours appeared in different groups that were fed the unprocessed variety of areca-nut preparations (Rao & Das, 1989).

Groups of 15 male and 15 female ICRC/HiCri mice, 6–8 weeks of age, received 25 or 50 mg per animal (quantities denote original dry weight of the product) ethanolic extract of *pan masala* (EPME; containing areca nut, catechu, lime flavouring agents and unspecified spices), a chewing mixture, by gavage in distilled water or distilled water alone five times per week for 6 months. No forestomach or oesophageal tumour was observed in mice that survived until the end of the experiment or died beforehand (Ramchandani *et al.*, 1998).

Groups of 54 male and 54 female Swiss S/RVCri mice, 6–7 weeks of age, were fed diets containing 0, 2.5 or 5% *pan masala* (containing areca nut, catechu, lime, spices and flavouring agents) in the diet for life. Animals were killed when moribund or at the end of 24 months. A significant decrease was observed in the overall survival rate of mice receiving 2.5% and 5% *pan masala* compared with the controls with or without adjustment for sex. Organs were excised and processed for histopathology. A total of 15 benign and 12 malignant tumours were observed in treated mice. The commonest benign tumour was liver haemangioma in 7/108 mice fed 2.5% *pan masala*. In the group fed 5%, more diverse types of benign tumour were found. Malignant tumours were observed in 5/108 and 7/108 mice fed 2.5% and 5% *pan masala*, respectively. Lung and liver adenocarcinomas were observed in 3/108 and 1/108 mice fed 2.5% *pan masala*, as well as one hepatoma. In the 108 mice fed 5%, five adenocarcinomas of the lung, one forestomach carcinoma and one testicular lymphoma were observed. No tumours were found in the 108 controls. A statistically significant positive trend ($p = 0.004$) with dose was observed in the number of mice with lung carcinoma (Bhisey *et al.*, 1999).

### 3.1.2 *Rat*

Groups of eight to nine male and eight female ACI rats, 6 weeks of age, were fed diets containing either 20% Indonesian areca nut or 20% Taiwanese betel-leaf powder for 480 and 300–327 days, respectively. A group of 11 males and eight females received a diet containing 20% Indonesian areca nut and 1% calcium hydroxide for 480 days. A group of nine males and 10 females served as untreated controls. At the end of the treatment periods, the animals were fed a normal diet and observed for life. No statistically significant difference in tumour incidence was observed between the treated and control groups. No tumours were observed in the oral cavity or gastrointestinal tract (Mori *et al.*, 1979). [The Working Group noted that addition of 20% (wt/wt) areca-nut powder to the diet results in severe caloric and nutritional imbalances, which may have affected the results. This could not be assessed because of inadequate reporting of the survival data for the various groups.]

The effect of marginal vitamin A deficiency on carcinogenicity was examined in 4–6-week-old male and female ACI rats. Group 1 (32 males and 27 females) was fed a marginally vitamin A-deficient diet (20 IU palmitate/100 g diet) mixed with 20% areca-nut powder and 1% calcium hydroxide; Group 2 (39 males and 28 females) received vitamin A-deficient diet; Group 3 (21 males and 21 females) was fed vitamin A-sufficient diet (1200 IU palmitate/100 g diet) containing 20% areca-nut powder and 1% calcium hydroxide; and Group 4 (20 males and 21 females) received vitamin A-sufficient diet alone. The experiment lasted for 647 days and 176/209 animals survived beyond 360 days. Two male and two female rats from each group were killed 30 weeks after the start of the experiment to determine vitamin A levels in serum and liver. All other animals were autopsied at natural death, when moribund or at 647 days. Liver tissues were processed for histology. In Group 1 (vitamin A-deficient + areca nut + calcium hydroxide), one papilloma of the tongue and one of the buccal mucosa in males and one papilloma of the tongue and one of the forestomach in females were observed. No upper aerodigestive tract tumour developed in Group 2 or Group 3. Two neoplastic liver nodules were observed in female rats of Groups 1 and 3 and one in Group 4. A solitary hepatocellular carcinoma developed in one female in Group 1. Other tumours that developed were: one spindle-cell carcinoma of the parotid gland in Group 1 males; two transitional-cell carcinomas and two squamous-cell carcinomas of the urinary bladder in Group 2 females; and two endometrial carcinomas, one leiomyosarcoma of the uterus and one mammary adenoma in Group 3 females. Group 4 rats did not develop tumours. The difference in tumour incidence in various groups did not reach statistical significance. Female susceptibility to tumour development could not be interpreted (Tanaka et al., 1983).

### 3.1.3 Hamster

Three groups of eight, eight and four Syrian hamsters (males and females approximately equally distributed), 6–7 weeks of age, were given distilled water containing 2% arecoline and 0.5% calcium hydroxide or 2% arecoline alone or were fed a diet that contained 0.1% arecoline with 2.5% calcium hydroxide, respectively, for life. Mean survival was 18 months, animals were killed when moribund or died spontaneously [no specific survival data given for the various experimental groups]. No tumours were observed in any of the treated animals. No tumours were found in four control Syrian hamsters (two males and two females) that ingested distilled water containing 0.5% calcium hydroxide or in four controls that were fed a diet containing 2.5% calcium hydroxide (Dunham et al., 1974). [The Working Group noted the small number of animals.]

Of a group of two males and two females, one male Syrian golden hamster, 25.5 months of age, developed a carcinoid tumour of the glandular stomach after being fed a diet containing 0.1% arecoline and 2.5% calcium hydroxide for 12 months from the age of 1.5 months (Dunham et al., 1975). [The Working Group noted the small number of animals used. Because of the lack of available data, a fortuitous finding cannot be excluded.]

In a study aimed at evaluating the effect of concomitant oral administration of areca nut and sodium nitrite, 120 Syrian golden hamsters, 8 weeks of age, were divided into four treatment groups, each consisting of 15 males and 15 females. Group I received a diet containing 0.2% sodium nitrite, group II a diet containing 2% powdered areca nut, group III a diet containing both the sodium nitrite and the areca nut powder added in doses as mentioned above, and group IV received a diet without additives once a day on 5 days a week. The experiment lasted until the animals died spontaneously or were killed when moribund. Controls were killed after the death of the last experimental animal. The group-based percentage of tumour-bearing animals and the total number of tumours were elevated [not statistically significantly] in animals fed areca nut alone or combined with nitrite as compared with the group fed nitrite only or control. Malignant tumours occurred three times more frequently in the group fed areca powder together with nitrite, but this increase did not reach statistical significance except for an increase in malignant lymphomas in male animals (5/15 versus 1/15; pairwise Fisher's exact probability test, $p < 0.05$). No statistical difference in survival time was seen for the various groups (Ernst et al., 1987).

## 3.2 Skin application

*Mouse*

A group of 12 Swiss mice [sex and age unspecified] received daily topical applications of an aqueous extract of betel quid (areca nut, stone lime and *gambir*) plus tobacco on the ears for 2 years; two animals developed squamous-cell carcinomas and one a benign squamous papilloma at the site of application (Muir & Kirk, 1960). [The Working Group noted that no controls were reported.]

Groups of 16–23 male and female C17 mice [sexes approximately equally distributed], 2–3 months of age, received thrice-weekly topical applications of 0.1 mL dimethyl sulfoxide (DMSO) extracts of tobacco (5 g ground tobacco in 20 mL DMSO), areca nut (30 g ground areca nut in 20 mL DMSO) or tobacco and areca nut, or applications of 0.1 mL DMSO alone on their backs for life. Animals were allowed to live their normal lifespan or were killed when they showed signs of debility. Skin papillomas were observed in 1/23 animals and epidermoid carcinomas were observed in 2/23 animals that received applications of combined tobacco and areca-nut extracts; no local tumour was observed in the other treatment groups (Ranadive et al., 1976).

## 3.3 Subcutaneous administration

### 3.3.1 *Mouse*

Groups of 10 male and 10 female Swiss mice, 2–3 months of age, were given subcutaneous injections of 0.2 mL hot or cold filtered aqueous areca-nut extracts (50 mg/mL) once a week for 6 weeks. Animals were allowed to live their normal lifespan or were killed when they showed signs of debility. Fibrosarcomas at the site of injection were observed in 14/20 and 10/20 mice treated with hot and cold areca-nut extracts, respectively; the first tumour appeared after 8 months. No local tumour was seen in a group of 13 male and 12 female controls receiving injections of distilled water for 10 weeks (Ranadive et al., 1976). [No further details on follow-up and survival were available.]

Effects on tumour development were investigated in male Swiss mice [age not specified] after subcutaneous injection of distilled water, an aqueous extract of areca nut, a polyphenol fraction of areca nut, a polyphenol-free fraction of areca nut, arecoline, an aqueous extract of areca nut and betel leaf, an aqueous extract of betel quid or an aqueous extract of betel quid and tobacco. Groups were treated as follows: Group 1 (controls; 20 mice) was injected with 0.1 mL distilled water; group 2 (12 mice) received injections of 0.1 mL of a 1:10 extract of areca nut (prepared by lyophilization of a 1% aqueous extract of areca nut dissolved in 10 mL distilled water); group 3 (20 mice) received injections of 0.1 mL of a polyphenol fraction of areca nut (prepared, concentrated to dryness and dissolved in 10 mL distilled water); group 4 (20 mice) received injections of 0.1 mL of a polyphenol-free fraction of areca nut (1:10 dilution obtained after extraction of ethyl acetate-extracted residue with distilled water, lyophilization and dissolution in 10 mL distilled water); group 5 (10 mice) received injections of 1.5 mg arecoline; group 6 (15 mice) received injections of 0.2 mL of aqueous extract of areca nut and betel leaf; group 7 (20 mice) received injections of 0.2 mL aqueous extract of betel quid; and group 8 (20 mice) received injections of 0.2 mL of aqueous extract of betel quid with tobacco. All groups received weekly injections for 13 weeks. Animals were killed when moribund and abnormal tissues were processed for histopathology. The incidence of tumours was: Group 1, 0/20 tumours; Group 2, two fibrosarcomas, two haemangiomas of the liver (4/12 mice; 33%); Group 3, 16/20 fibrosarcomas, one hepatoma, three lung adenocarcinomas (20/20; 100%); Group 4, 0/20 tumours; Group 5, 0/10 tumours; Group 6, 0/15 tumours; Group 7, 7/20 fibrosarcomas; Group 8, 2/20 tumours at the site of injection [histological identification not mentioned] (Shivapurkar et al., 1980).

### 3.3.2  Rat

A group of 15 male and 15 female outbred NIH Black rats, 1–2 months old, received weekly subcutaneous injections of 0.5 mL of a tannin-rich aqueous extract of areca nut for up to 56 weeks and were observed for a further 12 weeks. Injections were discontinued when the first tumour appeared. All treated animals developed fibrosarcomas at the injection site. No local tumour occurred in 15 male and 15 female controls receiving injections of saline (Kapadia et al., 1978).

### 3.4  Intraperitoneal administration

*Mouse*

Groups of 7–10 male Swiss mice, 6 weeks of age, received weekly intraperitoneal injections of 0.1 mL aqueous extract of areca nut (seven mice), betel leaf (10 mice) or the polyphenol fraction of areca nut (nine mice) [details of doses were insufficiently defined] for 13 weeks. Additional groups were injected with commercial tannin (10 mice), arecoline (1.5 mg; 10 mice) or distilled water (10 mice). All animals were observed for their entire lifespan. No tumour was observed in any of the groups (Shivapurkar et al., 1980). [The Working Group noted the small number of animals used, the poor definition of the substances tested and the absence of details on the methods used.]

## 3.5 Administration to the oral mucosa or cheek pouch

### 3.5.1 *Rat*

A group of 21 albino (Wistar strain) rats [sex not specified], 3–4 months of age, received applications to the palate and cheek mucosa of a paste (1 g) of *pan masala* [mode of preparation not described; exact site not described; method of application not described] administered every other day for 6 months. A group of 14 untreated animals served as controls. Biopsies were taken after 2, 4 and 6 months of application of *pan masala* and treatment was discontinued for 2 weeks after each biopsy to allow tissue healing. A biopsy was taken in the beginning and at the end of the experiment from control rats. After 6 months of treatment with *pan masala* paste, no tumour was observed; however, a high incidence of dysplastic epithelial changes (loss of nuclear polarity in 65% of animals after 6 months of application) was reported (Khrime *et al.*, 1991). [The Working Group noted that the duration of the experiment was only 6 months, and that the incidence of dysplasia is a matter for concern.]

A group of 14 male and 13 female Wistar rats, 2 months of age, received daily applications to the buccal and palatal surfaces of 2% ethanolic extract of arecoline for 2.5 (six animals), 3 (six animals) and 4.5 months (15 animals). Groups of six and 12 animals served as solvent and untreated controls, respectively. Animals were killed at the end of the experiment. Histologically, no tumour was observed (Sirsat & Khanolkar, 1962).

### 3.5.2 *Hamster*

Groups of 8–50 male and female Syrian golden hamsters, 1–2 months of age, received an implantation in the cheek pouch of a pellet of single beeswax containing 7–50% betel quid or its various components: betel leaf, areca nut, areca nut and betel leaf, or areca nut and tobacco. Animals were allowed to live their normal lifespan or were killed when moribund. Exposure varied from 1 to 35 months. No malignant tumour was observed at the implantation site in any of the groups (Dunham & Herrold, 1962). [The Working Group noted that only a single administration was given.]

A total of 65 male Syrian golden hamsters, 9 weeks of age, was divided into four groups of 11–21. Animals received topical applications on the cheek-pouch mucosa of DMSO extracts of areca nut, tobacco, areca nut plus tobacco or DMSO alone thrice weekly for 21 weeks, at which time all animals were killed. Local squamous-cell carcinomas and leukoplakia were seen in 8/21 and 19/21 of the animals treated with areca-nut extract, and in 16/21 and 18/21 of the groups treated with areca-nut and tobacco extract, respectively; no local tumour was seen in hamsters treated with tobacco extract alone, but 8/12 had leukoplakia. No local tumour was observed in the 11 DMSO-treated controls (Suri *et al.*, 1971). [The Working Group noted that development of cheek pouch tumours between 7 and 21 weeks was extremely unusual and would imply an exceedingly powerful carcinogenic effect.]

A group of nine Syrian golden hamsters, 6–7 weeks of age, received applications to the cheek pouch mucosa of 1.5% arecoline in water [quantity not specified] five times per week for life; about 30 mg of 0.5% calcium hydroxide was applied to the cheek pouch mucosa before treatment with arecoline. One papilloma developed in the upper third of the oesophagus in one 15-month-old female (Dunham et al., 1974). [The Working Group noted the small number of animals used.]

Groups of 12–14 male Syrian golden hamsters (total number, 38), 2–3 months of age, received applications to the cheek-pouch mucosa of DMSO extracts of tobacco, areca nut or tobacco plus areca nut thrice weekly for life. A solvent-control group of seven animals received applications of DMSO alone. The combination of tobacco and areca-nut extracts resulted in the development of lesions in the mucous membrane that were diagnosed as early malignant changes in 3/12 animals and in one stomach tumour. One stomach tumour was also found in the 12 animals treated with tobacco extract, but none were found in 14 animals treated with areca-nut extract alone (Ranadive et al., 1976). [The Working Group noted the small group size, the ambiguous description of the principal lesions reported and that histology of the stomach tumours was not provided.]

A total of 317 Syrian golden and white mutant hamsters [details on pheno- or genotype of the mutant not provided; sex and distribution of strains in each group unspecified], 2–3 months of age, were administered betel-quid ingredients separately or in various combinations in the cheek pouch, using the following modes: thrice-weekly applications of aqueous extracts of the test materials; deposition of replaceable wax pellets containing the test materials; introduction of gelatin capsules containing the powdered materials; or insertion of the natural components for direct exposure. Animals were killed at 6–12 or 13–14 months. A group of 64 animals served as controls: 25 received a placebo wax pellet, nine received a gelatin capsule and 30 were untreated. The incidences of cheek-pouch and forestomach carcinomas in animals receiving topical applications of the aqueous extracts of test materials are given in Tables 67 and 68. Of the group receiving implants of wax pellets containing betel quid, 4/18 and 8/18 developed cancers of the cheek pouch and forestomach, respectively. Cheek-pouch carcinomas [histology not specified] and forestomach squamous-cell carcinomas were observed in 3/21 and 8/21 (two of these eight carcinoms were located in the oesophageal region) animals receiving implants of wax pellets containing betel quid plus tobacco. The incidence of tumours in hamsters given betel-quid ingredients in their natural form was not markedly different from that seen after other modes of administration. Cheek-pouch carcinomas and forestomach carcinomas developed in 5/16 hamsters given cheek-pouch implantations of capsules containing areca-nut powder, tobacco and lime. Cheek-pouch carcinomas (4/19) and forestomach carcinomas (6/19) occurred in hamsters given capsules containing areca-nut powder (Ranadive et al., 1979). [The Working Group noted the lack of information on sex and strain distribution, the lack of data on the number of tumours per animal and the lack of details on the quantitative composition of the mixtures tested.]

A total of 243 male Syrian golden hamsters, 6–7 weeks of age, were divided into eight groups. Group 1 served as controls. In the other groups, the following test substances were

Table 67. Design and results of experiments in Syrian golden hamsters given topical applications of aqueous extracts of betel-quid ingredients on the cheek pouch

| Group | No. of hamsters at start | Age (months) | Cheek-pouch carcinoma | | Forestomach carcinoma | |
|---|---|---|---|---|---|---|
| | | | No. | %[a] | No. | %[a] |
| Control | 19 | 6–12 | – | | – | |
| | 11 | 13–21 | – | | – | |
| Areca-nut extract[a] | 6 | 6–12 | – | | 1 | 16.6 |
| | 15 | 13–21 | 1 | 6.6 | 3 | 20.0 |
| Polyphenol fraction of areca nut[b] | 4 | 6–12 | – | | – | |
| | 16 | 13–21 | 1 | 6.2 | 4 | 25.0 |
| Areca nut and tobacco extract[b] | 6 | 6–12 | – | 16.6 | – | |
| | 12 | 13–21 | 2 | | 3 | 25.0 |
| Betel-quid extract[c] | 16 | 6–12 | – | | 4 | 25.0 |
| | 4 | 13–21 | – | | 1 | 25.0 |
| Betel quid with tobacco extract[d] | 7 | 6–12 | – | | 1 | 14.2 |
| | 6 | 13–21 | – | | 3 | 50.0 |
| Areca-nut pieces with extract of areca nut[b] | – | 6–12 | – | | – | |
| | 13 | 13–21 | – | | 6 | 46.1 |
| Areca-nut pieces with extracts of areca nut and tobacco[b] | 4 | 6–12 | – | | 2 | 50.0 |
| | 10 | 13–21 | – | | 1 | 10.0 |

From Ranadive et al. (1979)
[a] Both hot and cold extracts of areca nut; filtered from an initial mixture of 0.5 g/mL
[b] Details of preparation not mentioned
[c] Filtered from a mixture containing betel leaf (0.5 mg/mL), areca-nut powder (0.2 mg/mL), slaked lime (0.01 g/mL) and catechu (0.01 g/mL)
[d] Filtered from a mixture containing betel leaf (0.5 mg/mL), areca-nut powder (0.2 mg/mL), slaked lime (0.01 g/mL), catechu (0.01 g/mL) and 0.04 g/mL tobacco

applied: liquid paraffin, liquid paraffin with 0.5% 7,12-dimethylbenz[a]anthracene (DMBA), DMSO, extract of cured tobacco, extract of Thai areca nut, extract of cured tobacco with Thai areca nut and extract of Indian areca nut. The mode of application was according to Salley (1954) and the extracts were prepared by the methods of Suri et al. (1971), with a remark that an additional 10 mL DMSO had to be added to the areca nut before the extract could be obtained by squeezing. Groups 1, 2 and 3 (six animals per group) were killed at week 16. Other groups (45 animals per group) were killed serially at 2-week intervals, from weeks 2 to 30. Squamous-cell carcinoma was seen in the

Table 68. Design and results of experiments in hamsters given implantations of wax pellets and capsules containing betel-quid ingredients[a] on the hamster cheek pouch

| Group | No. of hamsters at start | Age (months) | Cheek-pouch carcinoma | | Forestomach carcinoma | |
|---|---|---|---|---|---|---|
| | | | No. | % | No. | % |
| Wax pellet control | 20 | 6–12 | – | | – | |
| | 5 | 13–21 | – | | – | |
| Betel quid | 8 | 6–12 | 1 | 12.5 | 3 | 37.5 |
| | 10 | 13–21 | 3 | 30 | 5 | 50 |
| Betel quid + tobacco | 9 | 6–12 | – | | 1 | 11 |
| | 12 | 13–21 | 3 | 25 | 7[b] | 42 |
| DMBA (standard carcinogen control) | 15 | 6–12 | 12 | 80 | 7[b] | 33 |
| | 0 | 13–21 | – | | – | |
| Capsule control | 5 | 6–12 | – | | – | |
| | 4 | 13–21 | – | | – | |
| Areca-nut powder | 10 | 6–12 | 2 | 20 | 2 | 20 |
| | 9 | 13–21 | 2 | 22 | 4 | 44 |
| Areca-nut powder + tobacco powder + lime | 4 | 6–12 | 1 | 25 | 1 | 25 |
| | 12 | 13–21 | 4 | 33 | 4 | 33 |

From Ranadive et al. (1979)
DMBA, 7,12-dimethylbenz[a]anthracene
[a] Each pellet weighed 2–3 g and contained 0.82–1.3 g of test substance [proportion of the various components not mentioned].
[b] Two of the tumours were oesophageal carcinomas, and were not included in the percentages.

DMBA-treated group [number of tumours not stated]. No tumour was seen in any of the other groups (Weerapradist & Boonpuknavig, 1983).

In a study in which the tumour-promoting activity of arecaidine was tested in DMBA-treated hamster buccal pouches, 112 male adult Syrian hamsters, 10–12 weeks of age, were divided into 16 groups, each containing seven animals. Three of these groups received applications of 1000, 2000 or 3000 µg/mL arecaidine solutions six times per week for 12 weeks without DMBA pretreatment, and one group was untreated. [Arecaidine was obtained from Sigma but the chemical form was not provided.] At the end of 12 weeks, all animals were killed. In all four groups, no tumour was observed (Lin et al., 1996).

In an initiation–promotion study, 24 male Syrian golden hamsters, 8 weeks of age, received applications to the cheek pouch of 25 µg/mL arecaidine in distilled water thrice weekly for 12 weeks. Ten weeks later, 1% croton oil in acetone was applied thrice weekly to the cheek pouches of the 13 remaining animals for another 3 weeks, after which the animals were killed and the last three animals were killed 34 weeks after the start of the experiment. No tumours were found in any of the animals (MacDonald, 1986).

In a study of the tumour-promoting activity of betel quid on DMBA-treated hamster cheek pouches, two groups of male Syrian golden hamsters, about 6–8 weeks of age at the start of the experiment, received insertions of betel quid alone into the cheek pouch. Treatment with betel quid alone for 36 weeks (10 males) or 52 weeks (nine males) did not lead to tumour formation (Wong et al., 1992).

The tumour-promoting activity of betel quid on DMBA-treated hamster cheek pouch was tested in groups of 42 non-inbred male adult Syrian hamsters, 8–10 weeks of age, one group was tested with Taiwanese betel-quid extract alone, which was painted six times weekly. The quid extract consisted of the filtrate of a mixture of areca nut (450 g), 'unripe betel fruit' (120 g) [assumed to be inflorescence of *Piper betle* L.] and slaked lime (50 g) to which 300 mL DMSO were added as solvent. At the end of 2 weeks, six animals were taken from each group and killed; this was repeated after periods of 2 weeks each, thus enabling evaluation of the effect of treatment in relation to its duration. After 14 weeks, all animals had been killed. No tumours were seen in the group treated with betel quid alone (Lin et al., 1997).

Groups of 20 female Syrian golden hamsters, 6–7 weeks of age, received topical applications to the cheek pouch mucosa of aqueous extracts of tobacco (1 mg per pouch), areca nut (1 mg per pouch) or betel leaf (5 mg per pouch) twice a day for either 10 days or 6 months and were killed 6 months after the last treatment. In the short-term study, none of the animals developed any lesion. In the long-term study, one local squamous-cell papilloma and two local squamous-cell carcinomas of the cheek pouch developed in 3/20 animals in the tobacco-treated group and one local papilloma and one local squamous-cell carcinoma were found in 2/20 animals in the areca nut-treated group. No cheek-pouch tumour was observed in 20 animals treated with betel leaf or in 10 untreated or 10 vehicle controls (Rao, 1984).

Epithelial atypia only was observed in the cheek pouches of 3/6 male and female Syrian golden hamsters after repeated application of 250 mg calcium hydroxide once a day five times a week for 2 weeks and thereafter three times each week between the 2nd and 40th weeks of treatment. Treatment started when the hamsters were 3.5–4.5 weeks old and they reached an average age of 81 weeks. They were either killed when moribund or found dead (Dunham et al., 1966). [The Working Group noted the large amount of slaked lime.]

Eight Syrian golden hamsters (males and females), 6–7 weeks of age, received 0.5% calcium hydroxide in DMSO painted on the cheek pouch epithelium, without yielding any lesions [no data on frequency and duration of treatment mentioned] (Dunham et al., 1974).

Slaked lime either alone (38 animals) or with tobacco (24 animals) [concentrations not specified] was painted onto the cheek-pouch epithelium of 62 Syrian golden hamsters [sex unspecified] (initial weight, 40–50 g) thrice weekly until they were killed after 2, 4,

8, 16, 24 and 52 weeks of exposure. No tumours were observed (Kandarkar & Sirsat, 1977).

### 3.5.3 Baboon

Twelve young adult baboons (one male and 11 females) were divided into two groups and fed a diet intended to simulate protein deficiency. With this diet, the normal average serum protein level dropped from 7.4 to 6.4% and was maintained for over 3 years. Five animals received a basic betel quid (a freshly prepared ground mixture of betel leaves, areca nut and calcium hydroxide) and seven baboons received the basic quid with added Maharashtran tobacco. Thrice weekly, 3.5 g of the test substance were administered into a surgically created buccal mucosal pouch for 42 months. Biopsies were taken after 1, 6, 9, 12, 16, 23, 29, 34 and 42 months. Severe epithelial atypia was seen microscopically in 1/7 animals treated with betel quid with tobacco after 34 months of quid insertion and in 3/7 of the same group after 42 months. After 42 months of treatment with betel quid without tobacco, 5/5 baboons showed epithelial atypia but not to the degree observed in the group treated with betel quid and tobacco (Hamner, 1972).

## 3.6 Intravaginal instillation

*Mouse*

A group of 60 virgin female Swiss mice, about 40 days old, received daily instillation into the vagina of a betel-quid mixture (shell lime and areca nut) with tobacco for up to 380 days, at which time 13 animals were still alive. A group of 10 females received instillations of isotonic saline and served as controls. Of the 50 animals that survived for periods ranging from 324 to 380 days, seven developed carcinomatous changes in the vagina; no tumour was found in controls (Reddy & Anguli, 1967). [The Working Group noted the ambiguous description of the lesions and considered the study to be inadequate for evaluation.]

## 3.7 Administration with known carcinogens or modifiers of cancer risk

### 3.7.1 Mouse

The anticarcinogenic effect of betel-leaf extract on the development of benzo[*a*]pyrene-induced forestomach papilloma and oral neoplasia induced by the tobacco-specific carcinogenic nitrosamines $N'$-nitrosonornicotine (NNN)- and 4-(methylnitrosoamino)-1-(3-pyridyl)-1-butanone (NNK) was investigated. Groups of 20 inbred male Swiss mice, 8 weeks of age, were administered betel-leaf extract (1 mg/day; 5 days per week) by intragastric instillation for 2 weeks. Thereafter, animals received eight twice-weekly doses of 1 mg benzo-[*a*]pyrene in sesame oil by gavage for 4 weeks. The mice again received betel-leaf extract for 2 weeks following cessation of carcinogen treatment. In a second set of experiments, betel-leaf extract was given in drinking-water on 5 days per week (2.5 mg per day per mouse) during administration of NNN or NNK on the tongue of animals. Treatment with betel-leaf extract in drinking-water reduced the incidence and the yield (number per mouse) of benzo[a]pyrene-induced forestomach papilloma (4.9 ± 0.28 versus 0.9 ± 0.22; $p < 0.0005$). The decrease was statistically significant. Betel-leaf extract reduced the number of tumour-bearing mice in NNN- and NNK-treated animals from 49/82 to 23/80; the effect was pronounced in animals receiving low doses of NNN or NNK (Padma et al., 1989).

In order to test the chemopreventive efficacy of an extract of betel leaves on benzo-[a]pyrene-induced forestomach tumours, groups of 20 male Swiss mice, 6–8 weeks of age, were administered an extract of betel leaf or its constituents including eugenol, hydroxychavicol, β-carotene and α-tocopherol in drinking-water (2.5 mg per animal in 6 mL) for 2 weeks. From the 3rd week, the mice were administered eight doses of 1 mg benzo[a]pyrene in 0.1 mL peanut oil by gavage twice a week for 4 weeks. Betel-leaf extract or one of its constituents was continued for a further 2 weeks after the cessation of carcinogen treatment. Other groups were treated with betel-leaf extract or each of its constituents only and one group of animals served as peanut oil-vehicle controls. After completion of the treatment, animals were observed and killed at the age of 180 days. In studies on benzo[a]pyrene-induced forestomach neoplasia, treatment with betel-leaf extract or its constituents did not influence the number of animals with tumours. However, the average number of papillomas per mouse was significantly lower in mice treated with betel-leaf extract or its constituents. Maximal inhibition of papilloma development was observed in mice receiving hydroxychavicol (Bhide et al., 1991).

Effects of topically applied betel-leaf extract and its constituents, β-carotene, α-tocopherol, eugenol and hydroxychavicol, on DMBA-induced skin tumours were evaluated in two strains of mice. Betel-leaf extract, β-carotene and α-tocopherol significantly inhibited papilloma formation by 83, 86 and 86% in Swiss mice and by 92, 94 and 89% in male Swiss bare mice, respectively. Hydroxychavicol showed 90% inhibition in Swiss bare mice at 23 weeks of treatment. Eugenol showed minimal protection in both strains of mice. The mean latency period and survival in betel-leaf extract-, β-carotene-, α-tocopherol- and hydroxychavicol-treated groups were remarkably long compared with the group treated with DMBA alone (Azuine et al., 1991). [The results may have been confounded by low survival of the animals.]

A group of 12 male and 12 female C17 mice, 10–12 weeks of age, was fed a diet containing 10% (w/w) areca nut coated with saccharin [concentration not specified] for 40 weeks and also received 0.2 mL of a 0.1% solution of 1,4-dinitrosopiperazine per day by gavage. A group of 15 males and 14 females received 1,4-dinitrosopiperazine only. The animals were followed for life. In the group treated with 1,4-dinitrosopiperazine only, seven male and four female mice developed squamous-cell carcinomas of the forestomach. Five females also developed uterine malignancies. In the group treated with 1,4-dinitrosopiperazine and fed areca nut, six male and three female mice developed squamous-cell carcinomas of the forestomach and five females developed uterine malignancies. The authors concluded that treatment with areca nut did not potentiate the carcinogenicity of 1,4-dinitropiperazine (Pai *et al.*, 1981).

Groups of 20 male and female random-bred Swiss mice, 4 weeks of age, were initiated with topical applications of 50 µg DMBA in 0.1 mL acetone, treated 2 weeks later with twice-weekly topical applications of 0 or 1% croton oil for 18 weeks and fed diets containing 0 or 1% ripe, unprocessed, sun-dried areca nuts ground into a fine powder. No influence of areca nut on the incidence of skin papillomas was observed (Singh & Rao, 1995).

Groups of 15 male and 15 female ICRC-strain mice, 6–8 weeks of age, were administered a cumulative dose of 16 g/kg bw *N*-nitrosodiethylamine (NDEA) in the drinking-water for 4 days. One week later, mice were fed by gavage 12.5, 25 or 50 mg ethanolic *pan masala* extract, 5 nmol 12-*O*-tetradecanoylphorbol-13-acetate or distilled water on 5 days a week for 3 or 6 months to assess promoting–progression activity on the incidence of oesophageal and stomach tumours. The cumulative rate and yield of forestomach and oesophageal tumours (squamous-cell papillomas) increased significantly in animals treated with 25 mg ethanolic *pan masala* extract (Ramchandani *et al.*, 1998).

### 3.7.2 Rat

The effect of areca nut on chemical carcinogenesis in the upper digestive tract and liver was examined in two different experimental models using ACI rats. The incidences of neoplasms and preneoplastic lesions of the tongue in animals given [5 mg/L] 4-nitroquinoline-1-oxide (4NQO) in the drinking-water for 16 weeks followed by 20% areca nut in the diet for 40 weeks were significantly higher than those in the 14 animals given 4NQO alone. No enhancing effect from areca nut on the incidences of neoplastic and preneoplastic lesions in the upper digestive tract was found in animals administered 4NQO for 12 weeks (Tanaka *et al.*, 1986).

When an aqeous extract of the leaves of *Piper betle* was given orally at different dose levels during the initiation phase of DMBA-induced mammary carcinogenesis in rats, higher doses of the extract inhibited the emergence of tumours. However, when the extract was fed to the rats bearing DMBA-induced mammary tumours for 8 weeks, no appreciable degree of inhibition of tumour growth was noted. Betel-leaf extract at the dose levels used did not affect the body-weight gain of rats (Rao *et al.*, 1985).

### 3.7.3 Hamster

Groups of female Syrian golden hamsters, 6–7 weeks old, were treated with topical exposures to graded doses of benzo[*a*]pyrene (25 µg, 50 µg and 100 µg per pouch) thrice weekly either alone (20 animals per group) or combined with areca nut (1 mg per pouch; 25 animals per group) or betel leaf (5 mg per pouch; 25 animals per group) twice a day for 6 months and killed 6 months later. The incidence of squamous-cell papilloma or carcinoma in the group treated with the three different doses of benzo[*a*]pyrene alone was

20, 35 and 61%. In the animals treated with the three different doses of benzo[*a*]pyrene together with areca nut, tumour incidence was 26.1, 52.4 and 77.3%, respectively. In the animals treated with the three different doses of benzo[*a*]pyrene together with betel leaf, the tumour incidence was 12.5, 18.2 and 27.3% for the three groups (Rao, 1984).

In a short-term study, groups of 25 female Syrian golden hamsters, 6–7 weeks old, were treated with topical exposures to graded doses of benzo[*a*]pyrene (25 µg, 50 µg and 100 µg per pouch) daily either alone or combined with areca nut (1 mg per pouch) or betel leaf (5 mg per pouch) twice a day for 10 days and killed 6 months later. For the three different doses of benzo[*a*]pyrene, an incidence of squamous-cell papilloma or carcinoma of 4, 8.7 and 16.7%, respectively, was found. Addition of areca nut yielded tumour incidences of 0, 4.2 and 8.3%, respectively. In the animals that were treated with benzo[*a*]pyrene and betel leaf, tumour incidence was 0, 0 and 4.0% for the three groups, respectively (Rao, 1984).

The inhibitory effect of oral administration of betel-leaf extract and two of its constituents, β-carotene and α-tocopherol, as single agents or in combination with dietary turmeric, on methyl(acetoxymethyl)nitrosamine (DMN-OAC)-induced oral carcinogenesis was studied in 226 Syrian hamsters. DMN-OAC was administered twice monthly for 6 months. The chemopreventive effect of betel-leaf extract or its constituents with turmeric was determined by comparing tumour incidence observed in treated groups with that seen in control animals. The apparent site-specific chemopreventive effect of betel-leaf extract or its constituents was demonstrated by inhibition of tumour incidence, reduction of tumour burden, extension of the tumour latency period and regression of established, obvious tumours. The inhibitory effect of betel-leaf extract or its constituents combined with turmeric was higher than that of the individual constituents (see Table 69; Azuine & Bhide, 1992). [Data regarding survival were incomprehensible.]

The tumour-promoting activity of arecaidine on DMBA-treated hamster buccal pouches was tested in 112 male adult Syrian golden hamsters, 10–12 weeks of age. The animals were divided into 16 groups, each containing seven animals. The buccal pouch of each hamster was painted three times weekly for 12 consecutive weeks with a heavy mineral oil containing 0.5% DMBA in group 1, for 8 consecutive weeks followed by 4 weeks without any additional treatment in group 2, and for 8 consecutive weeks followed by application of 200, 300, 400 and 500 µg/mL arecaidine in polyethylene glycol, respectively, six times per week for 4 weeks in groups 3–6. In six additional groups, DMBA was painted thrice weekly for 4 weeks, without additional treatment in group 7 and with arecaidine solutions incremented from 600 to 1000 µg/mL applied six times per week for a further 8 weeks in groups 8–12. In groups 13–15, arecaidine in solutions of 1000, 2000 or 3000 µg/mL was applied six times a week for 12 weeks. Group 16 was untreated. At the end of 12 weeks, all animals were killed. In groups 2–4, 5/7 hamsters per group had tumours, with a total of seven, nine and eight tumours, respectively, whereas in groups 5 and 6, all hamsters (7/7 per group) had tumours (13 tumours in each of the groups). The increase in the number of tumours in groups 5 and 6 was statistically significant ($p < 0.05$, *t*-test). In groups 7–12, the number of hamsters with tumours

**Table 69. Effect of betel-leaf extract and its constituents on DMN-OAC-induced oral tumours in Syrian golden hamsters at 13 months**

| DMN-OAC[a] | Test compound[b] | Weight gain (g)[c] | Latency period (months) | Tumour incidence | | | | Tumour burden (mm$^3$)[c] |
|---|---|---|---|---|---|---|---|---|
| | | | | Overall | | At death | | |
| | | | | 5–13 months | % | 5–13 months | % | |
| + | – | 52 ± 2 | 5–10 | 14/15 | 93 | 14/15* | 93 | 600 ± 72 |
| + | BLE | 28 ± 2 | 6–11 | 4/15* | 27 | 4/15* | 27 | 1.4 ± 0.9* |
| + | β-Carotene | 35 ± 4 | 8–12 | 4/15* | 27 | 1/15* | 7 | 0.5 ± 0.0* |
| + | α-Tocopherol | 48 ± 3 | 9 | 1/15* | 7 | 1/5 | 7 | 4.2 ± 0.0* |
| – | – | 58 ± 2 | – | 0/15 | 0 | 0/15 | 0 | – |

From Azuine & Bhide (1992)
[a] DMN-OAC (methyl(acetoxymethyl)nitrosamine) at 2 mg/kg bw twice a month for 6 months
[b] BLE (betel-leaf extract; 2.5 mg), β-carotene (3.1 mg, 5.8 µM) and α-tochopherol (2.5 mg, 5.8 µM) administered daily in drinking-water 2 weeks prior to and simultaneously with DMN-OAC treatment and continued until the end of the experiment
[c] Results are mean ± SE.
* $p < 0.01$ as compared with DMN-OAC alone ($\chi^2$ for tumour incidence data and Student's $t$ test for the difference in total tumour burden between the control and treated groups)

in the various groups was 0/7, 5/7, 5/7, 4/7, 7/7 and 7/7, respectively, whereas the total number of tumours was zero, seven, eight, seven, 13 and 15, respectively ($p < 0.05$, $t$-test, for the number of tumours in the groups treated with 900 and 1000 µg/mL arecaidine). In groups 13–15, no tumour was observed (Lin et al., 1996).

Six groups of 10 male Syrian golden hamsters, 6–8 weeks of age, received topical applications of 0.5% DMBA three times per week for 2, 4 or 6 weeks, followed by insertion of Taiwanese betel quid, consisting of fresh unripe areca nut, betel stem, slaked lime and catechu, for 12 or 24 weeks. The betel quid was renewed twice a week for the duration of the experiment. The incidence of tumours in cheek pouches was recorded 6 weeks after removal of the insert. Six groups similarly treated with DMBA only served as concurrent control groups. The incidences of tumours (carcinomas) were significantly higher in the group treated with DMBA for 4 weeks followed by betel quid for 24 weeks and in the group treated with DMBA for 6 weeks followed by betel quid for 12 weeks than in their concurrent control groups (6/9 versus 1/9, $p < 0.05$ and 7/7 versus 1/9, $p < 0.01$, respectively) (Wong et al., 1992).

Groups of 10 male Syrian hamsters, 2 months of age, were used to test the promoting activity of the various components of Taiwanese betel quid. Following an initial application of 0.5% DMBA three times per week for 4 weeks, the animals remained untreated for 1 week. Twelve of the 13 groups served as the experimental groups and their buccal pouches were filled or painted [for further technical details on application, the authors refer to another publication (Wong et al., 1992)] with components of betel quid thrice weekly for 24 weeks. Thereafter, animals were untreated for a further 6 weeks before being killed. The 13th group that served as a control was left untreated after the initial 4-week application of DMBA and killed at the same time as the other groups. The following substances were applied: group 1, slaked lime; group 2, areca-nut fibre; group 3, *Piper betle*; group 4, *Piper betle* and slaked lime; group 5, hot aqueous extract of areca nut; group 6, hot aqueous extract of areca nut and slaked lime; group 7, cold aqueous extract of areca nut; group 8, cold aqueous extract of areca nut and slaked lime; group 9, hot aqueous extract of areca nut and *Piper betle*; group 10, cold aqueous extract of areca nut with *Piper betle*; group 11, hot aqueous extract of areca nut with *Piper betle* and slaked lime; and group 12, cold aqueous extract of areca nut with *Piper betle* and slaked lime. The incidence of tumours was significantly higher in groups exposed to dry areca-nut fibre (9/10; $p < 0.01$, two-tailed Student's $t$-test) and cold aqueous areca-nut extract only (7/10; $p < 0.05$, two-tailed Student's $t$-test) versus the control in which the tumour incidence was 2/9 (Jin et al., 1996).

Groups of 42 non-inbred male adult Syrian golden hamsters, 8–10 weeks old, received applications to the buccal pouch of 0.5% DMBA thrice weekly concurrently with betel-quid extract six times a week, DMBA alone or betel-quid extract alone. The betel-quid extract consisted of the filtrate of a mixture of areca nut (450 g), unripe betel fruit (120 g) and slaked lime (50 g) to which 300 mL DMSO was added as solvent. At the end of 2 weeks, six animals were taken from each group and killed; this was repeated after periods of 2 weeks each, thus enabling evaluation of the effect of treatment in relation to its duration. After 14 weeks, all animals had been killed. In three other groups, the treatment regimen was as follows: DMSO six times a week, mineral oil six times a week and no treatment at all. After 8 weeks of treatment, tumours occurred in the groups treated with DMBA alone and in the group treated with DMBA and concomitant betel quid. Both the number of tumours and their size were greater in the group with the combined treatment than in the group treated with DMBA alone ($p < 0.05$, two-tailed Student's $t$-test). No tumours were seen in any of the other groups (Lin et al., 1997).

DMBA-impregnated sutures (300–400 µg DMBA/cm suture) approximately 1.5 cm in length were placed in the buccal pouch of 165 adult Syrian golden hamsters [age and sex not specified]. The placement of the suture was confirmed every 2 weeks and replaced if lost. After 12 weeks, the DMBA-coated sutures were removed. The cheek pouches were painted with a solution of arecaidine (0.5 mg/mL mineral oil) thrice weekly for an additional 4 weeks or until tumours reached a size of 100 mm$^2$. With this protocol, all of 133 hamsters that were still alive after 16 weeks of initiation–promotion treatment developed squamous-cell carcinomas (Wani et al., 2001). [The Working Group noted that no animals treated with DMBA only were included.]

In a large experiment investigating 130 Syrian golden hamsters, aged 2 months, four males and four females received applications to the buccal pouch of 0.5% DMBA solution thrice weekly for 4 consecutive weeks and were then left untreated for 1 week. After this period, the buccal pouches were treated with slaked lime for 24 weeks and animals were left untreated for a further 6 weeks. No differences were seen between the group treated with slaked lime and the control that received DMBA only (Jin et al., 1996).

# 4. Other Data Relevant to an Evaluation of Carcinogenicity and its Mechanisms

## 4.1 Absorption, distribution, metabolism and excretion

### 4.1.1 *Humans*

(a) *Constituents of betel quid*

(i) *Areca nut*

Areca nut contains several alkaloids and tannins. Among the alkaloids, arecoline is most abundant, whereas arecaidine, guvacine and guvacoline occur in smaller quantities (see Figure 5).

**Arecoline**

*Absorption after dermal application*

Hayes et al. (1989) developed a gas chromatography–mass spectrometry (GC–MS) technique for quantitative analysis of arecoline in blood plasma, in the concentration range 1–50 ng/mL, which was used on plasma samples from healthy volunteers [number not given] who had received transdermal doses at 3 mg/h. The time–concentration profile showed a maximum plasma concentration of 4–5 ng/mL at 5–10 h after dermal application.

*Absorption after application in the buccal cavity*

Strickland et al. (2003) studied the influence of areca nut on energy, metabolism and hunger and also assessed the absorption of arecoline and its level in plasma among eight fasting men (20–29 years of age). Freshly dried areca nuts were pulverized and assayed for arecoline content (mean value, 0.17%); the powder was then suspended in bioadhesive gel and placed in the buccal cavity so as to deliver 0, 5, 10 or 20 mg arecoline. At 15, 155 and 365 min after placement, arecoline could be detected by GC–MS in blood plasma in amounts that increased with dose and time.

*Polyphenols*

Polyphenols constitute one of the most numerous and ubiquitous groups of plant metabolites and are an integral part of both human and animal diets. There is a vast amount of literature on the metabolism of polyphenols in humans. Important polyphenolic constituents of areca nut are catechin, tannin, caffeic acid and ferulic acid. For detailed information on absorption, distribution, metabolism and excretion of these substances, the reader is referred to a number of review articles (Stich et al., 1984a; Rosazza et al., 1995; Bravo, 1998; Miyazawa, 2000; Scalbert et al., 2002; Higdon & Frei, 2003).

## Figure 5. Relationship of areca-nut alkaloids to areca-nut-derived nitrosamines (formed by nitrosation) and a urinary metabolite of *N*-nitrosoguvacoline and *N*-nitrosoguvacine

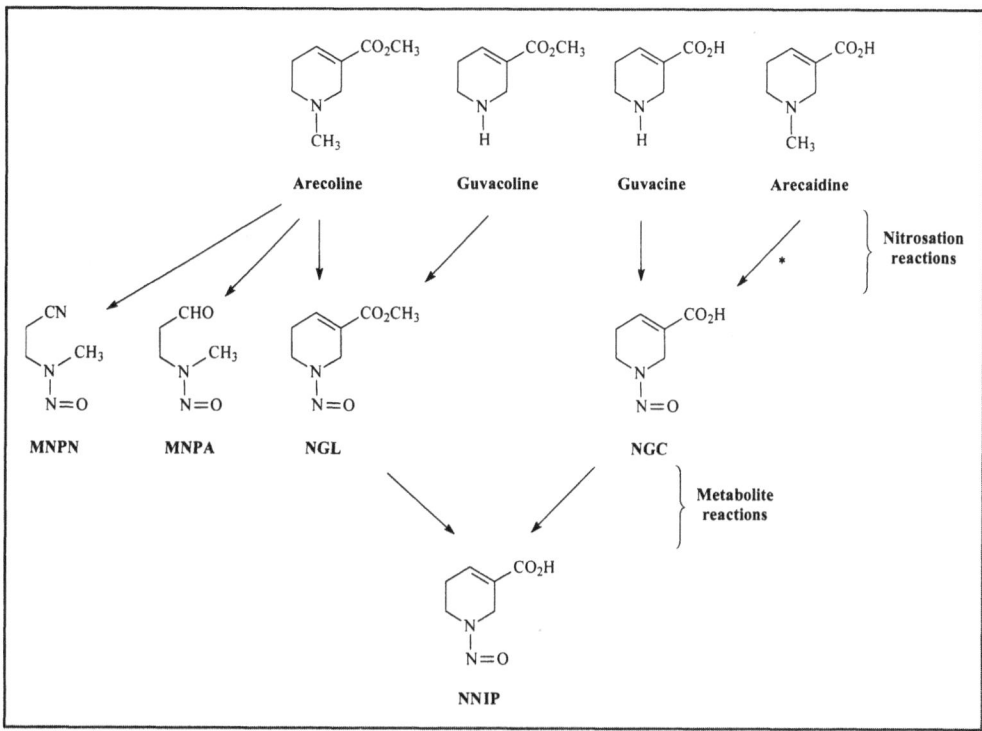

Adapted from Wenke & Hoffman (1983); Nair *et al.* (1985); Ohshima *et al.* (1989)
MNPN, 3-methylnitrosaminopropionitrile; MNPA, 3-methylnitrosaminopropionaldehyde; NGL, *N*-nitrosoguvacoline; NGC, *N*-nitrosoguvacine; NNIP, *N*-nitrosonipecotic acid
*It is likely that nitrosation of arecaidine would produce NGC but this has not been demonstrated.

*Areca-nut-derived nitrosamines*

The detection of areca-nut-derived nitrosamines in saliva and their formation during betel-quid chewing are discussed in Section 4.1.1(*a*) of this monograph; other data are reviewed in the monograph on areca-nut-derived nitrosamines.

(ii) *Betel leaf and betel inflorescence*

**Safrole** (IARC, 1976)

Chang, M.J.W. *et al.* (2002) developed a method to assess exposure to safrole based on HPLC analysis of its metabolites, dihydroxychavicol and eugenol (IARC, 1985b, 1987). The method was used to measure these compounds in 38 spot urine samples from Taiwanese betel-quid chewers and 115 samples from non-chewers. The urinary concentration of dihydroxychavicol was higher in non-chewers than in chewers, probably because safrole exists in many common species such as ginger and black pepper that are frequently used in Taiwanese cooking. However, the chewers had a higher urinary concentration of eugenol.

(iii) *Tobacco*

The components of tobacco, as part of betel quid, will be reviewed in a forthcoming monograph on smokeless tobacco products (see also IARC, 2004).

(b) *Biomarkers of constituents of betel quid*

(i) *Detection of* N-*Nitrosamines in saliva*

Carcinogens derived from tobacco and areca nut have been detected in the saliva (mixture of saliva with macerated betel-quid ingredients produced while chewing) of users of these products. The tobacco-specific nitrosamines, $N'$-nitrosonornicotine (NNN), 4-(methylnitrosamino)-1-(3-pyridyl)-1-butanone) (NNK) and $N'$-nitrosoanabasine (NAB) (see Figure 6 for the structures), as well as the volatile nitrosamines, $N$-nitrosodimethylamine and $N$-nitrosodiethylamine, were detected in the saliva of chewers of betel quid with tobacco. These volatile nitrosamines are probably also tobacco-derived. Three areca-nut-derived nitrosamines, $N$-nitrosoguvacoline (NGL), $N$-nitrosoguvacine (NGC) and 3-methylnitrosaminopropionitrile (MNPN), a rodent carcinogen (Figure 6), were detected in the saliva of chewers of betel quid with or without tobacco (Table 70).

The highest levels of tobacco-specific nitrosamines were detected in samples collected from India (Bhide *et al.*, 1986), whereas the highest levels of areca-nut-derived nitrosamines (NGL) were found in the sediment of saliva collected from Taiwanese betel-quid chewers (Stich *et al.*, 1986). NNN, NNK and NGL were reported in more than one study (Wenke *et al.*, 1984; Nair *et al.*, 1985; Bhide *et al.*, 1986; Nair *et al.*, 1986; Stich *et al.*, 1986), whereas NAB (Bhide *et al.*, 1986), MNPN (Prokopczyk *et al.*, 1987), NGC (Nair, J. *et al.*, 1985), and the volatile nitrosamines (Bhide *et al.*, 1986) were reported in single studies. One study that especially looked for MNPN failed to demonstrate its presence (Stich *et al.*, 1986). Concentrations of NGL in the saliva obtained from Taiwanese chewers were higher than those in saliva from Indian chewers (Stich *et al.*, 1986).

Volatile nitrosamines and tobacco-specific nitrosamines found in the saliva of chewers could result from the leaching of those present in tobacco or could be formed endogenously during chewing from abundant precursors (see Section 4.1.1(*b*)(ii)). Areca-nut-derived nitrosamines have not been reported to be components of areca nut or betel quid, except on one instance in which the presence of some NGC was noted. Hence their occurrence in the saliva of betel-quid chewers is most probably due to their formation during chewing.

In-vitro nitrosation of betel quid with nitrite and thiocyanate at neutral pH for 1 h generated NGL (Nair *et al.*, 1985). Nitrosation of arecoline at neutral pH yielded approximately four times more NGL than at acidic or alkaline pH (Wang & Peng, 1996).

**Figure 6. Structures of nitrosamines**

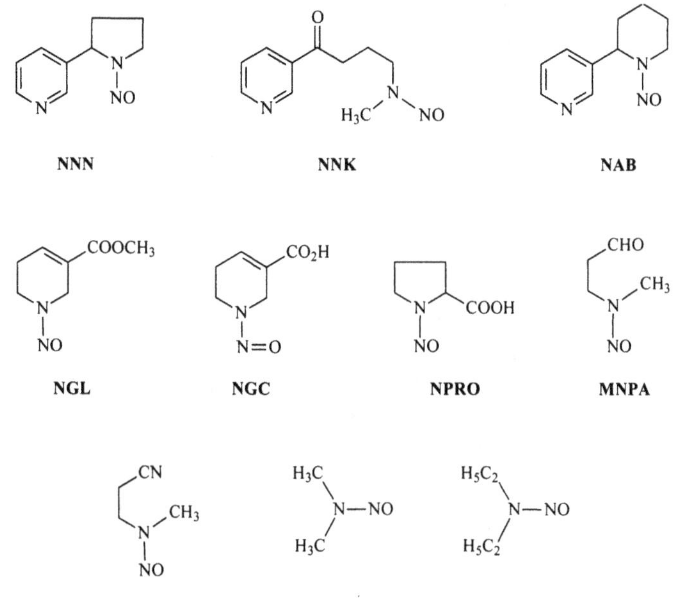

NNN, $N'$-nitrosonornicotine; NNK, 4-(methylnitrosamino)-1-(3-pyridyl)-1-butanone; NAB, $N'$-nitrosoanabasine; NGL, $N$-nitrosoguvacoline; NGC, $N$-nitrosoguvacine; MNPN, 3-methylnitrosaminopropionitrile; NDMA, $N$-nitrosodimethylamine; NDEA, $N$-nitrosodiethylamine; NPRO, $N$-nitrosoproline; MNPA, 3-methylnitrosaminopropionaldehyde

(ii)  *Formation of N-nitroso compounds in the oral cavity*

Areca nut and tobacco contain secondary and tertiary amines that can be nitrosated in the saliva during the chewing of betel quid when they react with available nitrite in the presence of nitrosation catalysts such as thiocyanate. Microgram per millilitre levels of nitrite and thiocyanate have been reported in the saliva of chewers of betel quid (Nair *et al.*, 1985; Nair, J. *et al.*, 1987). Using a modified *N*-nitrosoproline (NPRO) test (Ohshima & Bartsch, 1981), whereby 100 mg L-proline were added to the betel quid and saliva was collected from each subject 20 min later, it was clearly shown that NPRO (a non-carcinogenic compound) is formed during the chewing of betel quid with and without tobacco, although the extent of increased nitrosation varies among individual subjects (Nair, J. *et al.*, 1987).

The role of poor oral hygiene in the formation of *N*-nitroso compounds was investigated using the NPRO assay. Endogenous nitrosation is significantly higher in subjects with poor oral hygiene (determined by dental plaque) compared with those with good oral hygiene (Nair *et al.*, 1996). This implies that, on the basis of the availability of nitrosa-

Table 70. Levels (range, ng/mL) of nitrosamines detected in saliva of chewers of betel quid with tobacco (BQ + T) and without tobacco (BQ)

| Nitrosamine | BQ + T (*n*) | BQ (*n*) | Reference |
|---|---|---|---|
| *Volatile* | | | |
| NDMA | 0–35.5 (17) | NR | Bhide et al. (1986) |
| NDEA | 0–5.6 (17) | NR | Bhide et al. (1986) |
| *Tobacco-specific* | | | |
| NNN | 1.2–38 (6) | ND (5) | Wenke et al. (1984) |
| | 1.6–14.7 (12) | ND (12) | Nair et al. (1985) |
| | 3–85.7 (17) | NR | Bhide et al. (1986) |
| | 4.9–48.6 (10) | NR | Nair, J. et al. (1987) |
| NNK | 1–2.3 (6) | ND (5) | Wenke et al. (1984) |
| | 0–2.3 (12) | ND (12) | Nair et al. (1985) |
| | 0–14.3 (17) | NR | Bhide et al. (1986) |
| | 0–9.4 (10) | NR | Nair, J. et al. (1987) |
| NAB | 0–40[a] (17) | NR | Bhide et al. (1986) |
| *Areca nut-specific* | | | |
| NGL | 4.3–350 (5) | 2.2–9.5 (5) | Wenke et al. (1984) |
| | 0–7.1 (12) | 0–5.9 (12) | Nair, J. et al. (1985) |
| | NR | 0–142 (11) | Stich et al. (1986) |
| | 3.1–23.5 (10) | 0.6–8.8 (10) | Nair, J. et al. (1987) |
| NGC | 0–30.4 (6) | 0–26.6 (6) | Nair et al. (1985) |
| MNPN | NR | 0.5–11.4 (10) | Prokopczyk et al. (1987) |

[a] Detected in only three samples

NDMA, *N*-nitrosodimethylamine; NR, not reported; NDEA, *N*-nitrosodiethylamine; NNN, *N'*-nitrosonornicotine; ND, not detected; NNK, 4-(methylnitrosamino)-1-(3-pyridyl)-1-butanone; NAB, *N'*-nitrosoanabasine; NGL, *N*-nitrosoguvacoline; NGC, *N*-nitrosoguvacine; MNPN, 3-(methylnitrosamino)propionitrile

table amines from areca nut and tobacco, there is more extensive formation of nitrosamines in subjects with poor oral hygiene if they chew tobacco. The enhanced endogenous nitrosation in subjects with poor oral hygiene may be due to the increased conversion of nitrate to nitrite or bacterial enzyme-mediated formation of nitrosamines, or both (Calmels et al., 1988). Increased formation of nitrite and nitric oxide (NO) in the mouth has been reported during the formation of dental plaque (Carossa et al., 2001).

(iii) *Products of endogenous nitrosation*

Endogenous nitrosation in betel-quid chewers is significant. Many chewers swallow the quid that contains precursors of nitrosamines (nitrosatable amines, nitrite); these are then subjected to the acidic pH of the stomach, which is a more favourable condition for the nitrosation reaction of many secondary and tertiary amines. Urinary levels of NPRO, a marker for endogenous nitrosation, were ~6.5-fold higher in chewers of betel quid with tobacco following ingestion of L-proline compared with chewers not ingesting proline (mean, 0.28 versus 1.86 µg/24 h; $n = 5$). In groups with no chewing habit, this increase was only marginal (mean, 0.32 versus 0.55 µg/24 h; $n = 4$) (Nair et al., 1986). In another study, chewers of betel quid without tobacco also showed a significant ~2.4-fold increase in urinary excretion of NPRO following ingestion of L-proline compared with no ingestion of proline (2.60 versus 6.31 µg/24 h, $n = 8$), and the group with no chewing habit again had a marginal increase in NPRO excretion (1.92 versus 2.54 µg/24 h; $n = 9$). An increase in mean NPRO excretion was also measured in 6-h urine (µmol/mol creatinine) of chewers of betel quid with tobacco (2.2 versus 3.6; $n = 15$) and betel quid without tobacco (1.9 versus 4.7; $n = 18$) and only a marginal increase in those with no chewing habit (2.9 versus 3.3; $n = 18$) (Chakradeo et al., 1994). The above studies clearly demonstrate the potential of gastric nitrosation in betel-quid chewers. Using the NPRO assay, Stich et al. (1983) showed that the polyphenolic fractions of areca nut inhibited endogenous nitrosation in one male and one female volunteer following ingestion of sodium nitrate and L-proline.

(iv) *Formation of reactive oxygen species in the oral cavity*

Direct evidence that reactive oxygen species such as the hydroxyl radical (HO•) are generated in the oral cavity during betel-quid chewing was provided by measuring the formation of *ortho-* and *meta-*tyrosines from L-phenylalanine in human saliva by means of high-performance liquid chromatography (HPLC)-fluorescence detection (Nair et al., 1995; see Section 4.1.2 for in-vitro studies). Saliva from five Indian volunteers collected after chewing betel quid (consisting of betel leaf, areca nut, catechu and slaked lime but no tobacco) contained high concentrations of *para-*tyrosine, but no appreciable amounts of *ortho-* or *meta-*tyrosine. Saliva samples from the same subjects collected after chewing betel quid complemented with 20 mg phenylalanine contained 1010–3000 nM *ortho-*tyrosine and 1110–3140 nM *meta-*tyrosine. These levels were significantly higher ($p < 0.005$) than those detected in the saliva of subjects who kept L-phenylalanine in the oral cavity without betel quid (*ortho-*tyrosine, 14–70 nM; *meta-*tyrosine, 10–35 nM). These studies clearly demonstrate that the HO• radical is formed in the human oral cavity during betel-quid chewing and could contribute to the genetic damage observed in the oral epithelial cells of chewers. Using the same method, formation of the HO• radical was monitored in Taiwanese subjects who chewed unripe areca nut and lime with either *Piper betle* inflorescence ($n = 9$) or betel leaf ($n = 9$) (Chen et al., 2002). *ortho-* and *meta-*Tyrosines were detected at levels that were ~5–14 times lower than those detected in Indian chewers (Nair et al., 1995), which is probably due to differences in betel-quid ingredients.

4.1.2 *Experimental systems*

(a) *Areca nut/arecoline*

(i) *Metabolism*

In rats, arecoline is de-esterified in the liver to arecaidine, and both arecoline and arecaidine are excreted as the mercapturic acid, $N$-acetyl-$S$-(3-carboxy-1-methylpiperid-4-yl)-L-cysteine (Boyland & Nery, 1969).

According to Nery (1971), the metabolism of arecoline may be complex, with up to five major metabolic products being released from three different routes of metabolism: arecoline 1-oxide, arecaidine 1-oxide, arecaidine, $N$-acetyl-$S$-(3-carboxy-1-methylpiperid-4-yl)-L-cysteine and an unidentified product.

Arecoline is rapidly metabolized in both liver and kidney (essentially 100% and approximately 87%, respectively). Arecoline was not metabolized by either blood or brain homogenates to any significant degree. Using various enzymatic inhibitors, any significant involvement of monoamine oxidase or hepatic microsomal oxidative enzymes in the metabolism of arecoline was ruled out. However, the specific carboxylesterase inhibitors tri-*ortho*-tolylphosphate and tetraisopropyl pyrophosphoramide completely blocked arecoline metabolism in the liver homogenate. It was therefore suggested that a carboxylesterase (EC 3.1.1.1) is primarily responsible for the metabolism of arecoline in mice (Patterson & Kosh, 1993). The short half-life of arecoline has been attributed to the rapid in-vivo enzymatic hydrolysis of the ester functionality (Saunders *et al.*, 1988) to form the carboxylic acid derivative arecaidine which appears to be a major metabolic product of arecoline in mice (Nieshulz & Schmersahl, 1968).

(ii) *Influence of areca nut/arecoline on drug-metabolizing enzymes and cellular antioxidant profiles*

**In humans: in-vitro studies**

Jeng *et al.* (1996) studied the effect of arecoline on the intracellular antioxidant profile of glutathione (GSH) in human fibroblasts *in vitro*. At concentrations of 0.4 mM and 1 mM, arecoline depleted about 26% and 45% of GSH, respectively, after 2 h of incubation; control cells maintained their original GSH levels during the incubation period.

Chang, Y.C. *et al.* (1998) demonstrated that arecoline-induced cytotoxicity in human buccal fibroblasts *in vitro* could be inhibited by exposure to GSH. This cytotoxicity could also be inhibited by exposure to $N$-acetyl-L-cysteine, a glutathione synthesis precursor, and by exogenous addition of carboxylesterase (Jeng *et al.*, 1999a).

Chang, Y.-C. *et al.* (2001a) studied the effect of arecoline on glutathione $S$-transferase (GST) activity and lipid peroxidation in cultured human buccal mucosal fibroblasts. At concentrations higher than 50 µg/mL, arecoline significantly decreased GST activity in a dose-dependent manner. At concentrations of 100 and 400 µg/mL, arecoline reduced GST activity by approximately 21% and 46%, respectively, during a 24-h incubation period. However, it did not increase lipid peroxidation at any dose tested in this assay system. The adverse effect of arecoline on GST may increase the risk for oral cancer due to other chemical carcinogens such as tobacco products. Exposure to areca-nut extract and arecoline also gives rise to GSH depletion and mitochondrial dysfunction of oral keratinocyte KB epithelial cells (Chang, M.C. et al., 2001).

COX2, an inducible enzyme responsible for prostaglandin ($PGE_2$ and 6-keto-$PGF_{1\alpha}$) synthesis, plays an important role in certain inflammatory diseases and carcinogenesis. Areca-nut extract induced COX2 mRNA and protein expression and $PGE_2$ and 6-keto-$PGF_{1\alpha}$ in primary human gingival keratinocytes (Jeng et al., 2000); it was suggested that this stimulation of $PGE_2$ production could partly result from the up-regulation of COX2 mRNA expression.

Tsai et al. (2003) studied the influence of arecoline on the expression of COX2 in human buccal mucosal fibroblasts incubated for 2 h with different doses of arecoline (10–160 μg/mL) in vitro. COX2 mRNA increased approximately 1.5- and 2.7-fold after exposure to 20 and 160 μg/mL arecoline, respectively, and a peak level was induced by 80 μg/mL. In addition, pretreatment with the GSH precursor, 2-oxothioazolidine-4-carboxylic acid, led to a decrease in the induction of COX2 mRNA by arecoline, and the GSH synthesis inhibitor, buthionine sulfoximine, led to an increase, suggesting that regulation of COX2 expression induced by arecoline is critically dependent on cellular glutathione concentration.

Areca-nut extract (50–150 μg/mL) slightly enhanced the activity of COX (also called prostaglandin-endoperoxidase synthase (PHS)) in the human oral carcinoma cell line, OEC-M1, but inhibited its activity in KB cells (> 50 μg/mL) after 24 h of exposure (Yang et al., 2002).

## In animals: in-vivo studies

Mice given areca nut in the diet (0.25, 0.5 or 1.0%) for 5 or 36 weeks had significant increases in hepatic levels of cytochrome P450, cytochrome b5, malondialdehyde and GST, whereas hepatic content of sulfhydryl groups (-SH) was depressed (Singh & Rao, 1995a). Mice that had been on this diet for 45 days were supplemented during the last 10 days with mace (Myristica fragans), mustard seed (Brassica niger), garlic (Allium sativum L.) or butylated hydroxyanisole (BHA) — known chemopreventive agents; the levels of GST and -SH content normally induced by these agents were found to be decreased by areca nut. Conversely, levels of cytochrome P450 and cytochrome b5 normally induced by these agents were augmented following ingestion of an areca-nut diet (Singh & Rao, 1993a,b,c, 1995b,c).

Singh et al. (1996, 1997, 2000) studied the modulatory influence of intraperitoneal administration of arecoline on the chemopreventive efficacy of phytic acid, clocimum oil or chlorophyllin in lactating and suckling neonate mice. Phytic acid increased the hepatic levels of GST and -SH content in both lactating dams and suckling neonates whereas supplementation with arecoline inhibited these levels. Conversely, phytic acid elevated the levels of cytochrome P450 and cytochrome b5 in dams, and supplementation with arecoline further increased these elevated levels (Singh et al., 1997). Clocimum oil raised the hepatic levels of GST, -SH, cytochrome b5 and cytochrome P450 in lactating dams and suckling neonates; treatment with arecoline depressed the phase II enzyme and -SH content level but further raised the phase I enzyme levels (Singh et al., 2000). Arecoline treatment inhibited the levels of chlorophyllin-induced hepatic GST and -SH content in lactating females. Arecoline, whether given alone or concomitantly with chlorophyllin, elevated the levels of hepatic cytochrome b5 and cytochrome P450 to the same significance level compared to the untreated lactating dams (Singh et al., 1996).

(iii) *Effect of arecoline on TIMP and MMP*

Chang, Y.-C. et al. (2002a) hypothesized that oral submucous fibrosis is caused by increased or altered de-novo synthesis and deposition of extracellular matrix and/or altered fibrolysis, which, if unbalanced, may result in this fibrosis during betel-quid chewing. These authors attempted to assess the role of tissue inhibitors of metalloproteinases (TIMPs) and matrix metalloproteinases (MMPs) in the pathogenesis of OSF associated with chewing betel quid. Biopsy specimens were taken from buccal mucosal fibroblasts (BMFs) of six healthy individuals with no chewing habit and OSF of 10 male patients with betel-quid chewing habits. These biopsy specimens were used for preparation of fibroblast cultures and expression of TIMP-1 and production of MMP-2, which is the main gelatinolytic proteinase secreted by the human buccal mucosal fibroblasts, and were analysed by Western blot and gelatin zymography, respectively; OSF specimens were found to have higher TIMP-1 expression than BMFs. In-vitro exposure of human buccal mucosal fibroblasts to arecoline resulted in elevated TIMP-1 expression at concentrations below 20 µg/mL in a dose-dependent manner and inhibited MMP-2 secretion and production at higher concentrations (40 µg/mL), reducing MMP-2 activity by ~54% at 80 µg/mL. Arecoline acted not only as an inhibitor of gelatinolytic activity of MMP-2 but also as a stimulator for TIMP-1 activity, altering the balance between these two processes in favour of matrix stability. These synergistic effects may contribute to the accumulation of extracellular matrix components in betel quid-associated oral submucous fibrosis.

(b) *Betel leaf/hydroxychavicol/eugenol*

(i) *Metabolism*

Hydroxychavicol is a major phenolic compound in the leaf as well as the inflorescence of *Piper betle*. During its metabolism, an *ortho*-quinone is produced, which subsequently induces the production of reactive oxygen species via redox cycling (Iverson et al., 1995; Krol & Bolton, 1997). The reactive metabolites of hydroxychavicol such as quinones, quinone methide and imine methide enter into conjugation reactions with the reduced GSH (Iverson et al., 1995; Krol & Bolton, 1997; Nikolic et al., 1999). A similar pattern of metabolism was shown for eugenol (Bolton et al., 1992; Thompson et al., 1993).

(ii) *Influence on pro-oxidant and antioxidant mechanisms*

Chang, M.C. et al. (2002a) studied the effects of hydroxychavicol, which, like many phenolic antioxidants, can show pro-oxidant properties on oral KB carcinoma cells *in vitro*. Hydroxychavicol induced the intracellular production of reactive oxygen species at concentrations higher than 0.1 mM and depleted GSH. This compound acts as an antioxidant at low concentrations, whereas at high concentrations (> 0.1 mM), it may elicit intracellular accumulation of ROS and changes in redox status.

Choudhary and Kale (2002) evaluated the antioxidant properties of betel-leaf extract *in vitro* and *in vivo*. Male Swiss albino mice (7–8 weeks old) were given 1, 5 and 10 mg/kg bw betel-leaf extract orally for 2 weeks. The activity of superoxide dismutase (SOD) in liver increased in a dose-dependent manner. However, at 5- and 10-mg/kg dose levels, catalase activity was inhibited.

Panda and Kar (1998) studied the effect of betel-leaf extract (0.10, 0.40, 0.80 and 2.0 g/kg bw per day for 15 days) on the activities of catalase and SOD in the thyroid of male Swiss albino mice. Higher doses decreased the activities of catalase and SOD while increasing the level of lipid peroxidation. However, these effects were reversed with lower doses of the extract.

In a study to investigate its anticarcinogenic effect on tobacco carcinogens, 8-week-old inbred male Swiss albino mice were treated with betel-leaf extract (2.5 mg per mouse per day in drinking-water) for 10–16 months (13 mice) or 17–22 months (six mice). The concentrations of vitamin A and vitamin C (both strong antioxidants) in the liver were increased (Padma *et al.*, 1989a).

Jeng *et al.* (2002) showed that an aqueous extract of betel-leaf components contained potent scavengers of hydrogen peroxide ($H_2O_2$), superoxide ($O_2^{\bullet-}$) and hydroxyl radical ($HO^{\bullet}$) and was also an inhibitor of xanthine oxidase in a dose-dependent manner. In the presence of 10 and 20 µg/mL betel-leaf extract, about 95% of $O_2^{\bullet-}$ radicals were scavenged. Similarly, 20, 100 and 200 µg/mL betel-leaf extract inhibited $HO^{\bullet}$ by 47, 76 and 88%, respectively. The extract also effectively prevented $HO^{\bullet}$-induced DNA breaks on PUC18 plasmid DNA.

Patel and Rajorihia (1979) demonstrated that betel leaf has an antioxidative property that is much more effective than that of either BHA or butylated hydroxytoluene (IARC, 1986) *in vitro*.

(c) *Formation of nitrosamines*

(i) *Endogenous formation of areca-nut-derived nitrosamines in animals: in-vivo studies*

Ohshima *et al.* (1989) identified *N*-nitrosonipecotic acid (NNIP) (see Figure 5 for structure) as a major urinary metabolite of the areca-nut-derived nitrosamines, NGL and NGC, in BDIV rats. In a previous study, NNIP was detected in the urine of Syrian hamsters that were fed with powdered areca nut and sodium nitrite in the diet. Urine collected from control animals fed only areca nut or nitrite alone did not contain any NNIP (Ernst *et al.*, 1987). The authors concluded that the origin of this nitrosamine metabolite was from the endogenously formed areca-nut-derived nitrosamines, NGL and/or NGC.

(ii) *Formation of nitrosamines from arecoline and from betel quid: in-vitro studies*

In-vitro experiments with nitrite and the areca-nut alkaloid arecoline have shown the formation of at least three nitrosamines: NGL, MNPN and 3-methylnitrosaminopropionaldehyde (MNPA) (Wenke & Hoffmann, 1983). Nitrosation of arecoline at neutral pH yielded approximately four times more NGL than at acidic and alkaline pH (Wang & Peng, 1996). In-vitro nitrosation of betel quid without tobacco with nitrite and thiocyanate at neutral pH generated NGL, whereas similar nitrosation of betel quid with tobacco yielded NGL to a lesser extent and NGC (Nair *et al.*, 1985). The structure of the alkaloids and the nitrosamines derived from these alkaloids are given in Figure 5.

When the nitrosation reaction of betel quid with tobacco was carried out at acidic pH, formation of NNN and $N'$-nitrosoanatabine (NAT) was observed in addition to the formation of areca-nut-derived nitrosamines. NNK, MNPN and MNPA were not detected in any of the betel-quid samples nitrosated *in vitro* (Nair *et al.*, 1985). In-vitro nitrosation of betel quid with added L-proline yielded NPRO; addition of ascorbic acid with proline reduced the formation of NPRO in only one of three betel-quid samples tested (Nair, J. *et al.*, 1987). $N$-Nitrosopiperidine, $N$-nitrosopyrrolidine and $N$-nitrosomorpholine were detected in nitrite-treated aqueous extract of *Piper betle* L. fruit (Chen *et al.*, 1984).

(iii) *Modulation of nitrosamine formation by polyphenols from betel-quid ingredients*

Polyphenols have been shown to inhibit or enhance the nitrosation of amines (Pignatelli *et al.*, 1982; Walker *et al.*, 1982). Wang and Peng (1996) investigated the effect of crude phenolic extracts from areca fruit (areca nut) and the inflorescence and leaf of *Piper betle* on the formation of NGL from arecoline. They observed that low concentrations (< 60 mg/300 mL [< 0.2 mg/mL]) of polyphenolic extract from areca fruit and all tested concentrations of phenolics from *Piper betle* (up to ~530 mg/300 mL [~1.8 mg/mL]) inhibited the formation of NGL from arecoline, whereas higher concentrations of areca phenolics (> 260 mg/300 mL [> 0.86 mg/mL]) enhanced the formation of NGL. Hydroxychavicol, a polyphenol from betel leaf, has been shown to scavenge nitrite, thereby reducing the formation of $N$-methyl-$N$-nitrosourea, the mutagenic reaction product of nitrite plus methylurea (Nagabhushan *et al.*, 1989).

(*d*) *Formation of reactive oxygen species from betel-quid ingredients*

**Cell-free systems**

Several polyphenols including the tannin fraction of areca nut have been shown to be genotoxic at alkaline pH in *Saccharomyces cerevisiae* (Rosin, 1984). The genotoxicity of polyphenols was postulated to be attributable to the generation of $H_2O_2$ and free radicals as a result of rapid autoxidation under alkaline pH. The generation of superoxide anion ($O_2^{\bullet-}$) and $H_2O_2$ from aqueous extracts of areca nut and catechu at pH greater than 9.5 was demonstrated by Nair, U.J. *et al.* (1987) using a chemiluminescence technique. Of the various areca-nut extracts, the catechin fraction, at alkaline pH, was shown to be the most active producer of reactive oxygen species. The formation of $O_2^{\bullet-}$ was enhanced by $Fe^{2+}$, $Fe^{3+}$, $Mg^{2+}$ and $Cu^{2+}$ but inhibited by $Mn^{2+}$ and higher concentrations of $Mg^{2+}$ and $Cu^{2+}$. Tobacco extract failed to generate reactive oxygen species under similar conditions but showed formation of $O_2^{\bullet-}$ only in the presence of metal ions. Saliva inhibited both $O_2^{\bullet-}$ and $H_2O_2$ formation from betel-quid ingredients. Upon incubation of DNA at alkaline pH with areca-nut extract or catechu and $Fe^{3+}$, 8-OH-deoxyguanosine (8-OHdG) was formed as quantified by HPLC-electrochemical detection (Nair, U.J. et al., 1987).

Using 25 samples of slaked lime from Papua New Guinea, Nair et al. (1990) demonstrated that the free calcium hydroxide content and pH of slaked lime samples ($\geq 9.5$) were highly correlated with the generation of reactive oxygen species from areca-nut extract and DNA damage in vitro, as measured as 8-OHdG. The $Fe^{2+}$ and $Mg^{2+}$ levels in the lime samples were too low to modify the formation of reactive oxygen species, but the formation of 8-OHdG in DNA was enhanced by the addition of high concentrations of $Fe^{2+}$ and the formation of $H_2O_2$ was almost entirely inhibited by adding $Mg^{2+}$ to the reaction mixture. These results show the importance of pH for the formation of reactive oxygen species that is likely to occur via autoxidation of polyphenols, redox cycling via quinone semiquinone radicals and iron-catalysed Haber-Weiss and Fenton reactions (Figure 7).

**Figure 7. Scheme for the formation of reactive oxygen species from polyphenols present in the betel-quid ingredients, areca nut and catechu**

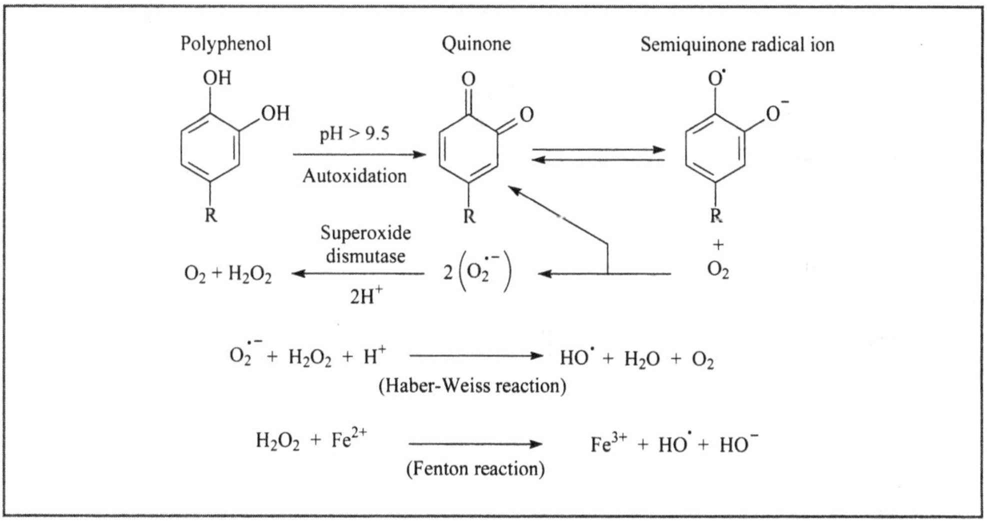

Adapted from Nair et al. (1996)

To determine whether hydroxyl radical (HO•) is generated while chewing betel quid, in-vitro studies were performed using L-phenylalanine with different reaction conditions. The formation of ortho- and meta-tyrosine from L-phenylalanine was measured as a marker of OH• radical generation. Both *ortho-* and *meta-*tyrosine were formed *in vitro* in the presence of extracts of areca nut and/or catechu, transition metal ions such as $Cu^{2+}$ and $Fe^{2+}$ and alkaline pH due to slaked lime or sodium carbonate. The omission of any of these ingredients from the reaction mixture significantly reduced the yield of tyrosines. HO• scavengers such as ethanol, D-mannitol and dimethylsulfoxide inhibited phenylalanine oxidation in a dose-dependent fashion (Nair *et al.*, 1995).

Iron and copper are involved in the catalysis of reactive oxygen species generation. Copper contents in various betel-quid ingredients are reported to be in the range 3–188 µg/g (areca nut) and 8–53 µg/g (*pan masala*) (Trivedy *et al.*, 1997; Ridge *et al.*, 2001), whereas the iron contents were 75 µg/g (areca nut), 171 µg/g (betel leaf), 5.2 mg/g (catechu), 190 µg/g (slaked lime) (Zaidi *et al.*, 2002) and 22–526 µg/L [89.6–2100 µg/g] (slaked lime) (Nair *et al.*, 1990).

In the presence of $FeCl_2$ (1–1000 µM) and under alkaline conditions, the reaction of tender (1 mg/mL) and ripe (1 mg/mL) areca-nut extracts with herring sperm DNA for 60 min produced more 8-OHdG than without iron (Liu *et al.*, 1996).

**Cultured cell systems**

Significant amounts of superoxide anion production (determined by the cytochrome c reduction assay) and lipid peroxidation (formation of thiobarbituric acid-reactive substances) were demonstrated in normal human oral keratinocytes treated with commercially available *gutka* and *pan masala* with or without saccharin (Bagchi *et al.*, 2002).

Exposure of Chinese hamster ovary (CHO)-K1 cells to ripe areca-nut extract (0.05–0.4 mg/mL) for 18 h induced a 1.2–2.8-fold increase in 8-OHdG formation. Tender areca-nut extract induced only a slight increase in 8-OHdG formation ($p > 0.05$). A 3.5-h exposure of CHO-K1 cells to areca nut produced marked formation of reactive oxygen species (hydrogen peroxide), as indicated by an increase in intracellular dichlorofluorescein fluorescence (Liu *et al.*, 1996).

(*e*)    *Antioxidant effects*

Lei *et al.* (2003) directly evaluated the antioxidative properties of aqueous extract of *Piper betle* inflorescence. It was an effective scavenger of reactive oxygen species, with a 50% inhibitory concentration ($IC_{50}$) of 80, 28 and 73 µg/mL towards $H_2O_2$, superoxide and hydroxyl radicals, respectively.

Aqueous extract of *Piper betle* leaf was also shown to be a potent scavenger towards reactive oxygen species such as hydroxyl radicals (> 15 µg/mL), superoxide radicals (> 10 µg/mL) and a xanthine oxidase inhibitor (> 50 µg/mL). It inhibited the rabbit platelet aggregation induced by arachidonic acid and collagen, possibly because of its antioxidative property and its inhibition of cyclooxygenase. *Piper betle* leaf extract also inhibited thromoxane $B_2$ and prostaglandin-$D_2$ production in platelet aggregates induced by collagen and arachidonic acid (Jeng *et al.*, 2002; Lei *et al.*, 2003), but had no effect on areca-nut-induced platelet aggregation (see Section 4.2.2(*b*)(iii)).

## 4.2 Physiological and toxic effects

### 4.2.1 *Humans*

#### (a) *Psychopharmacological effects*

Areca nut is the fourth most commonly used psychoactive substance in the world after tobacco, alcohol and caffeine-containing beverages (Sullivan & Hagen, 2002). It is described as a popular pleasure-giving substance in South Asia (Schneider, 1986) and chewed for its psychostimulating effects (Norton, 1998). Areca-nut chewing is reported to have varied and widespread, predominantly stimulant, effects (Chu, 2001, 2002).

'Betel-nut' (areca-nut) psychosis was originally described about 25 years ago in Papua New Guineans by Burton-Bradley (1977). He described how traditional healers challenged victims with so-called betel nut to induce insanity as a part of their diagnostic strategy. Psychosis, although rare, was described in predisposed people following abrupt cessation of the habit (Burton-Bradley, 1978). In Melanesia, other authors have also reported areca nut as producing altered status of consciousness and being capable of inducing intoxication (Cawte, 1985). More recently, so-called betelmania was reported among Cambodian refugee women living in the USA who were addicted to areca nut (Pickwell *et al.*, 1994).

Habituation and addiction to areca nut in Papua New Guineans has been reported (Burton-Bradley, 1978; Talonu, 1989). More recently, regular, daily use of areca nut at high frequency — on average 17.3 portions a day — was reported among aborigines of Taiwan (Yang, Y.-H. *et al.*, 2001). Winstock *et al.* (2000) described findings consistent with a dependence syndrome related to areca-nut use among regular users in the Gujarat community in the United Kingdom. Reported effects of areca-nut chewing were relaxation, improved concentration, mild lifting of the mood and enhanced satisfaction after eating. Withdrawal symptoms on trying to quit the habit were mood swings, anxiety, irritability, reduced concentration, sleep disturbance and craving for the nut. The mean severity of dependence score was 7.3 (range, 1–12), which is equivalent to problematic use of amphetamines. The majority of the users reported the development of tolerance to the effects of the nut.

In a preliminary study conducted in a hospital population in Sri Lanka, a higher proportion of patients diagnosed with schizophrenia chewed betel quid compared with control subjects, and the frequency of chewing betel quid was also higher among these patients (Kuruppuarachchi & Williams, 2003).

#### (b) *Effects on oral hard and soft tissues*

A growing body of evidence over the last five decades from epidemiological and experimental studies has shown that areca nut, even when consumed in the absence of tobacco or slaked lime, may have potentially harmful effects on the oral cavity (Trivedy *et al.*, 1999a).

(i) *Effects on hard tissues*

**Dental attrition**

The main effects of areca on the hard tissues are on the teeth. The habitual chewing of areca nut may result in severe tooth wear involving incisal and occlusal tooth surfaces, particularly the enamel covering. The loss of enamel exposes the underlying dentine which, as it is softer than enamel, wears away at an increased rate. The exposure of dentine may also result in dentinal sensitivity. The degree of attrition is dependent upon several factors, which include the consistency (hardness) of the areca nut, the frequency of chewing and the duration of the habit. Root fractures have also been demonstrated in chronic areca-nut chewers, which are probably a consequence of the increased masticatory load, and excessive and repetitive masticatory stress applied on teeth during chewing (Yeh, 1997; Gao *et al.*, 2001).

Extrinsic staining of teeth in the form of black or brown surface discoloration due to areca-nut deposits is often observed among areca-nut chewers, particularly when good oral hygiene prophylaxis is lacking and where regular dental care is minimal.

**Dental caries**

It has been suggested that areca-nut chewing may confer protection against dental caries. Epidemiological studies carried out in South-East Asia suggest that the prevalence of dental caries in areca-nut chewers is lower than that in non-chewers (Möller *et al.*, 1977; Schamschula *et al.*, 1977; Nigam & Srivastava, 1990). Some investigators, however, have shown that there is no difference in the prevalence of dental caries between areca-nut chewers and non-chewers in other Asian populations (Reichart & Gehring, 1984; Williams *et al.*, 1996). Although little is known about the cariostatic properties of areca nut, it has been suggested that the stain that often coats the surface of the teeth may act as a protective varnish (Howden, 1984).

(ii) *Effects on soft tissues*

**Gingivae and the periodontium**

A higher prevalence of gingivitis was recently reported among chewers of betel quid with tobacco (Amarasena *et al.*, 2003).

Ling *et al.* (2001) found that the levels of two periodontal pathogens, *Porphyromonas gingivalis* and *Actinobacillus actinomycetemcomitans*, are higher in betel-quid chewers who show a higher gingival index (an indicator of gingival inflammation) than in non-chewers.

It has been shown that loss of periodontal attachment and calculus formation is greater in areca-nut chewers (Ånerud *et al.*, 1991). [The Working Group noted that it is difficult to interpret these studies, as there are several confounding variables such as the level of oral hygiene, dietary factors, general health and dental status, and especially tobacco smoking, which may have a significant influence on periodontal status. It is therefore difficult to ascertain the biological effects of chewing areca nut on periodontal health.]

**Oral submucous fibrosis**

There has been recent interest in the role of copper in the pathogenesis of oral submucous fibrosis, and elevated copper concentrations have been found in products containing areca nut in comparison with other nut-based snacks (Trivedy et al., 1997). Chewing areca nut for up to 20 min releases significant amounts of soluble copper into the oral cavity (Trivedy et al., 1999b), and mucosal biopsies taken from oral submucous fibrosis patients contain higher concentrations of copper than those taken from healthy controls (Trivedy et al., 2000). This has led to the hypothesis that higher tissue concentrations of copper may increase the activity of the enzyme lysyl oxidase, an extracellular copper-dependent enzyme that catalyses the cross-linking of elastine and soluble collagen to form insoluble collagen in the extracellular matrix. Lysyl oxidase is implicated in the pathogenesis of several fibrotic disorders including oral submucous fibrosis (Ma et al., 1995; Trivedy et al., 1999c). Further support for this theory comes from in-vitro studies showing that inorganic copper salts significantly increase the production of collagen by oral fibroblasts (Trivedy et al., 2001).

As described in Section 4.1.2(a)(iii), Chang, Y.-C. et al. (2002a) hypothesized that oral submucous fibrosis is probably the consequence of a disturbance in the homeostatic equilibrium between synthesis and degradation of extracellular matrix and/or altered fibrolysis which may result in this fibrosis during betel-quid chewing, and attempted to assess the role of tissue inhibitors of metalloproteinase (TIMP) in the pathogenesis of this disease. Biopsy specimens of buccal mucosal fibroblasts were taken from six healthy individuals with no chewing habit and oral submucous fibrosis tissue from 10 men who chewed betel quid, and were used to prepare fibroblast cultures for the analysis of TIMP-1 expression by Western blot. Oral submucous fibrosis specimens were found to have higher TIMP-1 expression than fibroblasts derived from normal buccal mucosa. In this study, arecoline was found to increase TIMP-1 expression and to inhibit matrix metalloproteinases (MMP) in human buccal mucosal fibroblasts *in vitro*.

Cyclooxygenase (COX), an inducible enzyme responsible for prostaglandin synthesis, plays an important role in certain inflammatory diseases and carcinogenesis. Tsai et al. (2003) studied the influence of betel-quid (areca-nut) chewing on the expression of COX2 in six normal buccal mucosa specimens from persons who did not chew betel quid and in 15 oral submucous fibrosis specimens from betel-quid chewers; of the latter, 10 showed moderate fibrosis and five showed severe fibrosis. Immunohistochemical analysis showed that COX2 expression was significantly higher in oral submucous fibrosis specimens than in buccal mucosal fibroblasts. Strong immunostaining for COX2 was detected in epithelial cells, fibroblasts and inflammatory cells.

(c)  *Effects on various physiological systems*

(i)  *General physiological effects*

Dose-dependent increases in energy expenditure (varying with basal metabolism) and decreases in carbohydrate utilization (independent of variation in insulin secretion), together with increased hunger, were seen in a human volunteer when gels of betel extract were applied to the buccal sulcus after fasting. However, suppression of appetite after food intake was enhanced (Strickland & Duffield, 1997; Strickland et al., 2003). The four areca alkaloids have anti-muscarinic effects on smooth muscle and bind to γ-aminobutyric acid (GABA) receptors that are thought to contain chloride channels. These are similar to acetylcholine receptors and are found in many organs in the body, including the brain and pancreatic islets. Areca alkaloids can, therefore, be predicted to have widespread physiological effects (for a review, see Boucher & Mannan, 2002).

(ii) *Effects on the nervous and cardiovascular systems*

Areca nut contains a number of psychoactive alkaloids, one of which is arecoline, and affects the parasympathetic nervous system in intolerant users, inducing salivation and sweating. More importantly, areca-nut chewing also activates a sympathoadrenal response (Chu, 2002). Areca-nut chewing has been shown to cause a significant elevation in plasma concentration of adrenaline and noradrenaline (Chu, 1995a), but the sites of activation have not been defined. Chu (2001) hypothesized that these actions on the nervous system may be both central and peripheral. Arecoline readily crosses the blood–brain barrier (Asthana et al., 1996) and increases brain levels of acetylcholine in animals by 150–250% (Shannon et al., 1994). The areca-nut alkaloids, arecaidine and guvacine, are reported to be inhibitors of GABA-uptake (Johnston et al., 1975; Lodge et al., 1977). Thus, in addition to its stimulant effects, areca nut contributes to relaxation through its anxiolytic effects. This mixture of effects is common in other misused substances and supports earlier anecdotal reports claiming desirable effects by users. Arecoline and betel-quid use increase occipital α activity and generalized β activity on electroencephalograms (EEG), with reduction in θ activity, suggesting that areca alkaloids increase cerebral arousal and relaxation (Joseph & Sitaram, 1990; Chu, 1994). Short-term elevation in heart rate following administration of betel quid has been observed, indicating peripheral stimulation, but visual information processing is unaltered by areca nut (Frewer, 1990).

Betel quid reduces the severity of both positive and negative symptoms in schizophrenia but extrapyramidal symptoms (marked stiffness, tremor and distressing akathisia) are occasionally aggravated during heavy use in those on neuroleptic medication (Dealh, 1989). It is a risk factor for the movement disorder, Meige's syndrome (Behari et al., 2000). Betel-quid chewing increases central sympathetic activity in humans, leading to increased heart rate and increased blood flow through the common and external carotid arteries and facial-flush sensation (Chu, 2002; Lin, S.-K. et al., 2002).

Palpitations, sweating and facial flushing with sensations of skin warmth are early effects of areca chewing and skin temperature increases by 0.5–2 °C (Chu, 1993). Heart rates increase with or without habituation, but systolic blood pressure increases only in novice users (Chu, 1993). Betel leaves activate the sympathetic nervous system and increase the secretion of adrenal medullary catecholamine. Moderate areca-nut intake may activate the sympathetic nervous system and high doses activate both the sympathetic and parasympathetic nerves experimentally and *in vivo*. The effect on parasympathetic nerves reduces the RR interval variation (RRIV) as recorded on electrocardiograms of heavy areca-nut users during rest and hyperventilation (Chu, 1995b). In the presence of coronary artery disease, this could, with vasoconstriction caused by areca nut, increase the risk of heart attack, although few case reports suggest this possibility (Hung & Deng, 1998; Deng *et al.*, 2001). Elevated serum homocysteine is a risk factor for heart disease common among British Bangladeshis (Alfthan *et al.*, 1997; Obeid *et al.*, 1998) and increases in homocysteine levels related to smoking and areca-nut use were found to be as large as those related to folate deficiency in a study of Bangladeshis in the United Kingdom (Obeid *et al.*, 1998).

**Arterial plaque instability and fibrosis: role of matrix metalloproteinases**

Instability of arterial plaque is a major causal factor in myocardial infarction. It is associated with increases in MMP enzyme activity in active plaque, which destroys collagen and weakens the interstitium. High levels of circulating MMP-2 and MMP-9 are markers of coronary events (Galis *et al.*, 1994; Fabunmi, 1998; Kai *et al.*, 1998). Circulating TIMP-1 increases with the use of betel quid, independent of increases related to MMP-9 and other risk factors (Timms *et al.*, 2002a). It is not yet known whether the balance of these effects contribute to the risk for coronary heart disease or heart attack in areca-nut users.

Increases in TIMP-1 disproportionate to those in MMP-9, reported in areca-nut users, could contribute to the pathogenesis of diseases in which increased fibrosis is a feature, such as cirrhosis of the liver and hypertensive and left ventricular hypertrophy (Burt, 1993; Timms *et al.*, 1998, 2002a,b). Arecoline itself produces dose-dependent increases in TIMP-1 expression in human buccal fibroblasts together with inhibition of secretion of MMP-2 (Chang, Y.-C. *et al.*, 2002a), a phenomenon relevant to the risk for oral submucous fibrosis (see Section 4.1.2(*a*)(iii)).

(iii) *Effects on the respiratory system*

Arecoline has been known since 1912 to induce contraction of the bronchial muscles (Trendelenburg, 1912). Sufferers of asthma report worsening of their symptoms with areca-nut chewing: over 50% of those giving up the habit do so because of this effect. Minor reductions in forced expiratory volume in 1 s ($FEV_1$) are seen in non-asthmatics who chew areca nut. $FEV_1$ can improve by up to 10% in asthmatics using areca nut but reductions of ~22% are seen in those asthmatics who report worse asthma after chewing (Kiyingi, 1991; Kiyingi & Saweri, 1994). Arecoline causes dose-related constriction of bronchial smooth muscle *in vitro* and bronchoconstriction in most of the asthmatics studied who were not betel-quid users, some non-asthmatic controls and in betel-quid users with asthma. Reduction of $FEV_1$ (by up to 30%) may last several hours (Taylor *et al.*, 1992).

(iv) *Effects on the gastrointestinal system*

Users report that betel quid soothes the digestion and avoids constipation; colonic smooth muscle is stimulated through its muscarinic effects. Peptic ulceration, however, is increased in chewers of betel quid [with tobacco] (Ahmed *et al.*, 1993). Chewers secrete more saliva on chemical stimulation, diluting salivary amylase and potassium, and tobacco aggravates this effect (Reddy *et al.*, 1980). Areca-nut extracts reduce halitosis, probably by the reduction of the volatility of methyl mercaptan through arecal phenolic derivatives, and slaked lime plays an important role in this function (Wang *et al.*, 2001).

(v) *Effects on endocrine systems*

**Hyperglycaemic effects**

The neurotransmitter GABA is functional in insulin-secreting pancreatic $\beta$ cells; the GABA shunt enzyme, glutamate decarboxylase (GAD), is an autoantigen and GAD antibody formation is common in the development of the human type 1 diabetes, insulin-dependent diabetes mellitus (Martino *et al.*, 1991; Sorenson *et al.*, 1991). Areca alkaloids, which are inhibitors of the GABA receptor, block the inhibitory effects of GABA on the secretion of glucagon and somatotrophin, increasing their release. Glucagon release triggers the release of insulin resulting in short-term hypoglycaemia but long-term increases in glucagon cause diabetes. This provides a mechanism that could lead to diabetes in betel-quid chewers. At the same time, the inhibition of GABA reduces GAD activity and also, experimentally, the autoimmune response to GAD in rat pancreatic islets (Smismans *et al.*, 1997). It is not known whether this mechanism applies to humans, in whom it could reduce the risk of type 1 diabetes and also the risk of progression to insulin requirement in patients with type 2 diabetes.

In view of the diabetogenicity of areca nut in mice (see Section 4.2.2), glycaemia and anthropometric risk factors for type 2 diabetes were investigated in relation to use of *paan* quids in ~1000 adult Bangladeshis living in East London (1992–94) (Mannan *et al.*, 2000). Waist size and weight, major determinants of hyperglycaemia (Chan *et al.*, 1994), increased with increasing use of betel quid (approximately 80% of men aged 30–50 and 90% of women aged 40–60 were chewers), independent of established risk factors, such as central obesity, age, smoking and parity. Reductions in body mass index (with increases in resting metabolic rate) have also been reported with increasing use of betel quid but only at higher ambient temperatures in hot climates (Strickland & Duffield, 2003). The difference in findings may reflect the more temperate weather in the United Kingdom. Alternatively, vitamin D deficiency, which is common in British Asians, is known to reduce insulin secretion and to increase glycaemia and may have obscured the features related to the use of betel quid (Boucher *et al.*, 1995).

Recent work in Papua New Guinea, where vitamin D deficiency is less likely to be found, has shown that chewing betel quid without tobacco is the predominant independent risk factor for diabetes (diagnosed by fasting blood glucose $\geq$ 7.0 mmol/L), with age, body mass index and region of residence being the other relevant factors (odds ratio for diabetes in betel chewers, 3.4; 95% CI, 2.0–5.9) (Benjamin, 2001).

(vi) *Effects on the immune system*

## Betel-quid chewers and oral submucous fibrosis patients

*Antibodies*

Shah *et al.* (1994) and Gupta *et al.* (1985) found that oral submucous fibrosis patients ($n = 66$ and 10) had higher serum levels of immunoglobulin (Ig) G, IgM and IgA than controls ($n = 25$ and 5), whereas Canniff *et al.* (1986) found an increase in serum IgG levels in 30 oral submucous fibrosis patients relative to normal individuals, but no difference in IgM and IgA levels; and Rajendran *et al.* (1986) observed an increase in serum IgA, IgD and IgE concentrations in 50 oral submucous fibrosis patients compared with 50 controls.

Canniff *et al.* (1986) detected the presence of serum auto-antibodies such as gastric parietal cell antibody (GPCA), thyroid microsomal antibody, anti-nuclear antibody (ANA), anti-reticulin antibody and anti-smooth muscle antibody (SMA) in 38, 23, 8, 4 and 4% of 26 oral submucous fibrosis patients, respectively. [No report of a control group is given.] Chiang *et al.* (2002a) also studied serum auto-antibodies in 109 male oral submucous fibrosis patients, all of whom were betel-quid chewers. The frequencies of serum ANA (23.9%), SMA (23.9%) and GPCA (14.7%) in oral submucous fibrosis patients were higher than those in 109 controls (9.2%, 7.3% and 5.5%, respectively). The presence of serum GPCA ($p < 0.05$) and ANA ($p = 0.066$) in oral submucous fibrosis patients was associated with daily betel-quid consumption, but the presence of serum auto-antibodies in such patients showed little correlation with maximal mouth opening.

Balaram *et al.* (1987) found an increase in circulating immune complex (CIC) in the sera of 20 healthy betel-quid chewers compared with 50 controls. Forty betel-quid chewers with oral submucous fibrosis and 85 with oral cancer had showed even higher serum levels of CIC. Remani *et al.* (1988) evaluated levels of CIC and immunoglobulins in normal controls and patients with oral leukoplakia, oral submucous fibrosis and oral cancer ($n = 50$ for all groups). Clearly elevated levels of CIC, and of IgG and IgM in CIC, were found in both oral submucous fibrosis and oral cancer groups.

*Immune cells*

An impairment of natural killer-cell activity has been detected in patients with oral leukoplakia and oral submucous fibrosis, which can be improved by treatment with interferon-α (Pillai *et al.*, 1990).

In an earlier study, total leukocyte and lymphocyte counts in peripheral blood were decreased in 25 patients with oral cancer and 30 with oral precancerous lesions and conditions (including oral leukoplakia and oral submucous fibrosis) compared with 22 healthy controls, whereas an increase in the percentage of B lymphocytes was noted in precancer patients. (Pillai *et al.*, 1987) [no oral habit data given].

Using immunohistochemical staining, Haque *et al.* (1997) reported increased numbers of CD3 cells (T lymphocytes), CD4 cells (helper/inducer T lymphocytes) and HLA-DR cells and an increase in the ratio of CD4:CD8 (suppressor and cytotoxic T lymphocytes) cells in the epithelium and subepithelial connective tissues of oral submucous fibrosis patients compared with normal buccal mucosa. Chiang *et al.* (2002b) also noted a marked increase in the numbers of CD3 cells, CD20 cells (B lymphocytes) and CD68 cells (macrophages) and a predominance of CD4 lymphocytes over CD8 lymphocytes in the subepithelial connective tissue of 50 oral submucous fibrosis patients compared with 10 controls.

**Effects of tobacco/nicotine on the immune system**

Few data are available on the effects of chewing tobacco on the immune system in humans. Nicotine, however, has been reported to affect both humoral and cell-mediated immune responses (Johnson *et al.*, 1990; Geng *et al.*, 1995, 1996; Kalra *et al.*, 2000) and to produce an altered immune response that is characterized by a decline in inflammation, a reduction in antibody response and a decrease in T-cell receptor-mediated signalling (Sopori & Kozak, 1998). These findings suggest that nicotine is a potent immunopharmacological agent with regard to T-cell function (see IARC, 2004).

(*d*)    *Other effects*

Wu *et al.* (1996) reported cases with milk-alkali syndrome caused by betel-quid chewing. The patients showed the symptom of hypercalcaemia, metabolic alkalosis, nephrocalcinosis and renal insufficiency. Lin, S.-H. *et al.* (2002) also reported one case of milk-alkali syndrome who chewed 40 pieces of betel quid per day.

Winstock *et al.* (2000) found a decrease in vitamin $B_{12}$ level in 4 of 9 patients who had chewed betel quid for 35 years compared to historical reference range levels of supposed healthy non-chewers.

4.2.2    *Experimental systems*

(*a*)    *In-vivo studies*

(i)    *Chronic toxicity*

The chronic oral toxicity of *pan masala* was assessed in gavage studies in inbred male rats [strain not indicated]. The substance was ground, dispersed in water and given to the animals by gavage on 5 days per week for 6 months at 84, 420 or 840 mg/kg bw. The rats were killed 24 h after the last dose. Liver and serum enzymes (glutamic-oxaloacetic transaminase, glutamic-pyruvic transaminase and alkaline phosphatase) and organ weights were measured. The results showed that chronic feeding of *pan masala* impaired liver function at the highest dose, as indicated by changes in enzyme activity, and decreased relative weights of the brain at all doses tested (22% weight loss at the highest dose) (Sarma *et al.*, 1992).

(ii)    *Effect on oral soft tissues: induction of oral submucous fibrosis*

Earlier studies found that the application of arecoline to the palates of Wistar rats did not give rise to any features that were suggestive of oral submucous fibrosis (Sirsat &

Khanolkar, 1962). Application of arecaidine to hamster cheek pouch also failed to show any microscopic changes suggestive of fibrosis (MacDonald, 1987). The authors noted that the concentration chosen was too low to produce an effect *in vivo* and that the pH of the aqueous solution of aracaidine used was acid (pH 3), whereas in the human situation, the addition of lime to the betel quid would ensure an alkaline pH.

Paste made out of *pan masala* was painted onto the oral cavity (palate, cheek mucosa) of 21 Wistar albino rats on alternate days for a period of 6 months, except for a 2-week period after every biopsy. Biopsies were taken from the oral mucosa at the beginning of the study and every 2 months thereafter and were compared histopathologically with those obtained from a control group. Mild-to-moderate loss of nuclear polarity and increase in keratoses, parakeratoses, inflammatory cell infiltration and vascularity were noted compared with the controls. The increase in mitotic figures was not statistically significant and no definite changes in pigmentation or atypical cells were seen. Submucosal collagen increased sharply and steadily throughout the study. At the end of 6 months, 88% of biopsies showed thickened and condensed submucosal collagen, indicating submucous fibrosis (Khrime *et al.*, 1991).

(iii) *Neuropharmacological effects*

Arecoline, dissolved in saline, was given by subcutaneous injection to albino Swiss Nos mice at doses of 2 and 10 mg/kg bw. After 15 min, the animals were killed and the levels of acetylcholine, norepinephrine and dopamine in the cortex and subcortex (the remaining part of the brain) were studied. Arecoline at 10 mg/kg bw caused a reduction in levels of acetylcholine in the cortex and subcortex at the limit of statistical significance, and a statistically significant reduction in levels of norepinephrine. A statistically significant increase in the level of dopamine was observed only in the cortex after both doses of arecoline (Molinengo *et al.*, 1986).

The dichloromethane fraction from *Areca catechu* extraction was injected intraperitoneally into rats and mice at doses of 1–13 mg/kg bw 1 h prior to observation of antidepressant effects and analysis of monoamine oxidase A. Forced swim and tail-suspension test results indicated an antidepressant effect of the dichloromethane fraction, which was associated with inhibition of monoamine oxidase-A isolated from rat brain. No such inhibition was seen with various constituents of *areca catechu* such as arecoline, arecaidine catechin, gallic acid and few aminoacids (Dar & Khatoon, 2000).

(iv) *Neurocardiovascular effects*

Intravenous injections of eugenol, safrole or an aqueous extract of *Piper betle* inflorescence (containing 6.2% eugenol and 78.9% safrole) induced hypotensive and bradycardiac effects in male Wistar rats, whereas both intra-arterial and intrathecal injections of these substances resulted in hypotensive and tachycardiac effects. Moreover, the effects of intravenous injections of the extract were reversed or inhibited by pretreatment with bilateral vagotomy, or administration of atropine (1 mg/kg intraperitoneally) or capsaicin (100 mg/kg, subcutaneously). The tachycardia resulting from intrathecal injections of the extract was inhibited by pretreatment with propranolol (0.3 mg/kg intravenously). Eugenol and safrole induced the same pattern of changes in blood pressure and heart rate as the inflorescence extract. It was concluded that acute administration of extracts of betel inflorescence by different routes may activate C-fibre-evoked parasympathetic and sympathetic cardiovascular reflexes in rats (Chen et al., 1995).

Using normal and hypertensive rats as an experimental model, areca-nut components decreased blood pressure and inhibited angiotensin I- and angiotensin II-induced increases in blood pressure, but showed little effect on heart rate (Inokuchi et al., 1986). Oral intake of areca tannin (100–200 mg/kg) by hypertensive rats (6–8 per group) induced a long-lasting decrease in systolic blood pressure. Direct intravenous injection of areca tannin (10–15 mg/kg) led to hypotension (Inokuchi et al., 1986). A single intraperitoneal injection of arecoline (1 mg/kg) to Fischer 344 rats (4–5 per group) induced the incorporation of arachidonate into brain microvascular endothelial cells (Williams et al., 1998).

(v) *Effects on the gastrointestinal tract*

The effects of two Indian varieties of betel leaf (*Piper betle* L.), the pungent Mysore and the non-pungent Ambadi, on digestive enzymes of the pancreas and the intestinal mucosa, and on bile secretion were studied in rats. Betel leaves were despined, ground to a paste and given to female Wistar rats (eight per group) by gavage at doses of 40 and 200 mg/kg bw, comparable to one and five times the human consumption level. After 3 h, the pancreas and the small intestine were isolated and processed for assays of various enzymes. The betel leaves did not influence bile secretion or composition, but there was a significant stimulatory effect on pancreatic lipase activity. In addition, the Ambadi variety of betel leaf had a positive stimulatory influence on intestinal digestive enzymes, especially lipase, amylase and disaccharidases. A slight decrease in the activity of these intestinal enzymes was seen with the Mysore variety of the betel leaf, which also had a negative effect on pancreatic amylase. Both varieties caused a decrease in pancreatic trypsin and chymotrypsin activities (Prabhu et al., 1995).

Feeding male Wistar rats (10 per group) a diet containing betel quid (30%) or its components (30%) including areca nut, *gambir* and lime for 30 or 90 days increased gastric mucosal acid back-diffusion and reduced mucous secretion. These changes were seen with experimental haemorrhagic peptic ulceration and probably contributed to increased ulceration. Alkalinization with either antacids or therapeutic blockade of acid secretion by $NaHCO_3$ and cimetidine corrected these effects (Hung & Cheng, 1994). The acetylcholine-like effect of areca nut on the bowel was due mainly to arecoline and was mediated through neuroreceptors of the autonomic nerve plexus in the gut wall.

Daily oral administration of alcoholic and aqueous areca-nut extracts to male albino rats (100 mg/kg bw extract for 1 and 4 weeks; five rats per group) significantly decreased alkaline phosphatase, $Ca^{2+}$-$Mg^{2+}$-ATPase and sucrase activities in brush border. However, in-situ exposure of the intestine to aqueous areca-nut extract for 30 min activated brush border membrane enzyme, alkaline phosphatase, $Ca^{2+}$-$Mg^{2+}$-ATPase and sucrase activities, whereas alcoholic areca-nut extract did not produce any significant changes in the enzyme activities. Significant declines in brush border membrane constituents (total hexose, sialic acid and cholesterol) were also evident following continuous exposure to areca-nut extracts. These findings suggest that prolonged chewing of areca nut may cause significant functional alterations in the intestinal epithelial cell lining and could lead to malabsorption of nutrients (Kumar et al., 2000).

Feeding albino rats a diet containing 60–100% areca nut led to diarrhoea and even death of rats within 1–3 weeks. Histologically, splenomegaly, fatty liver changes, stunted skeleton and necrosis of buccal and intestinal mucosa were observed in dead rats. Diets containing 15% areca nut or more induced haemorrhagic and catarrhal enteritis (Saikia & Vaidehi, 1983).

### (vi) Lipid metabolism

Feeding Sprague-Dawley rats with areca nut for 6 days markedly decreased plasma cholesterol and triglyceride concentrations, and also the intestinal pancreatic esterase activity involved in the cholesterol absorption process (Jeon et al., 2000). Areca extracts reduce the absorption of triglycerides and cholesterol and subsequent blood levels of both through the inhibition of pancreatic cholesterol esterase, pancreatic lipase and intestinal acyl-co-enzyme A:cholesterol acyltransferase activities (Byun et al., 2001; Park et al., 2002).

### (vii) Diabetogenic effects

Young adult CD1 mice with a low spontaneous incidence of diabetes were fed areca nut in standard feed for 2–6 days. Single time-point (90 min) intraperitoneal glucose tolerance tests were used to follow glucose tolerance up to 6 months of age. Glucose intolerance was defined as more than 3 standard deviations (SD) above mean control values. Glucose intolerance was found in 3/51 male and 4/33 female adult mice fed the areca-nut diet ($p < 0.01$). The progeny of these mice were then studied. In Group 1, which comprised matings between parents fed areca nut, glucose intolerance was found in 4/25 male and 1/22 female $F_1$ offspring, with significant hyperglycaemia in $F_1$ males born to hyperglycaemic but not to normoglycaemic mothers ($p < 0.01$). In the $F_2$ generation, 4/23 males and 1/16 females and, in the $F_3$ generation, 1/16 males and 0/20 females were glucose intolerant. In Group 2, parents fed areca nut were mated with normal controls. Glucose intolerance was found in 10/35 male and 10/33 female $F_1$ progeny ($p < 0.005$). The glucose-intolerant animals fed areca nut or their offspring did not develop insulin dependence. These findings suggest that consumption of areca nut may be diabetogenic and induce a heritable abnormality (Boucher et al., 1994).

The possibility that betel chewing might be diabetogenic has been explored in CD1 mice (Boucher et al., 1994). Ground areca nut, bought in the United Kingdom and fed to young adults at 20% in a low nitrosamine feed (RM1 chow) for 5 days led to permanent diabetes in 8.3% of the animals (diagnosed by a 90-min plasma glucose concentration > 3 SDs above the mean for comparable pair-fed controls (with an incidence of spontaneous diabetes of 0.5%) at serial intraperitoneal glucose tolerance testing), in association with obvious central obesity and pancreatic islet enlargement. Islet histology was typical of human type 2 diabetes with enlargement and vacuolation of islet cells. The $F_1$ offspring of the animals fed areca nut, especially males, developed diabetes in 10.6–30% in the various litters (test parents mated with animals fed control diet or animals fed areca nut when they had not developed hyperglycaemia). Affected offspring were obese and had the same islet changes; further generations ($F_2$–$F_4$) showed the same phenomena. Diabetes appeared at a higher rate in the offspring of $F_0$ fathers fed areca nut than in those of $F_0$ mothers fed areca nut. The mechanism for the inheritance of this diabetes is unknown. Damage to sperm heads, apparent by light microscopy 30 days after completion of betel feeding, may be relevant (Muhkerjee et al., 1991). However, subcutaneous injection of 0.2 and 0.25 mg/kg bw arecoline into alloxan-induced diabetic male rabbits (four per group) resulted in a decrease in blood sugar of 52.1 and 49.7%, respectively, which lasted for 4–6 h (Chempakam, 1993).

Tap roots of *Potentilla fulgens*, often chewed with areca nut, are also a traditional remedy for diabetes and cause dose-dependent reductions in blood glucose in normal and alloxan-induced diabetic mice (Syiem et al., 2002).

(viii) *Effects on the immune system*

**Arecoline**

Shahabuddin et al. (1980) demonstrated the immunomodulatory influence of arecoline in mice, which, when injected subcutaneously with 0.5 mg arecoline twice daily for 34 days, showed suppression of both humoral and cell-mediated immunity.

Selvan et al. (1989) administered subtoxic doses (5, 10 and 20 mg/kg bw) of arecoline to male mice for 1, 2 and 3 weeks and found that there was a reduction not only in the weight of the thymus, spleen and mesenteric lymph nodes but also in cellularity. A marked reduction in cell numbers in the thymus and moderate effects on cellularity of the spleen and mesenteric lymph nodes were observed at a dose of 20 mg/kg bw arecoline. White and red blood cell counts decreased in a dose-dependent manner.

Selvan et al. (1991) explored the modulatory influence of arecoline on cell-mediated immune response. In-vivo effects of subtoxic concentrations of 5, 10 and 20 mg/kg bw arecoline given subcutaneously for 1, 2 or 3 weeks were evaluated. Delayed-type hypersensitivity (DTH) reaction to sheep red blood cells was not appreciable at the 5-mg/kg bw level, whereas at a dose of 10 mg/kg bw there was moderate reduction in DTH response. At 20 mg/kg bw given for 1, 2 or 3 weeks plus a 1-week no-exposure period, arecoline significantly suppressed the DTH reaction.

Selvan and Rao (1993) evaluated the modulatory action of arecoline on B cell-mediated immune response in male mice by administering subtoxic concentrations (5, 10 and 20 mg/kg bw) subcutaneously. After 1 week, control and experimental mice were immunized intraperitoneally with sheep red blood cells. The number of primary antibody-forming cells and haemagglutinating and haemolysis antibody titres to sheep red blood cells were assessed 4 days after immunization. Following exposure to arecoline for 1 week, there was a dose-dependent decrease in primary antibody-forming cells to sheep red blood cells, with maximum reductions at 20 mg/kg bw, moderate reductions at 10 mg/kg bw and no effect at 5 mg/kg bw; haemagglutinating and haemolysis antibody titres were also decreased. Exposure to arecoline (10 and 20 mg/kg bw daily for 4 days) following sheep red blood cell immunization exerted dose-dependent suppression of primary antibody response. Recovery experiments in mice revealed that arecoline-mediated suppression of antibody responses is reversible.

### Tobacco/nicotine

The effects of nicotine on the immune system in experimental animals have been studied extensively. Rats treated with nicotine showed a dose-dependent increase in interleukin-2 production and a suppressed splenic and peripheral blood lymphocyte response to mitogen (Caggiula *et al.*, 1992; Petro *et al.*, 1992). The latter effect has been attributed to the induction of a stage of anergy in these cells (McAllister-Sistilli *et al.*, 1998; IARC, 2004).

(ix) *Other biochemical effects*

### Glutathione status

Studies in male Sprague-Dawley rats fed low doses of betel quid (0.53 g dry aqueous extract/kg diet) showed significantly increased hepatic activities of GSH peroxidase and cytoplasmic GST. Feeding high doses of betel quid (26.5 g dry aqueous extract/kg diet) lowered the concentrations of GSH and total glutathione (GSH and two oxidized GSH (GSSG)) (Wang *et al.*, 1999).

### $Na^+$ and $Cl^-$ excretion

Subcutaneous administration of arecoline (1.25–3 mg/kg) to rats increases the amount of urine and urinary excretion of $Na^+$ and $Cl^-$ ions, which are associated with muscarinic receptor activation (Williams & Carter, 1965; Mujumdar *et al.*, 1979).

### Thyroxine and triiodothyronine

Panda and Kar (1998) studied the effects of betel-leaf extract on thyroid hormone concentrations in male Swiss albino mice treated with 0.1, 0.4, 0.8 and 2 g/kg bw per day for 15 days. At higher doses (0.8 and 2 g/kg plant extract), betel-leaf extract increased the serum concentration of thyroxine (T4), although at lower doses (0.1 and 0.4 g/kg plant extract), the concentration of T4 was decreased. Contrasting observations were made for triiodothyronine (T3) concentrations. [Such changes could lead to thyroid dysfunction in humans but have not been recognized as being clinically significant to date.]

### DNA and RNA synthesis

Male Swiss mice were given intraperitoneal injections of aqueous areca-nut extract (0.1 mL containing 1.5 mg alkaloids + 1.9 mg polyphenyl), a polyphenol fraction, tannic acid (1.9 mg per animal) or arecoline (0.06 mg/g bw). After 23 h, the mice received [$^3$H]-uridine or [$^3$H]thymidine by intraperitoneal injection and were killed 1 h later. Liver, lung, kidney and muscle tissues were isolated and analysed for RNAse and DNAse activity, and for incorporation of tritiated nucleosides in RNA or DNA. There was no effect of different constituents of areca nut on DNAse activity but they increased RNAse activity in different tissues. The polyphenol fraction and tannic acid did not affect the RNA content of any of the tissues studied. Areca-nut extract increased the incorporation of the radiolabel [$^3$H]uridine into RNA in liver and muscle tissue, but decreased it in kidney; DNA synthesis was higher in liver and muscle, with no effect in lung and kidney. Arecoline increased [$^3$H]thymidine incorporation in DNA only in liver and lung. It decreased the deoxynucleotide pool in liver and lung, but increased it in kidney and muscle. Areca-nut extract had no effect on the deoxynucleotide pool (Shivapurkar & Bhide, 1979).

An aqueous extract of dried areca nut was injected intraperitoneally into Swiss mice. The injected amount (0.1 mL) of the extract contained 1.5 mg arecoline and 1.9 mg polyphenols. Arecoline was injected for comparison. The animals were killed after 24 h and lung, liver, kidney and muscle tissues were isolated. The areca-nut extract increased the RNA content in liver and muscle, while arecoline decreased it in lung, kidney and muscle tissue. Areca-nut extract increased the DNA content in muscle and liver, whereas arecoline decreased it in kidney and muscle and increased it in liver and lung (Shivapurkar et al., 1978).

(b) *In-vitro studies*

(i) *Effects on oral hard and soft tissues*

**Oral hard tissues**

There is evidence *in vitro* suggesting that the tannin content of areca nut may have antimicrobial properties and this may contribute to the cariostatic role of areca nut (de Miranda et al., 1996).

**Biofilms**

Areca tannin (0.1–1 mg/mL) suppressed glucosyltransferase activity and consequently formation of dental plaque (Hada et al., 1989).

Exposure of human peripheral blood neutrophils to aqueous extracts of ripe areca nut without husk and fresh, tender areca nut with husk abolished their bactericidal activity against oral pathogens (*Actinobacillus* and *Streptococcus* species) and inhibited the production of bactericidal superoxide anion, as measured by ferricytochrome c reduction (Hung et al., 2000).

**Oral soft tissues**

*Periodontal tissues*

In-vitro studies have demonstrated that areca extracts containing arecoline inhibit growth and attachment of, and suppress protein synthesis in human cultured periodontal fibroblasts (Chang, M.-C. et al., 1998; Jeng et al., 1999b). Others have confirmed that areca-nut extracts also cause growth inhibition (van Wyk et al., 1996) and are toxic to human fibroblasts at a concentration of 300–500 µg/mL, leading to cell death (van Wyk et al., 1994).

Arecoline (0–200 µg/mL) depleted the intracellular thiols of human periodontal ligament fibroblasts *in vitro* in a dose-dependent manner. At concentrations of 25 and 100 µg/mL, depletion was approximately 18% and 56% ($p < 0.05$), respectively (Chang, Y.-C. et al., 2001b).

Components of areca nut stimulate the release of inflammatory mediators such as $PGE_2$, interleukin-6 (IL-6) and tumour necrosis factor α (TNF-α)) from primary cultured human oral keratinocytes. Co-incubation with aspirin, specific IL-6- or TNF-α-neutralizing antibodies does not protect the cells against areca-nut cytotoxicity, cell cycle arrest or apoptosis (Jeng et al., 2000, 2003).

*Buccal mucosa*

Early in-vitro studies showed that areca-nut alkaloids such as arecoline and arecaidine may stimulate proliferation and collagen synthesis in human cultured fibroblasts (Canniff & Harvey, 1981; Harvey et al., 1986), whereas in subsequent studies, arecoline did not have similar effects on cultured oral fibroblasts (Meghji et al., 1987; Jeng et al., 1994a; van Wyk et al., 1995). Furthermore, recent studies have shown that arecoline inhibits collagen synthesis and fibroblast proliferation *in vitro*, suggesting that it may have cytotoxic properties (Jeng et al., 1994a, 1996; van Wyk et al., 1996), and others have confirmed that areca-nut extracts also cause growth inhibition (Jeng et al., 1994a; van Wyk et al., 1996), and are toxic to human fibroblasts at a concentration of 300–500 µg/mL, leading to cell death (van Wyk et al., 1994). [The Working Group noted the inconsistent results between experiments.]

Flavanoids within the areca nut have been shown to increase the stabilization of collagen by enhancing its cross-linking, thereby increasing resistance to degradation by collagenase (Scutt et al., 1987). In addition, arecoline produces dose-dependent increases in TIMP-1 expression directly in human buccal fibroblasts together with reduced secretion of both MMP-2 and MMP-9 (Chang, Y.-C. et al., 2002a), a phenomenon that contributes to risk for submucosal fibrosis. Tsai et al. (1999) further found that fibroblasts cultured from human oral submucous fibrosis tissues showed a lower capacity to phagocytose collagen-coated beads than fibroblasts from healthy buccal mucosa, and that pretreatment with arecoline and arecaidine (10 and 50 µg/mL) markedly inhibited this phagocytosis.

Exposure of human buccal fibroblasts to arecoline stimulates the expression of vimentin (25–400 µg/mL) (Chang, Y.-C. et al., 2002b) and inhibits GST activity (50–400 µg/mL) but shows little effect on lipid peroxidation (25–200 µg/mL) (Chang, Y.-C. et al., 2001a).

Lysyl oxidase activity and basal collagen synthesis of fibroblasts cultured from oral submucous fibrosis patients are greater than those of fibroblasts from healthy buccal mucosa (Meghji et al., 1987; Ma et al., 1995). Production of type I collagen trimer (digested with difficulty by collagenase) by oral submucous fibrosis fibroblasts but not normal fibroblasts has also been reported (Kuo et al., 1995a).

(ii) *Effects on cultured human buccal epithelial cells*

**Cell survival and DNA repair capacity**

Exposure of buccal cell cultures to various organic or water-based extracts of products related to the use of tobacco and betel quid (bidi-smoke condensate, betel leaf, snuff, areca nut) decreased both cell survival (measured by reduction of tetrazolium dye) and activity of $O^6$-methylguanine–DNA methyltransferase (MGMT), enzyme that catalyses the repair of the premutagenic $O^6$-methylguanine lesion in DNA. Organic extracts of bidi-smoke condensate or betel leaf showed higher potency than those of tobacco or snuff. An aqueous snuff extract also decreased both parameters, whereas an aqueous areca-nut extract had no effect. While significant MGMT activity was demonstrated in buccal tissue specimens and in the major buccal mucosal cell types *in vitro*, inhibition of MGMT activity was observed in the buccal mucosa of tobacco and areca-nut chewers after exposure to complex mixtures present in the saliva (Liu *et al.*, 1997).

**Cell survival, membrane integrity and DNA breakage**

The pathobiological effects of an aqueous areca-nut extract, four areca-nut alkaloids and four areca-specific nitrosamines were investigated in cultured human buccal epithelial cells. Areca-nut extract decreased cell survival, vital dye accumulation and membrane integrity in a dose-dependent manner. Depletion of cellular free low-molecular-weight thiols also occurred, but at fairly toxic concentrations. Comparison of the areca nut-related $N$-nitroso compounds and their precursor alkaloids, at concentrations up to 5 mM, indicated that, on a molar basis, MNPA is the most potent at decreasing both cell survival and thiol content. Arecoline, guvacoline and NGL also decreased cell survival and thiol content, whereas arecaidine, guvacine, NGC and MNPN had only minor effects on these variables (Sundqvist *et al.*, 1989).

**Cell growth, differentiation and morphology**

The effects of an aqueous extract of areca nut on growth, differentiation, morphology and DNA damage were studied in cultured human buccal epithelial cells. Acute exposure (3 h) of the cells to the extract altered their morphology and induced ridges in the plasma membrane, with indications of internalization of extract particles. It also caused formation of DNA single-strand breaks, which accumulated during post-treatment culture, indicating continuous exposure to residual particles and/or the possibility of inhibited DNA repair. The extract accelerated terminal differentiation of the cells, measured as involucrin expression, at relatively non-toxic levels. The extract caused similar loss of colony-forming efficiency in normal cells and in a buccal carcinoma cell line (SqCC/YI), which was defective in its ability to undergo differentiation, indicating that extract toxicity could occur independently of this response. These findings *in vitro* suggest that betel-quid carcinogenesis in the human oral cavity may involve cytopathic alterations of normal cell morphology, growth and differentiation, by areca-nut-related agents extracted or formed in saliva (Sundqvist & Grafström, 1992).

(iii) *Effects on the cardiovascular system*

Exposure of isolated rat aorta to areca-nut extract, areca tannin or arecoline induces vasodilatation (Goto et al., 1997). Activation of muscarinic receptors by arecaidine propargyl ester induced 6-keto-$PGF_{1\alpha}$ and cGMP production in bovine aortic endothelial cells, but not in rabbit vascular aortic smooth muscle cells (Jaiswal et al., 1991).

Areca-nut extract stimulated rabbit platelet aggregation and thromboxane $B_2$ synthesis, which was inhibited by 1,2-bis(2-aminophenoxy)ethane-$N,N,N',N'$-tetraacetic acid, an intracellular calcium chelator, and neomycin, a phospholipase C inhibitor. Areca nut-induced platelet thromboxane production can be also inhibited by catalase, dimethylthiourea, two specific scavengers of reactive oxygen species and genistein (a tyrosine kinase inhibitor), indicating the participation of $H_2O_2$, hydroxyl radicals and tyrosine kinase activation. On the contrary, aqueous extracts of betel leaf and *Piper betle* inflorescence inhibited the aggregation and thromboxane synthesis of rabbit platelets. In addition, betel-leaf extract inhibited thromboxane $B_2$ production in platelet aggregates induced by collagen, arachidonic acid, thrombin or platelet activator factor (Jeng et al., 2002; Lei et al., 2003), but had no effect on areca nut-induced platelet aggregation (Jeng et al., 2002).

(iv) *Effects on the gastrointestinal system*

The aqueous fraction of betel-leaf extract (1–10 mg/mL) induced a spasmogenic effect in isolated guinea pig ileum, which was inhibited by atropine, a muscarinic receptor antagonist, and inhibited the spontaneous contraction of isolated rabbit jejunum at concentrations ranging from 0.03 to 3 mg/mL, indicating that it contains a potent spasmolytic component (Gilani et al., 2000).

Extracts of areca nut [10–1000 mg/mL] stimulated the contractile frequency of isolated colonic smooth muscle strips in rats dose dependently. This effect was partially inhibited by atropine (Xie et al., 2002).

(v) *Effects on the immune system*

**Betel quid**

Yang et al. (1979) studied the effect of areca-nut extract on the proliferation of phytohaemagglutinin-stimulated cultured human lymphocytes. At concentrations up to 2.5%, the extracts inhibited [$^3$H]thymidine incorporation by 10–100%, in a dose-dependent manner, demonstrating the adverse effect of areca-nut extract on cell proliferation.

Hsu et al. (2001) cultured peripheral blood mononuclear cells (PBMCs) from normal persons ($n = 10$) and betel-quid chewers with either oral submucous fibrosis ($n = 10$) or oral cancer ($n = 10$). The levels of IL-2, transforming growth factor β (TGF-β)) and interferon-γ (IFN-γ) production by peripheral blood mononuclear cells from betel-quid chewers with oral submucous fibrosis or oral cancer were lower than those from healthy individuals without these habits. Only peripheral blood mononuclear cells isolated from betel-quid chewers with oral cancer, and which were stimulated by arecoline, produced more IL-2.

**Arecoline**

Both dose-dependent and time-dependent cytotoxic effects were observed in spleen cells incubated with varying concentrations of arecoline. Arecoline ($10^{-6}$–$10^{-4}$ M) concomitantly with concanavalin A markedly inhibited both [$^3$H]-thymidine incorporation and IL-2 production in spleen cells (Selvan et al., 1991).

Concomitant treatment of IL-2-dependent murine cytolytic lymphocytes with arecoline ($10^{-4}$ M) and IL-2 decreased proliferative response up to 43% (Selvan et al., 1991). Arecoline at concentrations of $10^{-5}$ and $10^{-4}$ M added to spleen cells *in vitro* concomitantly with poke-weed mitogen inhibited the induced proliferative response by 17 and 21%, respectively (Selvan & Rao, 1993).

Exposure of oral KB cells to 1 and 100 µM of arecoline for 72 h stimulated IL-1β and IL-1α production and also intercellular adhesion molecule-1 expression (Cheng & Tsai, 1999). A 72-h exposure of KB cells to arecoline (1 and 100 µM) also stimulated IL-8 production, which was decreased by the addition of IL-1α and IL-1β antibodies, suggesting that IL-8 secretion by KB cells may be partially mediated by IL-1 (Cheng et al., 2000).

(vi) *Other effects*

Betel-quid components increased basal adrenal medullary catecholamine secretion in bovine chromaffin cells isolated from the adrenal glands but inhibited that induced by carbachol or potassium *in vitro* (Wang & Hwang, 1997).

## 4.3 Reproductive and developmental effects

### 4.3.1 *Humans*

The mean weight of newborn babies of 70 Indian tobacco chewers (the tobacco was either chewed or ingested alone or mixed with betel leaf or with lime) was 14% less than that of the babies of 70 matched controls (Verma et al., 1983).

de Costa and Griew (1982) carried out a study to determine whether betel chewing had any adverse effect on pregnancy outcome. The antenatal records of 400 Papua New Guinean women who had chewed betel quid throughout pregnancy were examined together with a control group of 400 pregnant women who did not smoke, drink or take any drugs and who had never chewed betel quid. At birth, body weight of the babies, stillbirths, neonatal deaths and abnormalities, if present, were recorded. Babies born to betel-chewing mothers had a mean weight of 2998.5 ± 492.5 g (SD), and non-chewing mothers gave birth to babies with a mean weight of 3079.5 g ± 464.1 g (SD); the difference was statistically significant ($0.02 > p < 0.01$). There were no outstanding differences between the two groups with regard to the occurrence of congenital abnormalities. Perinatal mortality rates were 25/1000 and 27.5/1000, respectively, in chewing and non-chewing groups. [The Working Group questioned the statistics applied.]

Betel-quid chewing is very common among the aboriginal tribes in southern Taiwan, China, and many women consume betel quid throughout pregnancy. Yang et al. (1999)

conducted a study to estimate the prevalence of substance use among aborigines during pregnancy, and to assess the extent of the adverse effects of betel-quid chewing on pregnancy outcomes. Betel quid consisted of areca nut, slaked lime and a piece of unripe fruit of Piper betle that contains safrole. Women of the Bunum tribe of aborigines, aged 15–50 years, were asked to participate in the study, and a group of 186 women was recruited consisting of 62 subjects who had experienced adverse pregnancy outcomes and 124 age-matched women who had had normal pregnancy outcomes (control group). The participants were interviewed using a questionnaire. Prevalence of the use of various substances in aborigines with adverse pregnancy outcomes was estimated as follows: alcohol, 43.6%; smoking, 14.5%; betel-quid chewing, 43.6%; and drug use, 4.8%. In the control group, the prevalence was: alcohol, 38.7%; smoking, 8.1%; betel-quid chewing, 28.2%; and drug use, 0%. Univariate analysis revealed that adverse pregnancy outcomes were associated with maternal betel-quid chewing, maternal illness during pregnancy and number of pregnancies (gravidity) experienced. After adjusting for maternal illness and number of previous pregnancies as covariates, the prevalence of adverse pregnancy outcome was computed to be 2.8-fold higher among women chewing betel quid compared with non-chewers (adjusted odds ratio, 2.8; 95% CI, 1.2–6.8). In addition to reductions in birth weight, the adverse pregnancy outcomes included spontaneous abortion, premature delivery, stillbirth and fetal malformation.

Yang, M.S. *et al.* (2001) studied adverse birth outcomes among pregnant aboriginal women who chewed betel quid. The study population comprised 32 cases and 197 controls. The betel quid consisted of three ingredients: areca nut, slaked lime and a piece of unripe fruit from *Piper betle*. A statistically significant association was found between low birth weight, pre-term birth and maternal betel-quid chewing. The mean birth weights for the neonates of betel-quid chewers and non-chewers were 3030 and 3200 g, respectively, the difference for which was statistically significant. The estimated odds ratio of adverse birth outcome was statistically significantly higher in women who were betel-quid chewers during their pregnancy (adjusted odds ratio, 5.0; 95% CI, 1.1–23.0). [The Working Group noted the limited size of the study.]

4.3.2 *Experimental systems*

(*a*) Pan masala

Mukherjee *et al.* (1991) studied the effect of one popular brand of *pan masala* on the germ cells of male mice that received 84, 420 and 840 mg/kg bw per day by intragastric intubation for 5 consecutive days. Sperm recovered from the tail of the epididymes showed significant ($p < 0.05$) increases in morphological abnormality.

Sarma *et al.* (1992) studied the effects of *pan masala* in different organs including testes in male rats. *Pan masala* was fed at dose levels of 84, 420 or 840 mg/kg bw per day for 6 months (5 days per week). Statistical evaluation of data on organ weight showed no significant difference from the control group (untreated rats) except for a decrease in absolute weight of testis ($p < 0.05$) at all dose levels.

(b) *Areca nut*

Sinha and Rao (1985a) investigated the effect of areca nut on the intrauterine development of mice. Extracts of processed and unprocessed varieties of areca nut (1, 3 or 5 mg) were given daily to pregnant mice from day 6 through day 15 of gestation. Animals were killed on day 17 of gestation, and fetal anomalies were assessed. Pregnant dams exposed to either variety of areca nut showed an increase in the percentage of resorption as well as dead, macerated fetuses, clearly indicating embryotoxicity of areca-nut extract. The percentage of dead fetuses per litter in all test groups was dose-dependent. Another very significant ($p < 0.01$) effect of the administration of areca-nut extract was a dose-related decrease in the average total body weight per litter, especially in the group receiving unprocessed areca nut. There was also a decrease in the ossification of coccygeal vertebrae, which was dose-dependent and was more pronounced after exposure to unprocessed areca nut.

Paul *et al.* (1996) studied the teratogenicity of processed areca-nut extract in chick embryos. Different doses (0.001, 0.1, 0.25 and 0.5 mg) were injected into the yolk sac of 4-day-old embryos and the latter were killed after 14 days of incubation. Higher doses caused dose-dependent mortality, with a significant effect at doses of 0.1, 0.25 and 0.5 mg per egg. Fetuses had reduced body size. In another experiment, Paul *et al.* (1997) injected 5-day-old chick embryos with different (0.015–0.375 mg per egg) doses of areca-nut extract. The embryos were killed after 8 days of incubation. Reduced body weight, abnormal hindlimb digits and everted viscera were prominent. Mortality rates were dose related. Paul *et al.* (1999) studied the teratogenicity of arecoline hydrobromide (0.25, 0.50, 0.75 and 1.0 mg per egg) given at 2, 3 or 4 days of incubation. On day 14 of incubation, the experiment was terminated and fetal anomalies were recorded. The rate of anomalies was greatest for embryos injected on day 2 of incubation. Developmental defects included reduced body size, sparse feathering, everted viscera, shortened lower beak and arthrogryposis. Unossified vertebrae, missing or unossified ribs, shortening of long bones and unossified phalanges also occurred.

(c) *Arecoline*

Anisímov (1978) studied the influence of arecoline on compensatory ovarian hypertrophy in rats. After unilateral ovariectomy, rats were given different doses (0.15, 0.5, 5.0 mg/kg bw) of arecoline for 7 days, and it was found that higher doses suppressed compensatory hypertrophy.

Sinha and Rao (1985b) investigated the influence of arecoline on the morphology of sperm in mice. Intraperitoneal injections of arecoline at doses of 20, 40 and 80 mg/kg bw was given for 5 consecutive days and mice were killed 35 days after the first injection. Sperm was recovered from the tail of the epididymes. A linear increase in the percentage of abnormal sperm was observed following exposure to arecoline, and treatment with arecoline increased unscheduled DNA synthesis response in the germ cells of mice.

Intraperitoneal administration of arecoline at three dose levels (20, 40 and 80 mg/kg bw) to Swiss albino mice on day 17 of gestation resulted in a significant increase in the frequency of micronucleated polychromatic erythrocytes in fetal mouse blood compared with that of control animals, which was found to be dose-dependent (Sinha & Rao, 1985c).

(d)  Stems of Piper betle

Adhikary et al. (1990a,b) studied the effect of oral administration of extracts of *Piper betle* stems on the reproductive function of female and male rats. In female rats, the treatment caused disturbance in estrus cycle, inhibition of fertility in a dose-dependent manner, reduction in implantation at higher doses, reduction in ovarian and uterine weights at higher doses and a fall in $\Delta^5$-3β-hydroxysteroid dehydrogenase activity (Adhikary et al., 1990a). In male rats, significant reduction in fertility and in the number and motility of sperm were observed at the higher doses, as well as a reduction in the relative weight of the testis and accessory sex organs of treated animals.

Another study by Adhikary et al. (1989) revealed the antigonadal property of extracts of *Piper betle* stems in rats. Following subcutaneous injection for 21 days with either extract or vehicle, males and females were allowed to mate; *Piper betle*-stem extract caused a 100% reduction in male fertility and a 63% reduction in female fertility when mated with fertile partners. A reduction in the weight of gonads and other reproductive organs was also observed. Sarkar et al. (2000) studied the antifertility effect of an alcoholic extract of air-dried leaf stem of *Piper betle* in male mice. The weights of the reproductive organs (testes, epididymes, seminal vesicles and prostate) of the treated animals decreased, and a decrease in the sperm count and sperm motility was also observed. Recovery experiments revealed that these effects were reversible.

[The Working Group noted that the stem is usually removed from the betel leaf before preparation of the betel quid in the Indian subcontinent.]

(e)  Nicotine

There is a vast literature on the effects of nicotine on reproductive and developmental systems in experimental animals of different species and during different stages of gestation. Examples are the delay in ovum cleavage and implantation (Yoshinaga et al., 1979), the interference with fetal brain differentiation and development (Slotkin et al., 1986; Slotkin, 1992; Slotkin et al., 1993) and with fetal testosterone levels (Lichtensteiger & Schlumpf, 1985), adverse effects on the adrenal glands (Monheit et al., 1983), an increase in the number of stillbirths (Arbeille et al., 1992) and impairment of cardio-respiratory defence to hypoxia (Hafström et al., 2002). The reader is referred to the monograph on tobacco smoking (IARC, 2004) and references therein.

**4.4  Genetic and related effects**

4.4.1  *Humans*

(a)  *Genotoxicity and mutagenicity*

(i)  *DNA adduct*

DNA extracted from exfoliated oral mucosal cells collected from Canadian non-smoking controls ($n = 19$), Indian areca-nut chewers ($n = 22$), Filipino inverted smokers (who smoke with the burning end of the cigar in their mouth; $n = 15$) and Indian *Khaini* tobacco chewers ($n = 22$) was used for analysis of aromatic DNA adducts by the $^{32}$P-post-labelling technique. Differential amounts of five aromatic DNA adducts were found within these four groups, but there were no differences among the groups (tobacco chewing, betel-quid chewing or smoking) (Dunn & Stich, 1986).

In Taiwan, China, Chen *et al.* (1999) identified several safrole-like DNA adducts from 77% (23/30) of tissues from oral squamous-cell carcinomas obtained from betel-quid chewers and 97% (29/30) of tissues from adjacent non-cancer areas, whereas no such adducts were identified in squamous-cell carcinomas obtained from non-chewers. Six of seven (86%) oral submucous fibrosis tissues obtained from betel-quid chewers also exhibited the same safrole-like DNA adducts.

(ii)  *Micronuclei, chromosomal aberrations and sister chromatid exchange*

In a multicountry study, Stich *et al.* (1986) scored scraped or brushed [erroneously referred to in the literature as exfoliated] micronucleated epithelial cells from oral mucosa. The number of betel quids consumed was an average of 44 quids each day in Taiwan, China, compared with an average of 20 quids per day in India (Stich *et al.*, 1982). Betel-quid chewers ($n = 36$) in Orissa (India) who regularly chewed dried areca nut, slaked lime, betel leaf, tobacco and catechu had the highest frequencies of micronucleated cells (6.1%), followed by those in Khasis (4.7%) (India, who chewed fresh areca nut [husk removed], slaked lime and betel leaf), the Philippines (3.9%) (fresh areca nut [husk removed], betel leaf, slaked lime and tobacco), Guam (1.8%) (fresh green areca nut with husk, slaked lime and betel leaf) and Hualien (1.7%) (Taiwan, China, fresh areca nut with husk, slaked lime and betel leaf).

Stich *et al.* (1984b,c, 1988, 1989, 1991) explored the possibility of reversal of the formation of micronuclei in the oral cavity (shown in exfoliated cells) using vitamin A and/or β-carotene. The treatment decreased the frequency of micronuclei in users of betel quid with tobacco. However, the reappearance of micronucleated cells was noted after termination of the treatment (Stich *et al.*, 1991).

Dave *et al.* (1991) compared 30 healthy controls and 15 *pan-masala* consumers with respect to cytogenetic effects in peripheral blood lymphocytes and exfoliated cells from buccal mucosa. Sister chromatid exchange and chromosomal aberrations of peripheral blood lymphocytes were more frequent in cells of *pan-masala* chewers' than in those isolated from control subjects. The percentage of micronucleated cells in exfoliated buccal mucosal cells was also higher in *pan-masala* consumers than in healthy controls [population size seems too small: $n = 5$ for *pan masala* + tobacco, $n = 10$ for *pan masala*, $n = 15$ for controls]. Consistently, the frequencies of micronuclei in exfoliated mucosal cells were shown to be higher in chewers (with or without oral submucous fibrosis) of tobacco plus slaked lime, *mava* (areca nut, slaked lime and tobacco), *tamol* (raw fermented areca nut, betel leaf and slaked lime) and areca nut in different regions of India compared with healthy individuals with no habit ($n = 10–36$ for each group) (Kayal et al., 1993).

Nair et al. (1991) reported that the frequency of micronuclei in exfoliated human oral mucosa cells was $4.83 \pm 0.7$ per 1000 cells in chewers of betel quid with tobacco ($n = 35$; tobacco, areca nut, betel leaf, slaked lime and catechu) and $5.2 \pm 0.66$ per 1000 cells in chewers of tobacco and slaked lime ($n = 35$), whereas the frequency in the control group ($n = 27$) was $2.59 \pm 0.37$ per 1000 cells. No correlation between the frequencies of micronucleated cells and the duration or frequency of the chewing habit was noted.

Adhvaryu et al. (1986) compared the frequency of sister chromatid exchange in cultured lymphocytes isolated from controls ($n = 15$), tobacco chewers ($n = 10$) and oral submucous fibrosis patients ($n = 10$) who chewed a combination of tobacco, areca nut and slaked lime. Marked elevation of sister chromatid exchange frequency in lymphocytes cultured from tobacco chewers and oral submucous fibrosis patients was noted. Moreover, Adhvaryu et al. (1991) further analysed sister chromatid exchange and chromosomal aberrations in peripheral lymphocytes and micronuclei in exfoliated mucosal cells in healthy *mava* (tobacco, areca nut and lime) chewers, *mava* chewers with oral submucous fibrosis and *mava* chewers with oral cancer ($n = 15$ for all groups). Chromosomal aberrations and sister chromatid exchange were significantly higher for all three groups of chewers than for controls. The frequencies of micronuclei were higher in healthy chewers and oral submucous fibrosis patients. The micronucleus assay was not conducted in oral cancer patients.

Desai et al. (1996) further analysed the frequencies of micronuclei in exfoliated oral mucosa cells and sister chromatid exchange in lymphocytes isolated from healthy volunteers, and patients with oral submucous fibrosis, oral leukoplakia and oral lichen planus. These patients chewed *pan masala*, areca nut, areca nut plus tobacco, betel quid plus tobacco or had mixed habits. The number of micronuclei in exfoliated cells was elevated from 1.9/1000 cells (normal) to 11.6, 10.8 and 11.7/1000 cells in patients with oral submucous fibrosis, oral leukoplakia and oral lichen planus, respectively. A large number of micronucleated cells was also seen in circulating lymphocytes obtained from these three groups.

Dave et al. (1992a) evaluated cytogenetic effects in controls ($n = 15$), healthy areca-nut chewers ($n = 10$), areca-nut chewers with oral submucous fibrosis ($n = 10$) and areca-nut chewers with oral cancer ($n = 8$). All three groups of areca-nut chewers showed significantly large numbers of chromosomal aberrations and sister chromatid exchange in peripheral blood mononuclear cells and the frequencies of micronucleated exfoliated buccal cells increased by approximately 3.8-fold.

(b) *Genomic instability*

Analysis of cytogenetic changes in betel quid- and tobacco-associated oral squamous-cell carcinomas showed most common gains in chromosomes 8q, 9q, 11q, 17q and 20q and most frequent losses in chromosome arms 3p (genes *FHIT*, *RARβ* and *VHL*), 4q, 5q, 9p21–23 and 18q, a high frequency of breakage and exchanges at the 1cen-1q12 region and allelic imbalance in short tandem repeat markers (Rupa & Eastmond, 1997; Mahale & Saranath, 2000; Lin, S.-C. *et al.*, 2002; Pai *et al.*, 2002). Loss of 3p was significantly associated with poor survival of patients (Lin, S.-C. *et al.*, 2002). Lee, H.-C. *et al.* (2001) showed mitochondrial DNA (mtDNA) deletions (4977-bp deletion) in oral squamous-cell carcinomas of betel-quid chewers. This study revealed that, irrespective of the history of betel-quid chewing, the mtDNA deletions detected in oral tumours were less abundant than those in the surrounding non-tumorous tissues. Moreover, betel-quid chewing significantly enhanced the accumulation of mtDNA deletions in non-tumorous oral tissues. Collectively, these observations are consistent with the mutagenic effects of betel quid and tobacco.

(c) *Oncogenes and tumour-suppressor genes*

Analyses of *TP53* mutations in oral carcinomas associated only with betel-quid chewing are limited. These studies demonstrate infrequent *TP53* mutations in oral cancers in South-East Asia including Sri Lanka, Taiwan, China, and India, as well as in Papua New Guinea (summarized in Table 71) (Chiba *et al.*, 1998; Hsieh *et al.*, 2001).

No *TP53* mutations were observed in oral leukoplakia or squamous-cell carcinomas of chewers of betel quid without tobacco ($n = 6$) in Indian populations (Heinzel *et al.*, 1996; Ralhan *et al.*, 2001), or in 48 cases of oral tumour from eastern India in chewers of betel quid with tobacco (Patnaik *et al.*, 1999). However, in Sri Lankan populations, Chiba *et al.* (1998) reported *TP53* mutations in 10/23 (43%) oral squamous-cell carcinomas in betel-quid chewers. [The Working Group noted that 7/10 cases harbouring *TP53* mutations had been betel-quid chewers and smokers for 10–30 years.]

In oral squamous-cell carcinomas associated with betel-quid chewing and tobacco smoking, *TP53* mutations were clustered in exons 5, 7 and 8 comprising A:T→T:A transversions or G:C transitions, G:C→A:T transitions and G:C→T:A transversions (Table 71) (Thomas *et al.*, 1994; Heinzel *et al.*, 1996; Chiba *et al.*, 1998; Wong *et al.*, 1998; Hsieh *et al.*, 2001; Ralhan *et al.*, 2001). In addition to point mutations in G + C-rich regions, small deletions or insertions were also observed (Chiba *et al.*, 1998). The G:C→C:G transversions were observed in betel-quid chewers or smokers, and codons 135 and 136 were frequently mutated (G→T; A→G) in oral squamous-cell carcinomas associated with betel-quid and tobacco consumption (Chiba *et al.*, 1998; Hsieh *et al.*, 2001; Ralhan *et al.*, 2001).

*TP53* mutations were reported in 8/36 (22%) Taiwanese betel quid/tobacco smoking-associated oral squamous-cell carcinomas (Wong *et al.*, 1998), and in oral preneoplastic lesions (leukoplakia) in betel-quid and tobacco consumers (Ralhan *et al.*, 2001).

**Table 71. Analysis of *TP53* alterations in human oral premalignant and malignant lesions**

| Total no. of cases | Exons analysed | *TP53* mutations | Population | Betel quid without tobacco | | Betel quid + tobacco smoking/chewing | | Betel quid + tobacco smoking/chewing + alcohol | | *TP53* mutational analysis | Reference |
|---|---|---|---|---|---|---|---|---|---|---|---|
| | | | | Total cases | *TP53* mutation cases | Total cases | *TP53* mutation cases | Total cases | *TP53* mutation cases | | |
| 5 SCCs | 5–9 | 0 | Sri Lankan | – | – | 5 | 0 | – | – | ND | Ranasinghe et al. (1993a) |
| 30 SCCs | 5–9 | 3 | Papua-New Guinean | – | – | 5[a] | 1 | 17[a] | 2 | Exon 6 codon 193 (C→T) (2 cases) Exon 7 codon 248 (G→A) | Thomas et al. (1994) |
| 23 SCCs | 5, 7 | 4[b] | Indian | 6 | 0 | 2 | 1 | – | – | Exon 5 codon 153 (C→T) (non-user) codon 158 (G→A) smoker codon 176 (T→C) (unknown) Exon 7 codon 239 (A→G) (betel-quid chewer + smoker) | Heinzel et al. (1996) |
| 23 SCCs 7 leukoplakia 2 OSF | 5–8 | 10 0 0 | Sri Lankan | 9 2 | 3 ND | 14 4 2 | 7 ND ND | – – – | – – – | Exon 5 codon 130 C deletion codon 135 (G→T) codons 144–148 deletion (2 cases) codon 164 (G→T) codons 172–187 deletion codon 176 (C→G) Exon 7 codon 245 (G→A) codon 248 (G→A) codon 250 C insertion | Chiba et al. (1998) |

**Table 71 (contd)**

| Total no. of cases | Exons analysed | TP53 mutations | Population | Betel quid without tobacco | | Betel quid + tobacco smoking/chewing | | Betel quid + tobacco smoking/chewing + alcohol | | TP53 mutational analysis | Reference |
|---|---|---|---|---|---|---|---|---|---|---|---|
| | | | | Total cases | TP53 mutation cases | Total cases | TP53 mutation cases | Total cases | TP53 mutation cases | | |
| 50 SCCs | 5–9 | 12 | Taiwanese | – | – | 36 | 8 | – | – | Exon 5 codon 161 (C→A)<br>Exon 5 codon 175 (G→A)<br>Exon 6 codon 222 (C→G)<br>Exon 7 codon 255 (A→T)<br>Exon 8 codon 266 (G→T)<br>Exon 8 codon 273 (C→T), 273 (G→T)<br>Exon 8 codon 277 (G→A) (2 cases), 277 (T→C)<br>Exon 8 codon 282 (C→T) (2 cases) | Wong et al. (1998) |
| | | | | | | 1 | | | | Allelic deletion of TP53 | |
| 37 SCCs | 5–8 | 2 | Taiwanese | 3 | – | 14<br>23 | 3<br>2 (1 smoker, + 1 non-user) | – | – | Exon 5 codon 177 (C→T)<br>Exon 8 codon 266 (G→A) | Kuo et al. (1999a) |
| 48 oral tumours | 5–8 | 0 | Indian | – | – | – | – | 48[c] | 0 | Rearrangement | Patnaik et al. (1999) |
| 187 SCCs | 5–9 | 91 | Taiwanese | 7 | 4 | 51 | 15 | 75 | 43 | Predominantly GC→AT in betel-quid chewers alone<br>Exon 5 codon 135 (G→T)<br>Exon 6 codon 195 deletion<br>Exon 8 codon 267 (G→C)<br>codon 273 (C→T) | Hsieh et al. (2001) |

**Table 71 (contd)**

| Total no. of cases | Exons analysed | TP53 mutations | Population | Betel quid without tobacco | | Betel quid + tobacco smoking/chewing | | Betel quid + tobacco smoking/chewing + alcohol | | TP53 mutational analysis | Reference |
|---|---|---|---|---|---|---|---|---|---|---|---|
| | | | | Total cases | TP53 mutation cases | Total cases | TP53 mutation cases | Total cases | TP53 mutation cases | | |
| 30 SCCs | 5–9 | 7 | Indian | 6 | ND | 12 | 8 | – | – | Predominantly missense (5) Exon 5 codons 126 (C→G), 136 (A→G), 174 (G→T) Exon 7 codons 233 (CA→TC), 234 (TAC→AAA) Exon 8 codon 267 (G→C), 270 (T→A) | Ralhan et al. (2001) |
| 30 leukoplakia | | 5 | | 6 | ND | 13 | 6 | – | – | Predominantly missense (3 missense, 2 nonsense) Exon 5 codons 126 (C→G), 136 (A→G) (2 cases), 174 (G→T) Exon 6 codon 196 (C→T) | |

SCC, squamous-cell carcinoma; ND, not detected; OSF, oral submucous fibrosis
[a] Includes four former alcohol consumers
[b] Patients with TP53 mutations: one was a non-user and data on betel/tobacco habit were not available for the other case.
[c] Patients were chewers of betel quid with tobacco and tobacco paste; no information about alcohol consumption was available.

Hsieh *et al.* (2003) reported that polymorphism in the DNA repair gene *XRCC1,399 Gln/Gln* phenotype showed an independent association with the frequency of *TP53* mutations (after adjustment for smoking, areca-quid chewing and alcohol drinking) in oral cancer patients in Taiwan, China. [The Working Group noted that, in absence of specific information on betel quid and tobacco consumption habits of oral squamous-cell carcinoma patients, the data from the reports of Chang *et al.* (1992), Munirajan *et al.* (1996), Ravi *et al.* (1996, 1999), Saranath *et al.* (1999), Tandle *et al.* (2001), Nagpal *et al.* (2002a) and Pande *et al.* (2002) were not included.]

Several studies reported a high incidence of p53 protein expression in oral premalignant lesions and squamous-cell carcinomas from betel quid and/or tobacco consumers (summarized in Table 72).

Comparison of p53 protein expression in 22 baseline biopsies of oral precancerous lesions that transformed to cancer 4–25 years later with that in 68 similar lesions that did not transform over the same period did not show a significant relationship between p53 protein expression and malignant transformation (Murti *et al.*, 1998). All cancers were detected among betel-quid chewers who included tobacco in their quid and/or smoked. However, the acquisition of p53 protein expression in 9/10 biopsies that did not show p53 expression at baseline occurred once they had undergone progression to squamous-cell carcinoma.

Cox and Walker (1996) reported p53 protein accumulation in 14/20 (70%) and proliferative cell nuclear antigen (PCNA) in 31.8% of Nepalese oral submucous fibrosis patients. Trivedy *et al.* (1998) reported p53 protein expression in 15/20 (75%) oral submucous fibrosis cases, 3/6 (50%) squamous-cell carcinomas arising from oral submucous fibrosis and 15/21 (67%) squamous-cell carcinomas not arising from this disease. Alterations in *TP53* were reported in 13/21 cases of oral submucous fibrosis and 15/27 cases of squamous-cell carcinoma, showing a concordance between results from immunocytochemistry and single-strand conformation polymorphism results in a majority (33/48) of cases. Chiang *et al.* (2000a,b) reported a significant increase in PCNA and p53 expression in oral submucous fibrosis, epithelial hyperplasia and epithelial dysplasia compared with normal oral mucosa in a population in Taiwan, China, population. However, no association was observed between PCNA and p53 expression in oral submucous fibrosis lesions associated with areca chewing and tobacco smoking. Srinivasan and Jewell (2001a) showed higher expression of the proliferation markers, epidermal growth factor receptor, TGF-α, PCNA and one genomic marker, *c-myc*, in oral submucous fibrosis lesions of betel quid and tobacco consumers compared with normal oral mucosa (Srinivasan & Jewell, 2001b). [The Working Group noted the absence of detailed information on betel quid and tobacco consumption habits of patients in these studies.]

Thongsuksai and Boonyaphiphat (2001) showed no independent association of betel-quid chewing with p53 expression. Moreover, the lack of correspondence between p53 protein expression and *TP53* mutations (Ranasinghe *et al.*, 1993a,b) suggests other pathways of p53 inactivation. The pathways identified include interaction of p53 with other cellular proteins: murine double minute 2 (MDM2), 70-kDa heat shock protein (HSP70)

Table 72. Analysis of p53 protein expression in human oral premalignant and malignant lesions

| Total cases | Total p53-positive cases | Population | Betel quid without tobacco | | Betel quid + tobacco smoking/chewing | | Reference |
|---|---|---|---|---|---|---|---|
| | | | Total cases | p53-Positive cases | Total cases | p53-Positive cases | |
| 34 SCCs | 25 | Indian | 5 | 3 | 14 | 13 | Kaur et al. (1994) |
| 27 leukoplakia | 15 | | 3 | 1 | 9 | 9 | |
| 30 SCCs | | Papua New Guinean | – | – | 21[a] | 5 | Thomas et al. (1994) |
| 23 SCCs | 13 | Indian | – | – | 20 | 13 | Kuttan et al. (1995) |
| 60 SCCs | 27 | Taiwanese | 44[b] | 17 | – | – | Yan et al. (1996) |
| 145 SCCs | 102 | Indian | 12 | 5 | 59 | 51 | Kaur et al. (1998a) |
| 75 leukoplakia | 39 | | 8 | 2 | 33 | 22 | |
| 48 SCCs | 22 | Indian | – | – | 48 (TC)[c] | 22 | Baral et al. (1998) |
| 81 SCCs | 47 | Taiwanese | 1 | 1 | 56 | 29 | Chiang et al. (1999) |
| 38 SCCs | 4 | Sri Lankan | – | – | 38 | 4 | Ranasinghe et al. (1993b) |
| 50 oral submucous fibrosis | 30 | Taiwanese | – | – | 50 | 30 | Chiang et al. (2000a) |
| 10 hyperplasia | 4 | | – | – | 10 | 4 | |
| 10 dysplasia | 4 | | – | – | 10 | 7 | |
| 10 normal mucosa | 0 | | – | – | 3[d] | 0 | |
| 106 SCCs | 74 | Thai | 64 | 42 | – | – | Kerdpon et al. (2001) |

Table 72 (contd)

| Total cases | Total p53-positive cases | Population | Betel quid without tobacco | | Betel quid + tobacco smoking/chewing | | Reference |
|---|---|---|---|---|---|---|---|
| | | | Total cases | p53-Positive cases | Total cases | p53-Positive cases | |
| 156 SCCs | 58[e] | Thai | 29 | 11 | 36 | 9 | Thongsuksai & Boonyaphiphat (2001) |
| 232 OELs | | Taiwanese | | | | | Chang, K.-C. et al. (2002) |
| 25 verrucous hyperplasia[f] | 0 | | 23 | 0 | — | — | |
| 13 dysplasia | 3 | | 10 | 3 | — | — | |
| 6 verrucous carcinoma[g] | 0 | | 5 | 0 | — | — | |
| 7 epithelial hyperplasia | 1 | | 7 | 1 | — | — | |
| 10 keratosis | 1 | | 9 | 1 | — | — | |
| 10 squamous papillomas | 0 | | 10 | 0 | — | — | |
| 5 verruca vulgaris | 0 | | 5 | 0 | — | — | |
| 104 SCCs | 37[h] | | 87 | 33 | — | — | |

SCC, squamous-cell carcinoma; ND, not detected; OEL, oral epithelial lesion
[a] Include 17 alcohol consumers
[b] Some of the patients were smokers, data not available
[c] TC, tobacco chewers
[d] Smokers only
[e] Data on other habits not included here
[f] Betel quid/tobacco habit data unknown for two cases
[g] Betel quid/tobacco habit data unknown for one case
[h] Four p53-positive cases were SCC unrelated to betel quid.

or E6 protein of human papilloma virus (HPV) (Kaur & Ralhan, 1995; Agarwal et al., 1999; Nagpal et al., 2002b).

[The Working Group noted the lack of information on specific *TP53* mutations associated with the habit of chewing betel quid without tobacco.]

High incidences of H-*ras* mutations (codons 12, 13 or 61) and loss of allelic heterozygosity were reported in oral squamous-cell carcinomas in Indian populations in comparison with populations in the West (Saranath et al., 1991a,b; Munirajan et al., 1998). [The Working Group noted that betel-quid chewing with or without tobacco is a common habit in this population. However, detailed data on chewing habits were not given in these studies.] Ki-*ras* codon 12 mutations or p21 ras protein accumulation have been observed in areca-quid chewing- and tobacco smoking-related oral squamous-cell carcinomas in a population in Taiwan, China (Kuo et al., 1994, 1995b).

Mutations and/or alterations in the expression of cancer-related genes (*MTS1*/p16, pRb, *FHIT*, *APC*, H-*ras*, Ki-*ras*, cyclin D1, MDM2, c-myc, p21$^{WAF1}$, Stat-3, p27$^{kip1}$, Bcl-2, Ets-1, RARβ, RARα and HSP70) associated with betel-quid chewing with or without tobacco have been observed in oral squamous-cell carcinomas (summarized in Table 73 and Figure 8).

A high prevalence of HPV-16 infection in 13/17 (76.4%) oral squamous-cell carcinomas was reported in betel-quid chewers and smokers in a Taiwanese population (Chang et al., 1989). A high prevalence of HPV-18 in addition to HPV-16 was also reported in 67/91 (74%) oral squamous-cell carcinomas in betel-quid chewers and smokers in an Indian population (Balaram et al., 1995). A lower prevalence of HPV infection (37/110; 33.6%) was observed in oral squamous-cell carcinomas associated with reduced frequency of Pro/Pro allele frequency at codon 72 of *TP53* in an eastern Indian population consuming betel quid and chewing tobacco (Nagpal et al., 2002a).

(*d*)  *Polymorphism in carcinogen-metabolizing enzymes*

Several isozymes of cytochrome P450 (CYP) are involved in the metabolic activation of polycyclic aromatic hydrocarbons and nitrosamines, while phase II enzymes such as GST are predominantly involved in detoxification. Numerous alleles that cause defective, qualitatively altered, diminished or enhanced rates of drug metabolism have been identified for many of the phase I and phase II enzymes and can result in marked interindividual differences in carcinogen metabolism. The underlying molecular mechanisms of a number of these genetic polymorphisms have been elucidated (reviewed in Vineis et al., 1999; Nair & Bartsch, 2001).

(i)  *Oral cancer and oral lesions* (Table 74)

The association between *CYP2E1*, *GSTM1* and *GSTT1* polymorphisms and oral cancer was reported in Taiwan, China, in a small case–control study of 41 male oral cancer cases from the National Taiwan University Hospital and 123 healthy controls taken among residents living in Taipei City and Taipei County and frequency-matched for ethnicity, sex and age (Hung et al., 1997). Cigarette smoking, alcohol drinking and betel-quid

Table 73. Analysis of cancer-related genes/proteins in premalignant and malignant oral lesions

| Gene/protein | Population | Total cases | Total altered | Betel quid without tobacco | | Betel quid + tobacco smokers/chewers | | Alteration | Reference |
|---|---|---|---|---|---|---|---|---|---|
| | | | | Total cases | Cases altered | Total cases | Cases altered | | |
| MTSI/p16 | Taiwanese | 110 SCCs | 7 | – | – | 77 | 7 | Mutations exon 2 intron 1/exon 2 splice site | Lin et al. (2000a) |
| | | | 15 | | | 56 | 15 | Methylation of promoter region exon 1 | |
| MTSI/p16 | Indian | 23 SCCs | 3 | 6 | – | 2 | 1 | 2 mutations exon 2, 1 deletion | Heinzel et al. (1996) |
| p16 | Indian | 23 SCCs | 22 | – | – | 31 | 22 | Loss of p16 expression | Pande et al. (1998) |
| | | 22 leukoplakia | 13 | – | – | 19 | 13 | | |
| pRb | Indian | 35 SCCs | 23 | – | – | 31 | 23 | Loss of pRb expression | Pande et al. (1998) |
| | | 22 leukoplakia | 14 | – | – | 19 | 14 | | |
| FHIT (exon 3–10) | Taiwanese | 39 SCCs | 3 | – | – | 39 | 3 | Deletion/mutation | Chang, K.W. et al. (2002) |
| | | | 8 | | | 29 | 8 | Promoter methylation | |
| | | | 11 | | | 31 | 11 | Aberrant transcription | |
| | | | 26 | | | 63 | 26 | Abnormal immunoreactivity | |
| APC (codon 279–1673) | Taiwanese | 40 SCCs | 6 | 6 | – | 21 | 6 | 5 missense mutations 1402 G→A 1367 A→G 1382 T→C 1352 T→C 1652 C→T 1 base pair deletion 1593 A<u>A</u>GC→AGC | Kok et al. (2002) |
| H-ras | Indian | 57 SCCs | 20 | – | – | 57 | 20 | Mutations Codon 12 G→T, G→A Codon 13 G→A Codon 61 A→G, A→T, G→T | Saranath et al. (1991a) |

**Table 73 (contd)**

| Gene/protein | Population | Total cases | Total altered | Betel quid without tobacco | | Betel quid + tobacco smokers/chewers | | Alteration | Reference |
|---|---|---|---|---|---|---|---|---|---|
| | | | | Total cases | Cases altered | Total cases | Cases altered | | |
| Ki-*ras* | Taiwanese | 33 SCCs | 6 | 28 | 6 | – | – | Codon 12 G→A, G→T | Kuo et al. (1994) |
| Ki-*ras* | Taiwanese | 51 SCCs[a] | 47 | 32 | 32 | 47 | 47 | p21 ras expression | Kuo et al. (1995b) |
| | | 4 dysplasia | 4 | – | – | 4 | 4 | | |
| | | 7 hyperplasia | 7 | – | – | 7 | 7 | | |
| | | 6 normal | 6 | – | – | 6 | 1 | | |
| Cyclin D1 | Taiwanese | 88 SCCs | 73 | 1 | 1 | 62 | 54 | Overexpression | Kuo et al. (1999b) |
| MDM2 | Indian | 65 SCCs | 51 | – | – | 50 | 40 | Overexpression | Agarwal et al. (1999) |
| | | 33 leukoplakia | 17 | – | – | 27 | 15 | | |
| MDM2 and p53 | Indian | 65 SCCs | 39 | – | – | 50 | 31 | Overexpression | Agarwal et al. (1999) |
| | | 33 leukoplakia | 16 | – | – | 27 | 14 | | |
| MDM2 | Taiwanese | 52 SCCs | 36 | 1 | 1 | 31 | 25 | Overexpression | Huang et al. (2001) |
| MDM2 | Japanese | 40 SCCs | 29 | – | – | 40 | 29 | Overexpression | Shwe et al. (2001) |
| MDM2 and p53 | Japanese | 40 SCCs | 25 | – | – | 40 | 25 | Overexpression | Shwe et al. (2001) |
| c-myc | Indian | 48 SCCs | 27 | – | – | 48 (TC)[b] | 27 | Overexpression | Baral et al. (1998) |
| c-myc and p53 | Indian | 48 SCCs | 9 | – | – | 48 (TC)[b] | 9 | Overexpression | Baral et al. (1998) |
| p21[WAF1] | Taiwanese | 43 SCCs | 31 | 1 | 1 | 29 | 20 | Overexpression | Kuo et al. (2002a) |
| Stat-3 | Indian | 90 SCCs | 74 | – | – | 90 (TC)[b] | 74 | Overexpression | Nagpal et al. (2002b) |
| p27[Kip1] | Taiwanese | 63 SCCs | 47 | 3 | 2 | 44 | 33 | Loss of expression | Kuo et al. (2002b) |
| Bcl-2 | Indian | 87 SCCs | 87 | – | – | 87 | 87 | Overexpression | Ravi et al. (1999) |
| | | 38 leukoplakia | 15 | – | – | 38 | 15 | | |
| Ets-1 | Indian | 100 SCCs | 62 | 14 | 8 | 32 | 25 | Overexpression | Pande et al. (2001) |

## Table 73 (contd)

| Gene/protein | Population | Total cases | Total altered | Betel quid without tobacco | | Betel quid + tobacco smokers/chewers | | Alteration | Reference |
|---|---|---|---|---|---|---|---|---|---|
| | | | | Total cases | Cases altered | Total cases | Cases altered | | |
| RARβ | Taiwanese | 38 SCCs[c] | 16 | 25 | 13 | 34 | – | Loss of expression | Kao et al. (2002a) |
| RARβ | Indian | 64 SCCs | 18 | – | – | 64 | 18 | Overexpression | Chakravarti et al. (2001) |
| | | 45 leukoplakia | 18 | – | – | 45 | 18 | | |
| RARα | Indian | 64 SCCs | 43 | – | – | 64 | 43 | Overexpression | Chakravarti et al. (2001) |
| | | 45 leukoplakia | 18 | – | – | 45 | 18 | | |
| RARα | Indian | 115 SCCs | 67 | 26 | 14 | – | – | Overexpression | Chakravarti et al. (2003) |
| HSP70 | Indian | 125 SCC | 92 | 9 | 4 | 52 | 48 | Overexpression | Kaur et al. (1998b) |
| | | 64 leukoplakia | 38 | 6 | 2 | 28 | 21 | | |

SCC, squamous-cell carcinoma

[a] Some chewers of betel quid were also tobacco smokers; detailed habit data not available; four SCC patients with negative p21 ras staining were nonsmokers and non-chewers of betel quid
[b] TC, tobacco chewers
[c] Data on betel quid users only were included.

**Figure 8. Molecular targets affected by chewing betel quid with tobacco, often in combination with smoking**

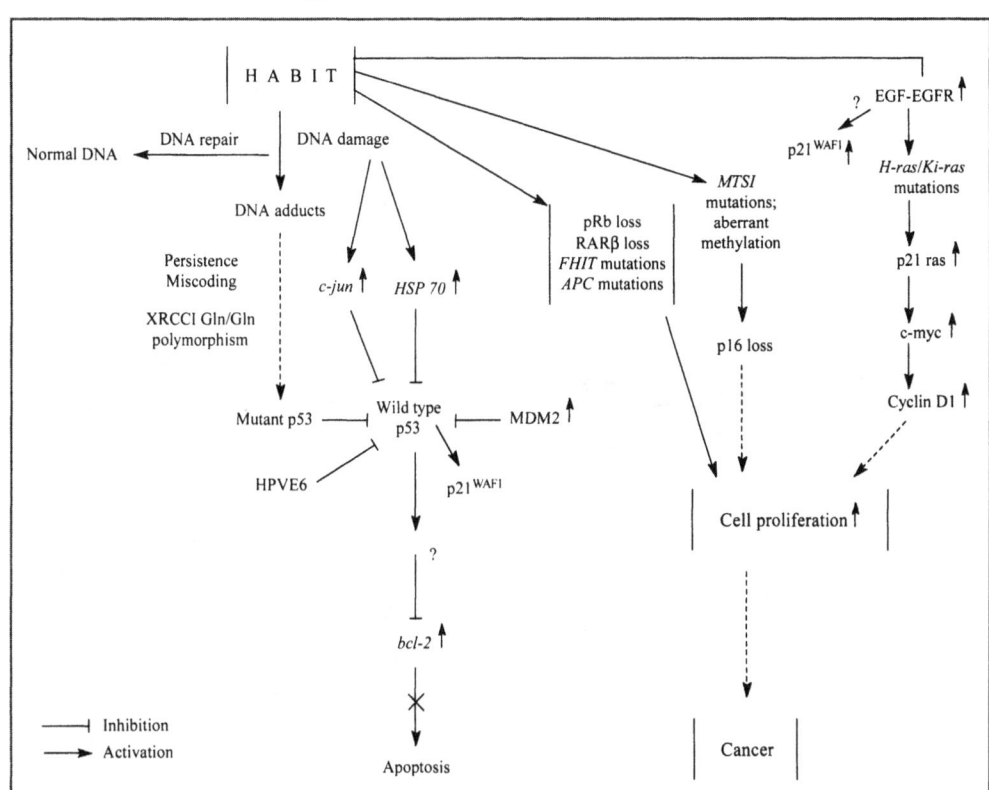

[The Working Group noted that in almost all cases, betel-quid chewing was combined with smoking.]

chewing were significantly associated with the risk for oral cancer and a dose–response relationship was observed. All betel-quid chewers also smoked cigarettes (30 cases and 15 controls). In the multiple logistic regression analysis, individuals with null genotypes of *GSTM1* and/or *GSTT1* had an increased risk for oral cancer compared with those who had non-null genotypes of both *GSTM1* and *GSTT1*, showing a multivariate-adjusted odds ratio of 4.6 (95% CI, 0.9–23.7). The *CYP2E1 c1/c2* and *c2/c2* genotypes were associated with a significantly increased risk for oral cancer compared with the *c1/c1* genotype among those who did not chew betel quid (odds ratio, 4.7; 95% CI, 1.1–20.2). This association was not observed among betel-quid chewers. [However, no adjustment was made in this study for cigarette smoking as a potential confounder as all betel-quid chewers were also smokers. Therefore, the relative importance of betel-quid chewing and smoking as risks for oral cancer could not be determined in this study.]

The effect of genetic variants of *GSTM1* and *GSTT1* on modifying the risk for oral leukoplakia was ascertained in genomic DNA from biopsies taken from 98 oral leuko-

Table 74. Genetic polymorphism and oral cancer

| Gene | Mutation/allele | Country/ethnicity | No. of cases/controls | Significance: odds ratio (95% CI) | Comments | Site | Reference |
|---|---|---|---|---|---|---|---|
| CYP2E1 | RsaI | Taiwan Chinese: 71% Fukienese 7% Hakka 22% mainland | 41/123 | NS: c1/c2+c2/c2 vs c1/c1 Among non-chewers only, S: 4.7 (1.1–20.2) n = 7/40 | Cases all men, age and ethinicity adjusted | Oral cancer | Hung et al. (1997) |
| GSTM1 GSTT1 | Gene deletion | | 98/82 | NS: GSTM1 and/or GSTT1 | NS: combination with GSTM1 and/or GSTT1 | Oral cancer | Hung et al. (1997) |
| GSTM1 GSTT1 | Gene deletion | India | 98/82 | S: GSTM1 null, 22 (10–47) S: GSTT1 null, 11 (5–21) | Association significantly higher for non-homogenous than homogenous leukoplakia | Oral leukoplakia | Nair et al. (1999) |
| GSTM1 GSTT1 | Gene deletion | Thailand | 53/53 | S: GSTM1 null, 2.6 (1.04–6.5) NS: GSTT1 null | | Oral cancer | Kietthubthew et al. (2001) |
| CYP1A1 | MspI RFLP, *2A Exon 7 Ile/Val, *2C | Taipei (Taiwan) | 166/146 (106 SCC, 60 OPL) | S: ile/val vs ile/ile OSCC, 5.1 (2.6–9.76); OPL, 2.67 (1.32–5.4) val/val vs ile/ile SCC, 18.86 (3.61–98.52); OPL, 15.23 (2.8–83.98) NS: MspI RFLP genotype A, B or C | Predominantly men No statistically significant difference in genotypes A (m1/m1), B (m1/m2) or C (m2/m2) between cases and controls | Oral cancer and oral premalignant lesions | Kao et al. (2002b) |
| CYP2A6 | Wild-type *1A Conversion type *1B Gene deletion *4C | Sri Lanka | 286/135 (15 SCC, 62 OSF, 209 leukoplakia) | S: *1B/*4C vs *1A/*1A, 0.2 (0.05–0.88) *4C/*4C vs *1A/*1A, 0.14 (0.03–0.72) | Hospital controls Only 5% SCC cases | Oral lesions | Topcu et al. (2002) |
| GSTM1 | Gene deletion | | | NS: GSTM1 null | S: Combination of CYP2A6 deletion allele and GSTM1 null | | Topcu et al. (2002) |

CI, confidence interval; S, significant; NS, not significant; SCC, oral squamous-cell carcinoma; OPL, oral precancerous lesion; OSF, oral submucous fibrosis plakia patients and exfoliated cells from 82 healthy controls from India (Nair et al., 1999). Most leukoplakia cases were heavy chewers (betel quid with or without tobacco; 15–20 quids per day), whereas the chewers among controls were regular but not heavy chewers (betel quid with or without tobacco; 1–2 quids per day). *GSTM1*-null genotype was found in 81.6% of cases compared with 17% of controls and was significantly associated with risk for oral leukoplakia [odds ratio, 22; 95% CI, 10–47]. Similarly, *GSTT1*-null genotype was found in 75.5% of cases and 22% of controls and was also significantly associated with risk for leukoplakia (odds ratio, 11; 95% CI, 5–22). Combined null genotypes of *GSTM1* and *GSTT1* prevailed in 60.2% of the cases with none detected in controls. Although the low prevalence of null genotypes in the control population may have contributed to the high relative risks observed, this study suggested an extremely strong association between null genotypes of *GSTM1* and *GSTT1* singly or in combination with high risk for oral leukoplakia.

Another population-based case–control study of 53 matched pairs conducted in Thailand (Kietthubthew et al., 2001) assessed the risk for oral cancer in relation to genetic polymorphism of the GST genes in cigarette smokers, alcohol drinkers and betel-quid chewers. The *GSTM1*-null genotype was found in 56.6% of cases compared with 30.2% of controls and was significantly associated with risk for oral cancer for each habit (odds ratio, 2.6; 95% CI, 1.04–6.5). Among the null *GSTM1* individuals, smoking (odds ratio, 4.0; 95% CI, 1.2–13.7), alcohol consumption (odds ratio, 7.2; 95% CI, 1.5–33.8) and/or betel-quid chewing (odds ratio, 4.4; 95% CI, 1.1–17.8) resulted in a significantly increased risk for oral cancer. Interactions between any two of the lifestyle habits for oral cancer risk, however, were not found. The frequency of the *GSTT1*-null genotype was 34.0% among cases and 47.2% among controls. No association was observed between the *GSTT1*-null allele and risk for oral cancer. This study indicates that *GSTM1*-null genotype predisposes towards oral cancer in individuals exposed to cigarette smoke, alcohol and betel quid.

The impact of *GSTM1*-null genotype on oral cancer risk was also analysed in separate groups of individuals from India with different tobacco habits (297 cancer patients and 450 healthy controls). The odds ratios associated with *GSTM1*-null genotype was 3.7 (95% CI, 2.0–7.1) in chewers of tobacco with lime or with betel quid, 3.7 (95% CI, 1.3–7.9) in bidi smokers and 5.7 (95% CI, 2.0–16.3) in cigarette smokers. Furthermore, increased lifetime exposure to tobacco chewing appeared to be associated with a twofold increase in oral cancer risk in *GSTM1*-null individuals (Buch et al., 2002). [Gene–environment interaction was not estimated for chewing betel quid with or without tobacco.]

The effect of *CYP2A6* and *GSTM1* genes on susceptibility to oral lesions among habitual betel-quid chewers was investigated in a Sri Lankan population in a hospital-based case–control study (Topcu et al., 2002). Of a total of 286 cases, 15 had oral squamous-cell carcinoma, 209 had leukoplakia and 62 had oral submucous fibrosis. The control group of 135 subjects was composed of patients who visited the hospital for clinical reasons other than oral cancer and had no oral lesions. The frequency of homozygotes for *CYP2A6\*4C*, a gene deletion polymorphism, was significantly lower in the cases compared with controls and a reduced risk was observed in the group with this deletion genotype (odds ratio, 0.1; 95% CI, 0.03–0.7). While all subjects were betel-quid chewers, 68% of cases and 45% of controls were also smokers. The significant association was stronger in nonsmoking betel-quid chewers than in those with both habits. Further, the *GSTM1*-null genotype had no effect on risk, but was more frequently found in cases with the susceptible genotype of *CYP2A6* than among controls.

The effect of *CYP1A1* polymorphisms on susceptibility to oral lesions associated with betel-quid use was investigated in an Indian population in a hospital-based case–control study (Kao et al., 2002). The percentage of betel-quid users was 62.3% in cases of oral squamous-cell carcinoma, 75% in cases of oral precancerous lesions and 15% among controls. No significant difference was observed for CYP1A1 Msp1 (*2A) polymorphism between cases and controls. However, the frequence of CYP1A1 *Ile/Val* and *Val/Val* genotypes in exon 7 of cases with squamous-cell carcinoma (79.2 and 7.6%) and oral precancerous lesions (68.3 and 10%) was significantly higher than that in controls (53.2 and 1.4%). The study of the genetic polymorphism of CYP1A1 and risk for cancer associated with the duration of betel-quid use has shown no statistically significant difference for squamous-cell carcinoma. Although the *Val/Val* genotype in betel-quid chewers of the oral precancerous lesions group had a history of betel use much shorter than that of other genotypes, no statistically significant difference could be found due to the small number of *Val/Val* genotype ($n = 2$) betel chewers. [The Working Group noted that all betel users were also smokers.]

(ii) *Oesophageal cancer* (Table 75)

Alcohol dehydrogenase-2 (ADH2) converts ethanol to acetaldehyde and aldehyde dehydrogenase-2 (ALDH2) converts acetaldehyde to acetate. The association of lifestyle habits and polymorphism of *ADH2* and *ALDH2* genes with the risk for oesophageal cancer was investigated in a Thai population (Boonyaphiphat et al., 2002) in a hospital-based case–control study of 202 cases and 261 controls. The results of multivariate logistic analysis showed that alcohol consumption (> 60 g per day), smoking (> 10 cigarettes per day) and chewing betel (≥ 10 quids per day) significantly increased the risk (odds ratios, 5.8; 95% CI, 3.2–10.9; 4.7 (2.0–10.8) and 4.7 (2.1–10.7), respectively). *ADH2\*1/\*1* also increased the risk significantly (odds ratio, 1.6; 95% CI, 1.01–2.4); *ALDH2* resulted in a similar but statistically non-significant odds ratio (odds ratio for *ALDH2\*1/\*2*, 1.6; 95% CI, 0.9–2.8). The combined genotypes, *ADH2\*1/\*1* and *ALDH2\*1/\*2*, increased the risk fourfold. In addition, significant gene–environment interaction was found for heavy drinkers (> 60 g per day) with *ADH2\*1/\*1* or *ALDH2\*1/\*2* genotype who had an 11-fold increased risk. [Gene–environment interaction was not estimated for chewing betel quid with tobacco.]

To assess the risk of *CYP1A1* polymorphisms on oesophageal cancer, a study was conducted using 146 cases of oesophageal squamous-cell carcinoma and 324 malignancy-free controls from three hospitals in Taiwan, China (Wu et al., 2002). Habitual use of cigarettes, alcohol and areca nut provided the most significant predictors of oesophageal cancer risk. The proportion of areca-nut chewers was 21.2% in cases and 9.3% among controls

Table 75. Genetic polymorphism and oesophageal cancer

| Gene | Mutation/allele | Country/ethnicity | No. of cases/controls | Significance: odds ratio (95% CI) | Comments | Reference |
|---|---|---|---|---|---|---|
| ADH2 ALDH2 | ADH2*2 ALDH2*2 | Thailand | 202/261 | S: *ADH2\*1/\*1*, 1.6 (1.01–2.4) NS: *ALDH2\*1/\*2* S: Combined *ADH2\*1/\*1* + *ALDH2\*1/\*2*, 4.4 (1.8–10.8) | Mixed ethnicity Significant gene interaction with heavy drinking; gene interaction with betel-quid chewing not estimated | Boonyaphiphat et al. (2002) |
| CYP1A1 | MspI RFLP, *2A exon 7 *ile/val*, *2C | Taiwan | 146/324 | S: *val/val* vs *ile/ile*, 2.5 (1.2–5.3) | 91% of cases and 92% of controls were men. Adjusted for age, education, ethnicity, smoking, alcohol and areca consumption | Wu et al. (2002) |
| SULT1A1 | *arg/his*, G→A, codon 213 | Taiwan | 187/308 | *arg/his* vs *arg/arg*, 3.5 (2.1–5.9) Positive association stronger in no-habit group, adjusted odds ratios, 4.0 for non-chewers, 4.5 for non-drinkers and 4.8 for nonsmokers | Men only Adjusted for age, education, ethnicity, smoking, alcohol and areca consumption | Wu et al. (2003) |

CI, confidence interval; S, significant; NS, not significant [data on mixed habits not shown]. No significant difference was observed for the *CYP1A1* MspI polymorphism between carcinoma cases and controls. However, the frequency of wild-type *Ile/Ile*, *Ile/Val* and mutant *Val/Val* in exon 7 was 46.6% (68/146), 42.5% 62/146) and 11.0% (16/146) in carcinoma cases and 55.3% (179/324), 39.2% (127/324) and 5.6% (18/324) in controls, respectively. Patients with *Val/Val* showed a 2.5-fold (95% CI, 1.2–5.3) greater risk for developing oesophageal cancer than those with *Ile/Ile* after adjustment for age, ethnicity, education, and cigarette, alcohol and areca habits. A slightly (not significantly) greater risk was identified in subjects with *Ile/Val* (odds ratio, 1.3; 95% CI, 0.9–2.1). These findings suggest that an exon 7 polymorphism, not a MspI polymorphism, in *CYP1A1* may be pivotal in the development of oesophageal cancer.

The association between the sulfotransferase *SULT1A1 arg/his* genotype and oesophageal cancer in men was studied in 187 cases of oesophageal squamous-cell carcinoma and 308 controls enrolled from three medical centers in Taiwan, China (Wu et al., 2003). [The population appears to overlap with that of Wu et al. (2002)]. The frequencies of *SULT1A1 arg/his* heterozygote cases (27.8%) and controls (11.0%) were significantly different ($p < 0.0001$). No subjects carried the *his/his* genotype. After adjusting for age, ethnicity, education and cigarette, alcohol and areca habits, individuals with the *arg/his* genotype had a 3.5-fold (95% Cl, 2.1–5.9) higher risk of developing oesophageal cancer than those with *arg/arg* genotype. Remarkably, this positive association was found to be even stronger among non-smokers, non-drinkers and non-chewers. Among the 163 non-substance users, 35.4% (17/48) of the cases and 8.7% (10/115) of the controls carried the *arg/his* genotype. Adjusted for age, education and ethnicity, the odds ratio was 5.7 (95% CI, 2.3–13.9). [The Working Group noted that data are not given regarding mixed-habit groups.]

(iii) *Other susceptibilities and polymorphisms*

As oral submucous fibrosis is a collagen-related disorder induced by cumulative exposure to betel-quid chewing, Chiu et al. (2002) investigated polymorphisms of six collagen-related genes, collagen 1A1 and 1A2 (*COL1A1* and *COL1A2*), collagenase-1 (*COLase*), transforming growth factor β1 (*TGF-β1*), lysyl oxidase (*LYOXase*) and cystatin C (*CST3*), among patients with low and high exposure to betel quid [tobacco content not specified]. The subjects comprised 166 patients with oral submucous fibrosis from a medical center in Taiwan, China, and 284 betel-quid chewers free of the disease and oral cancer from the same hospital and five townships. Polymerase chain reaction-restriction fragment length polymorphism assays were used to genotype the genes situated on different chromosomes. Genotypes associated with the highest risk for oral submucous fibrosis for *COL1A1*, *COL1A2*, *COLase*, *TGF-β1*, *LYOXase* and *CST3* were CC, AA, TT, CC, AA and AA, respectively, for the low-exposure group, and TT, BB, AA, CC, GG and AA, respectively, for the high-exposure group. A trend was noted for an increased risk for oral submucous fibrosis with increasing number of high-risk alleles for those with both high and low exposures to betel quid. The results imply that susceptibility to oral submucous fibrosis could involve multigenic mechanisms modified by the dose of exposure to betel quid.

The secretion of TIMP-1 in response to increases in circulatory MMP-9 in humans varies with the *Taq 1* polymorphism of the vitamin D receptor (VDR) gene (*Taq 1 VDR* genotypes) and also increases in relation to areca-nut consumption (Timms *et al.*, 2002a). No study of this polymorphism as a possible risk factor for submucosal fibrosis and/or cancer has been carried out.

A study on an ethnic Chinese population in Taiwan, China, was conducted to investigate the effect of DNA-repair *XRCCI* genes on susceptibility to oesophageal cancer (Lee, J.-M. *et al.*, 2001). *XRCCI* polymorphisms at codons 194, 280 and 399 were genotyped in 105 patients with oesophageal squamous-cell carcinoma and 264 healthy controls matched for age (± 3 years), sex and ethnicity. The distribution of the three genotypes was not significantly different among patients and controls. However, among alcohol drinkers, the *XRCCI399 Arg/Arg* genotype was frequently found in patients with oesophageal cancer. After adjustment for other potential environmental confounders, the odds ratio for the genotype of *XRCCI399 Arg/Arg* was 2.8 (95% CI, 1.2–6.7) compared with the *XRCCI399 Arg/Gln* and *XRCCI399 Gln/Gln* genotypes in alcohol drinkers. Similar trends, not reaching significance, were observed among cigarette smokers (adjusted odds ratio for *XRCCI399 Arg/Arg*, 1.7; 95% CI, 0.7–3.9) and areca chewers (adjusted odds ratio for *XRCCI399 Arg/Arg*, 2.8; 95% CI, 0.5–16.7).

4.4.2 *Experimental systems*

(*a*) *Genotoxicity and mutagenicity* (see Table 76 for details and references)

(i) Pan masala

Aqueous, aqueous/ethanolic and hot chloroform extracts of *pan masala* were not mutagenic to *Salmonella typhimurium* TA98 or TA100 in the presence or absence of an exogenous metabolic activation system in one study, but the aqueous extract induced mutation in these two strains both in the absence or presence of exogenous metabolic activation in another study. Only the ethanolic extract showed mild direct mutagenicity toward *S. typhimurium* TA98. These extracts were still not mutagenic to TA98 or TA100 even after addition of an exogenous metabolic system or after nitrosation at acidic pH (pH 3) with nitrite (Bagwe *et al.*, 1990). In another study, aqueous extract of *pan masala* was positive in *S. typhimurium* TA98 with or without bioactivation.

Aqueous extracts of both *pan masala* and *pan masala* with tobacco induced chromosomal aberrations, sister chromatid exchange and micronucleated cells in Chinese hamster ovary (CHO) cells in the presence and absence of an exogenous metabolic system, although metabolic activation markedly inhibited the chromosomal damaging effect, implicating the presence of direct-acting mutagens and clastogens (Jaju *et al.*, 1992). The clastogenic effect of *pan masala* towards CHO cells was evaluated in the presence of ethanol, which markedly decreased the mitotic index of CHO cells from 4.3

Table 76. Genetic and related effects of components of pan masala, betel quid and areca nut

| Test system | Result[a] Without exogenous metabolic system | Result[a] With exogenous metabolic system | Dose[b] (LED or HID) | Reference |
|---|---|---|---|---|
| **Pan masala** | | | | |
| *Salmonella typhimurium* TA100, TA98, reverse mutation, aqueous extract | – | – | 154 mg/plate | Bagwe et al. (1990) |
| *Salmonella typhimurium* TA100, TA98, reverse mutation, aqueous/ethanol extract | – | – | 37.5 mg/plate | Bagwe et al. (1990) |
| *Salmonella typhimurium* TA100,TA98, reverse mutation, hot chloroform extract | – | – | 1.4 mg/plate | Bagwe et al. (1990) |
| *Salmonella typhimurium* TA100, reverse mutation, aqueous extract | (+) | + | 100 μg/plate | Polasa et al. (1993) |
| *Salmonella typhimurium* TA98, reverse mutation, ethanol extract | (+) | – | 25 mg/plate | Bagwe et al. (1990) |
| *Salmonella typhimurium* TA98, reverse mutation, aqueous extract | + | + | 100 μg/plate | Polasa et al. (1993) |
| Sister chromatid exchange, Chinese hamster ovary cells *in vitro*, aqueous extract with or without tobacco | + | (+) | 5 μL/mL | Jaju et al. (1992) |
| Sister chromatid exchange, Chinese hamster ovary cells *in vitro*, DMSO extract with or without tobacco | + | (+) | 5 μL/mL | Patel et al. (1994a) |
| Sister chromatid exchange, Swiss albino mouse bone-marrow cells *in vivo*, aqueous suspension | + | | 25 mg/kg ip | Mukherjee & Giri (1991) |
| Micronucleus formation, Chinese hamster ovary cells *in vitro*, aqueous extract with or without tobacco | + | (+) | 5 μL/mL | Jaju et al. (1992) |
| Micronucleus formation, Chinese hamster ovary cells *in vitro*, DMSO extract with or without tobacco | + | (+) | 5 μL/mL | Patel et al. (1994a) |
| Chromosomal aberrations, Chinese hamster ovary cells *in vitro*, aqueous extract with or without tobacco | + | (+) | 5 μL/mL | Jaju et al. (1992) |
| Chromosomal aberrations, Chinese hamster ovary cells *in vitro*, DMSO extract with or without tobacco | + | (+) | 5 μL/mL | Patel et al. (1994a) |
| Chromosomal aberrations, Chinese hamster ovary cells *in vitro*, aqueous extract with or without tobacco plus ethanol | + | NT | 5 μL/mL + 1 or 2% ethanol | Patel et al. (1994b) |

Table 76 (contd)

| Test system | Result[a] | | Dose[b] (LED or HID) | Reference |
|---|---|---|---|---|
| | Without exogenous metabolic system | With exogenous metabolic system | | |
| **Betel quid** | | | | |
| *Salmonella typhimurium* TA100, TA1535, reverse mutation, aqueous BQ extract | + | + | 10 µg/plate | Shirname *et al.* (1983) |
| *Salmonella typhimurium* TA100, TA1535, reverse mutation, aqueous BQ + tobacco extract | + | + | 5 µg/plate | Shirname *et al.* (1983) |
| *Salmonella typhimurium* TA100, TA1535, reverse mutation, aqueous BQ + tobacco extract | – | + | 1 µg/plate | Shirname *et al.* (1983) |
| *Salmonella typhimurium* TA100, TA98, reverse mutation, aqueous BQ extract | – | – | 100 µg/plate | Wang *et al.* (1999) |
| Gene mutation, Chinese hamster V79 cells *in vitro*, aqueous BQ extract | – | – | 10 µg/mL | Shirname *et al.* (1984) |
| Gene mutation, Chinese hamster V79 cells *in vitro*, aqueous BQ + tobacco extract | + | + | 5 µg/mL | Shirname *et al.* (1984) |
| Sister chromatid exchange, Chinese hamster ovary-K1 cells *in vitro*, aqueous BQ extract | (+) | – | 100 µg/mL | Wang *et al.* (1999) |
| Micronucleus formation, Swiss mouse polychromatic erythrocytes *in vivo*, aqueous BQ extract | – | | 2 mg, ip × 2 | Shirname *et al.* (1984) |
| Micronucleus formation, Swiss mouse polychromatic erythrocytes *in vivo*, aqueous BQ + tobacco extract | + | | 0.3 mg ip × 2 | Shirname *et al.* (1984) |
| Chromosomal aberrations, Chinese hamster ovary-K1 cells *in vitro*, aqueous BQ extract | – | – | 1000 µg/mL | Wang *et al.* (1999) |
| **Areca nut** | | | | |
| *Salmonella typhimurium* TA100, TA1535, reverse mutation, aqueous areca-nut extract | + | + | 10 µg/plate | Shirname *et al.* (1983) |

**Table 76 (contd)**

| Test system | Result[a] | | Dose[b] (LED or HID) | Reference |
|---|---|---|---|---|
| | Without exogenous metabolic system | With exogenous metabolic system | | |
| *Salmonella typhimurium* TA100, TA98, reverse mutation, aqueous extract of *Supari* | (+) | + | 200 µg/plate | Polasa *et al.* (1993) |
| *Saccharomyces cerevisiae*, mitotic conversion, aqueous phenolic extract and tannin fraction | + | NT | 3 mg/mL (pH > 10) | Rosin (1984) |
| DNA strand breaks, mouse kidney cells *in vitro*, aqueous areca-nut extract | + | NT | 100 µg/mL | Wary & Sharan (1988) |
| Gene mutation, Chinese hamster V79 cells *in vitro*, aqueous areca-nut extract | + | + | 5 µg/mL | Shirname *et al.* (1984) |
| Sister chromatid exchange, Chinese hamster ovary cells *in vitro*, aqueous areca-nut extract | + | NT | 2.5 µL/mL | Dave *et al.* (1992b) |
| Sister chromatid exchange, Swiss albino mouse bone-marrow cells *in vivo*, aqueous ripe sun-dried areca-nut extract | + | | 12.5 mg/kg × 5, 10 or 15 d | Panigrahi & Rao (1986) |
| Chromosomal aberrations, Chinese hamster ovary cells *in vitro*, aqueous areca-nut extract | + | NT | 8 mg/mL | Stich & Dunn (1986) |
| Chromosomal aberrations, Chinese hamster ovary cells *in vitro*, aqueous areca-nut extract | + | NT | 5 mg/mL | Stich & Tsang (1989) |
| Chromosomal aberrations, Chinese hamster ovary cells *in vitro*, aqueous areca-nut extract | + | NT | 5 µL/mL | Dave *et al.* (1992b) |
| Cell transformation, mouse C3H10T1/2 cells *in vitro*, aqueous extract | + | NT | 0.6 mg/mL | Stich & Tsang (1989) |
| DNA strand breaks, DNA–protein cross-links, human primary buccal epithelial cells *in vitro*, aqueous areca-nut extract | + | NT | 300 µg/mL | Sundqvist *et al.* (1989) |
| DNA strand breaks, human oral mucosal fibroblasts *in vitro*, aqueous areca-nut extract | + | NT | 3 mg/mL | Jeng *et al.* (1994a) |
| Unscheduled DNA synthesis, human Hep 2 laryngeal carcinoma cells *in vitro*, aqueous, acetic acid, hydrochloric acid and ethanol areca-nut extracts | + | NT | 10–25 µg/mL | Sharan & Wary (1992) |

**Table 76 (contd)**

| Test system | Result[a] Without exogenous metabolic system | Result[a] With exogenous metabolic system | Dose[b] (LED or HID) | Reference |
|---|---|---|---|---|
| Unscheduled DNA synthesis, human primary gingival keratinocytes *in vitro*, aqueous areca-nut extract | + | NT | 200 µg/mL | Jeng *et al.*, (1999b) |
| Micronucleus formation, fibroblasts from healthy subjects *in vitro*, aqueous areca-nut extract | + | NT | 2.6 mg/mL | Yi *et al.* (1990) |
| Micronucleus formation, fibroblasts from ataxia telangiectasia patients *in vitro*, aqueous areca-nut extract | + | NT | 1.3 mg/mL | Yi *et al.* (1990) |
| Micronucleus formation, Swiss mouse bone-marrow cells *in vivo*, areca-nut extract | + | | 20 mg ip × 2 | Shirname *et al.* (1984) |
| Micronucleus formation, hamster cheek pouch buccal epithelial cells *in vivo*, areca-nut extract with catechu and lime | + | | 1 mg + 1 mg catechu + 2 mg lime, cpp × 5 | Nair *et al.* (1992) |
| Micronucleus formation, hamster cheek pouch buccal epithelial cells *in vivo*, areca-nut extract with lime and without catechu | + | | 1 mg + 2 mg lime, cpp × 5 | Nair *et al.* (1992) |
| **Areca alkaloids** | | | | |
| *Escherichia coli* PQ37, SOS induction (chromotest), arecoline | − | − | 156.8 µg/assay | Kevekordes *et al.* (1999) |
| *Salmonella typhimurium* TA100, TA1535, reverse mutation, arecoline | + | + | 10 µg/plate | Shirname *et al.* (1983) |
| *Salmonella typhimurium* TA100, TA1535, reverse mutation, arecaidine | + | + | 100 µg/plate | Shirname *et al.* (1983) |
| *Salmonella typhimurium* TA100, reverse mutation, crude alkaloid extracts | − | (+) | 4 mg/plate | Wang & Peng (1996) |

Table 76 (contd)

| Test system | Result[a] Without exogenous metabolic system | Result[a] With exogenous metabolic system | Dose[b] (LED or HID) | Reference |
|---|---|---|---|---|
| *Salmonella typhimurium* TA100, reverse mutation, oil arecoline | + | + | 6.5 µmol [1 mg]/plate] | Wang & Peng (1996) |
| *Salmonella typhimurium* TA98, reverse mutation, crude alkaloid extracts | – | – | 4 mg/plate | Wang & Peng (1996) |
| *Salmonella typhimurium* TA98, reverse mutation, oil arecoline | – | – | 26 µmol [4 mg/plate[c]] | Wang & Peng (1996) |
| DNA strand breaks, mouse kidney cells *in vitro*, arecoline | + | NT | 10 µg/mL | Wary & Sharan (1988) |
| Gene mutation, Chinese hamster V79 cells *in vitro*, arecoline | + | + | 5 µg/mL | Shirname et al. (1984) |
| Gene mutation, Chinese hamster V79 cells *in vitro*, arecaidine, | – | + | 10 µg/mL | Shirname et al. (1984) |
| Sister chromatid exchange, Chinese hamster ovary cells *in vitro*, arecoline | + | NT | 12.5 µg/mL | Dave et al. (1992b) |
| Sister chromatid exchange, Chinese hamster ovary cells *in vitro*, arecoline | + | NT | 12.5 µg/mL | Trivedi et al. (1993) |
| Micronucleus formation, Chinese hamster ovary cells *in vitro*, arecoline | + | NT | 0.2 µM | Lee et al. (1996) |
| Chromosomal aberrations, Chinese hamster ovary cells *in vitro*, arecoline | + | NT | 50 µg/mL | Dave et al. (1992b) |
| Chromosomal aberrations, Chinese hamster ovary cells *in vitro*, arecoline | – | NT | 12.5 µg/mL | Trivedi et al. (1993) |
| DNA strand breaks, human primary buccal epithelial cells *in vitro*, four areca alkaloids | – | NT | 5 mM | Sundqvist et al. (1989) |
| DNA strand breaks, human buccal mucosal fibroblasts *in vitro*, arecoline | – | NT | 400 µg/mL | Jeng et al. (1994a); Chang, Y.-C. et al. (1998) |
| Unscheduled DNA synthesis, human Hep 2 laryngeal carcinoma cells *in vitro*, arecoline | + | NT | 5 µg/mL | Sharan & Wary (1992) |

Table 76 (contd)

| Test system | Result[a] | | Dose[b] (LED or HID) | Reference |
|---|---|---|---|---|
| | Without exogenous metabolic system | With exogenous metabolic system | | |
| Unscheduled DNA synthesis, primary human gingival keratinocytes in vitro, arecoline | – | NT | 1.6 mM | Jeng et al. (1999a) |
| Micronucleus formation, human lymphocytes in vitro, arecoline | + | + | 12.5 μM [3 μg/mL] for 20 h | Kevekordes et al. (2001) |
| Micronucleus formation, human hepatoma cell line Hep-G2 in vitro, arecoline | + | + | 25 μM [6 μg/mL] for 24 h | Kevekordes et al. (2001) |
| Unscheduled DNA synthesis, Swiss albino mouse early spermatids in vivo, arecoline | + | | 20 mg/kg ip | Sinha & Rao (1985b) |
| Sister chromatid exchange, Swiss albino mouse bone-marrow cells in vivo, arecaidine | + | | 100 mg/kg ip × 5 or 10 | Panigrahi & Rao (1984) |
| Sister chromatid exchange, Swiss albino mouse bone-marrow cells in vivo, arecoline | + | | 20 mg/kg ip | Deb & Chatterjee (1998) |
| Sister chromatid exchange, Swiss albino mouse bone-marrow cells in vivo, arecoline | + | | 40 mg/kg ip × 1, 5 or 15 d | Chatterjee & Deb (1999) |
| Sister chromatid exchange, Swiss albino mouse bone-marrow cells in vivo, arecoline | + | | 170 μg/mL po × 1, 5 or 15 d | Chatterjee & Deb (1999) |
| Micronucleus formation, Swiss mouse bone-marrow polychromatic erythrocytes in vivo, arecoline | + | | 2 mg/animal/d ip × 2 | Shirname et al. (1984) |
| Micronucleus formation, Swiss mouse bone-marrow polychromatic erythrocytes in vivo, arecaidine | (+) | | 14 mg/animal/d ip × 2 | Shirname et al. (1984) |
| Micronucleus formation, pregnant Swiss albino mouse fetal polychromatic erythrocytes in vivo, arecoline | + | | 20 mg/kg ip | Sinha & Rao (1985b) |
| Chromosomal aberrations, Swiss albino mouse bone-marrow cells in vivo, arecoline | + | | 20 mg/kg ip | Deb & Chatterjee (1998) |

Table 76 (contd)

| Test system | Result[a] | | Dose[b] (LED or HID) | Reference |
|---|---|---|---|---|
| | Without exogenous metabolic system | With exogenous metabolic system | | |
| Chromosomal aberrations, Swiss albino mouse bone-marrow cells *in vivo*, arecoline | +[d] | | 40 mg/kg ip × 1, 5 or 15 d | Chatterjee & Deb (1999) |
| Chromosomal aberrations, Swiss albino mouse bone-marrow cells *in vivo*, arecoline | + | | 170 µg/mL po × 1, 5 or 15 d | Chatterjee & Deb (1999) |
| **Inflorescence *Piper betle*** | | | | |
| DNA strand breaks, human oral mucosal fibroblasts *in vitro*, aqueous extract | + | NT | 3 mg/mL | Jeng et al. (1994a) |
| Unscheduled DNA synthesis, primary human gingival keratinocytes *in vitro*, aqueous extract | – | NT | 1600 µg/mL | Jeng et al. (1999b) |
| **Piper betle leaf** | | | | |
| *Salmonella typhimurium* TA100, TA1535, reverse mutation, aqueous extract | – | – | 200 µg/plate | Shirname et al. (1983) |
| *Salmonella typhimurium* TA100, TA1535, TA1537, TA98, reverse mutation, aqueous and acetone extract | – | – | 200 µg/plate | Nagabhushan et al. (1987) |
| Micronucleus formation, human lymphocytes *in vitro*, acetone/ether extract | – | NT | 200 µg/mL | Ghaisas & Bhide (1994) |
| Micronucleus formation, Swiss albino mouse bone-marrow cells *in vivo*, extract | – | | 250 mg/kg × 2 | Amonkar et al. (1989) |
| **Eugenol and hydroxychavicol** | | | | |
| *Salmonella typhimurium* TA100, TA1535, TA1537, TA1538, TA98, reverse mutation, eugenol | – | – | 600 µg/plate | Amonkar et al. (1986) |
| *Salmonella typhimurium* TA100, TA1535, TA1538, TA98, reverse mutation, hydroxychavicol | – | – | 300 µg/mL | Amonkar et al. (1986) |

Table 76 (contd)

| Test system | Result[a] Without exogenous metabolic system | Result[a] With exogenous metabolic system | Dose[b] (LED or HID) | Reference |
|---|---|---|---|---|
| *Salmonella typhimurium* TA100, TA98, TA97, reverse mutation, hydroxychavicol | − | − | 100 μg/plate | Lee-Chen et al. (1996) |
| *Salmonella typhimurium* TA102, reverse mutation, hydroxychavicol | + | − | 0.1 μg/plate | Lee-Chen et al. (1996) |
| Micronucleus formation, Chinese hamster ovary-K1 cells *in vitro*, hydroxychavicol | + | NT | 20 μM | Lee-Chen et al. (1996) |
| Chromosomal aberrations, Chinese hamster ovary-K1 cells *in vitro*, hydroxychavicol | + | NT | 20 μM | Lee-Chen et al. (1996) |
| DNA strand breaks, human oral mucosal fibroblasts *in vitro*, eugenol | − | NT | 3 mM | Jeng et al. (1994b) |
| **Catechu** | | | | |
| *Salmonella typhimurium* TA100, TA1535, TA1538, TA98, reverse mutation, ethyl/alcohol extract and catechin | − | − | 250 μg/plate | Nagabhushan et al. (1988) |
| Micronucleus formation, human lymphocytes *in vitro*, acetone/ether extract | − | NT | 200 μg/mL | Ghaisas & Bhide (1994) |
| Sister chromatid exchange, Swiss albino mouse bone-marrow cells *in vivo*, extract | + | | 3 mg/kg ip × 1 | Giri et al. (1987) |

[a] +, positive; (+), weakly positive; −, negative; NT, not tested; BQ, betel quid
[b] LED, lowest effective dose; HID, highest ineffective dose unless otherwise stated; in-vitro tests, μg/mL; in-vivo tests, mg/kg bw/day; ip, intraperitoneal; cpp, cheek pouch buccal painting; po, oral
[c] The highest ineffective dose with an exogenous metabolic system is 39 μmol/plate (6 mg/plate), but this dose was not tested without an exogenous metabolic system.
[d] Chromosomal aberrations induced after 5 or 15 days of intraperitoneal treatment with arecoline were not statistically significant.

to 2.1 (Patel et al., 1994b). Exposure of CHO cells to extract of *pan masala/pan masala* with tobacco plus ethanol also increased the frequency of chromosomal aberrations. A dimethyl sulfoxide (DMSO) extract of *pan masala* with and without tobacco induced chromosomal aberrations and sister chromatid exchange and raised the frequency of micronuclei in CHO cells without metabolic activation. In the absence of an exogenous metabolic activation system, the genotoxic effect of the two extracts was markedly increased, indicating the content of direct-acting mutagens. The decrease in genotoxic response in the presence of an exogenous metabolic system is probbly due to detoxification of mutagens by microsomal enzymes (Patel et al., 1994a) [cytotoxicity data and the concentration of the extract of *pan masala* and *pan masala* with tobacco were not given].

Intraperitoneal injection of *pan masala* suspensions into Swiss albino mice *in vivo* induced sister chromatid exchange in bone-marrow cells. Higher doses resulted in delay in cell cycle progression of bone-marrow cells as revealed by a decrease in the proliferation rate index (Mukherjee & Giri, 1991).

(ii) *Betel quid*

Betel-quid extract was mutagenic to *S. typhimurium* TA100 and TA1535 in the presence or absence of metabolic activation in one study, but not to TA100 or TA98 in another. Betel quid plus tobacco induced stronger mutagenicity towards TA100 and TA1535.

Betel-quid extract did not induce 8-azaguanine gene mutation in Chinese hamster V79 cells in the presence or absence of an exogenous metabolic activation system, whereas betel quid plus tobacco did. Exposure of Chinese hamster ovary (CHO)-K1 cells to betel-quid extract resulted in a weak induction of sister chromatid exchange in the absence of an exogenous metabolic system and no change in chromosomal aberrations compared with unexposed cells.

Intraperitoneal injection of betel-quid extract into Swiss mice induced only a slight non-significant increase in micronucleated cells of polychromatic erythrocytes in the bone marrow, whereas injection of an extract of betel quid plus tobacco induced a greater increase ($p < 0.05$).

(iii) *Areca nut*

Areca-nut extract was mutagenic to *S. typhimurium* TA100 and TA1535 in the presence and absence of an exogenous metabolic activation system. Aqueous extract of *Supari* (processed areca nut with or without flavourings) was weakly positive in *S. typhimurium* TA100 and TA98 in the absence of bioactivation but clearly induced mutation in the presence of an exogenous metabolic activation system. Exposure to aqueous areca-nut extract and tannin induced mitotic gene conversion in *Saccharomyces cerevisiae* at pH values higher than 10.

Exposure of mouse kidney cells in culture to aqueous extract of ripe areca nut (after removal of coated fibres) induced a low but significant level of DNA strand breaks, but reduced cell cycle time [single dose tested only] (Wary & Sharan, 1988). Areca-nut extract induced 8-azaguanine gene mutation in Chinese hamster V79 cells, which was enhanced by the presence of exogenous metabolic activation [exposure time not given]. Continuous or pulse treatment of Chinese hamster ovary (CHO) cells with aqueous extract of ripe and sun-dried areca nut increased the frequency of sister chromatid exchange and chromosomal aberrations in a dose-dependent fashion. Chromatid-type aberrations were more frequent than the chromosomal type (Dave et al., 1992b). Although clinically β-carotene treatment may decrease the frequency of micronucleated buccal epithelial cells in betel-quid/tobacco chewers (Stich et al., 1984b,c), a 48-h pretreatment of CHO cells with β-carotene showed little protective effect against gallic acid (12 μg/mL)-, tannic acid (60 μg/mL)-, aqueous areca-nut extract (8 mg/mL)- and $H_2O_2$ (5–25 μM)-induced chromosomal aberrations and micronucleus formation. The last end-point was not analysed for aqueous areca-nut extract (Stich & Dunn, 1986) [only a single dose of β-carotene was used in this study; no cytotoxicity data on CHO cells were given]. In another study, aqueous areca-nut extract (5 mg/mL) induced a significant number of chromosomal aberrations in CHO cells.

Transfection of mouse C3H/10T1/2 cells with a plasmid containing bovine papillomavirus DNA (*pdBPV-1*) induced transformed foci. When transfection of C3H/10T1/2 cells by the plasmid *pdBPV-1* was followed by exposure to areca-nut extract (0.6–2.5 mg/mL) for 7 days, an observable elevation of transformed foci was noted (Stich & Tsang, 1989).

Areca-nut extract induced DNA strand breaks in human oral mucosal fibroblasts *in vitro*. Aqueous areca-nut extract induced DNA strand breaks and DNA–protein cross-links in human primary buccal epithelial cells *in vitro*. Exposure of Hep 2 human laryngeal carcinoma cells to aqueous, acetic acid, hydrochloric acid or ethanol extracts of areca nut induced unscheduled DNA synthesis [the assay seems unable to discriminate between total DNA synthesis and unscheduled DNA synthesis; no negative control data were given in the unscheduled DNA synthesis assay. This assay cannot distinguish between synthesis by induction of S-phase arrest by arecoline and areca nut and that due to DNA damage and subsequent DNA repair.] An aqueous areca-nut extract induced unscheduled DNA synthesis in human primary gingival keratinocytes *in vitro*. Arecoline (0.042–0.339 mM) [6.5–52.5 μg/mL] and sodium nitrite (0.145 mM) [10 μg/mL] showed additive cytotoxicity to cultured Hep 2 cells in the presence of an exogenous metabolic system at pH 4.2, with an exposure time of 30 min (Wary & Sharan, 1991). Four strains of fibroblasts cultured from ataxia telangiectasia patients were exposed to $H_2O_2$ or aqueous areca-nut extract and showed a stronger response in the cytokinesis-block micronucleated cell assay than control fibroblasts. This effect could be partially prevented by addition of catalase (100 U/mL) to the fibroblasts, indicating the involvement of $H_2O_2$ (Yi et al., 1990).

Chang, M.C. et al. (2002b) reported that areca-nut extract (1200 μg/mL)-induced unscheduled DNA synthesis in human gingival keratinocytes can be prevented by *N*-acetyl-L-cysteine (NAC, 1 and 3 mM), GSH (1 and 3 mM) and vitamin C (200 μg/mL), but not by specific reactive oxygen species scavengers such as DMSO (2%), SOD (50, 200 U/mL) or catalase (200, 400 U/mL).

Intraperitoneal administration of aqueous extracts of ripe and sun-dried areca nut to Swiss albino mice induced sister chromatid exchange in bone-marrow cells. However, areca-nut tannin induced only a mild elevation of sister chromatid exchange (Panigrahi & Rao, 1986). Intraperitoneal administration of areca-nut extract to Swiss mice increased the frequencies of micronuclei in bone-marrow polychromatic erythrocytes from 0.27 to 0.73% (Shirname et al., 1984). Painting of hamster cheek pouch with lime (50 µL, 4%, w/v) [2 mg] and areca-nut extract [50 µL of a 20 mg/mL solution; 1 mg] plus catechu extract [50 µL of a 20 mg/mL solution; 1 mg] increased the frequency of micronucleated cells of the cheek pouch. Painting of hamster cheek pouch with ripe and tender areca-quid extract (areca nut plus lime, 125 µL [concentration not given]) for 14 days induced a significantly higher amount of 8-OHdG formation in the buccal pouch than was seen in untreated control mucosa (Chen et al., 2002).

(iv) *Areca alkaloids*

Arecoline did not elicit SOS induction in *Escherichia coli* PQ37. Arecoline and arecaidine induced reverse mutation in *S. typhimurium* TA100 and TA1535 in the presence and absence of an exogenous metabolic activation system. Crude areca alkaloid extracts were not mutagenic to *S. typhimurium* TA98 but were weakly mutagenic to *S. typhimurium* TA100 in the presence but not in the absence of metabolic activation. Oily arecoline isolated from areca nut was not mutagenic to *S. typhimurium* TA98 but was mutagenic to TA100.

Arecoline induced DNA strand breaks in mouse kidney cells *in vitro* and inhibited the proliferation of these cells (Wary & Sharan, 1988). It induced gene mutation in Chinese hamster V79 cells, which was greater in the presence of an exogenous metabolic activation system (Shirname et al., 1984). Arecaidine was also mutagenic to V79 cells but only in the presence of metabolic activation. Arecoline induced sister chromatid exchange and the formation of micronuclei in Chinese hamster ovary (CHO) cells. It also impaired the division of CHO cells at concentrations equal to or higher than 2 µM (Lee et al., 1996). Arecoline induced chromosomal aberrations in Chinese hamster ovary cells in one study but not in another. Addition of nicotine plus arecoline showed synergistic effects in inducing chromosomal aberrations and sister chromatid exchange in CHO cells (Trivedi et al., 1993).

Arecoline did not induce DNA strand breaks in human buccal mucosal fibroblasts. It induced unscheduled DNA synthesis in human Hep 2 laryngeal carcinoma cells but not in primary human gingival keratinocytes. [Arecoline is cytotoxic to Hep 2 cells at concentrations greater than 10 µg/mL. No negative control data are given in the unscheduled DNA synthesis assay in human Hep2 laryngeal carcinoma cells.] Exposure of cultured human peripheral blood lymphocytes and the human hepatoma cell line Hep-G2 to arecoline induced micronucleus formation.

After intraperitoneal injection, arecoline induced unscheduled DNA synthesis in early spermatid cells, and sister chromatid exchange, micronucleus formation and chromosomal aberrations in the bone-marrow cells of Swiss mice *in vivo*. Intraperitoneal injection of arecaidine induced sister chromatid exchange and micronucleus formation in Swiss albino mouse bone-marrow cells *in vivo*.

(v) Piper betle *inflorescence*

Aqueous extract of *Piper betle* inflorescence (> 2 mg/mL) induced DNA breaks in human oral mucosal fibroblasts but did not stimulate unscheduled DNA synthesis in primary human gingival keratinocytes *in vitro* (< 1.6 mg/mL).

(vi) Piper betle *leaf*

Extract of *Piper betle* was not mutagenic to *S. typhimurium* TA100, TA1535, TA1537 or TA98 in the presence or absence of an exogenous metabolic activation system.

An acetone/ether extract of *Piper betle* leaf did not induce micronucleated cells in cultured human peripheral blood lymphocytes *in vitro*.

Administration of betel-leaf extract to Swiss albino mice twice failed to induce micronucleated bone-marrow cells.

(vii) *Eugenol and hydroxychavicol*

In the absence but not in the presence of an exogenous metabolic activation system, hydroxychavicol was mutagenic to *S. typhimurium* TA102, but not to TA100, TA98 or TA97. Eugenol and hydroxychavicol were not mutagenic to *S. typhimurium* TA100, TA1535, TA1537, TA1538 or TA98, even after metabolic activation. Catalase and SOD showed a protective effect towards hydroxychavicol-induced mutation in *S. typhimurium* TA102, indicating the participation of $H_2O_2$ and superoxide radicals in mediating these events (Lee-Chen *et al.*, 1996).

Hydroxychavicol induced DNA strand breaks in the presence of transition metal. Reaction of hydroxychavicol with supercoiled pRSVcat plasmid DNA in the presence of copper (100 μM) for 30 min induced DNA breaks. At concentrations ranging from 6.25 to 100 μM [1–15 μg/mL], hydroxychavicol dose-dependently induced oxidative damage with the addition of metal ions, as shown by the formation of 8-OHdG in CHO-K1 cells (Lee-Chen *et al.*, 1996).

Eugenol did not induce DNA strand breaks in human oral mucosal fibroblasts. Chen *et al.* (2000) found that hydroxychavicol was cytotoxic to human hepatoblastoma HepG2 cells at concentrations higher than 50 μM [7.5 μg/mL]. Pretreatment for 24 h with buthionine sulfoximine (BSO; 25 μM [49 μg/mL]), an inhibitor of γ-glutamyl cysteine synthetase, enhanced the cytotoxicity of hydroxychavicol. Hydroxychavicol weakly induced 8-OHdG formation, apoptosis and DNA fragmentation in HepG2 cells, which were enhanced by BSO. Catalase at a high dose (1000 U/mL) suppressed BSO/hydroxychavicol-mediated apoptosis (Chen *et al.*, 2000).

Exposure of Chinese hamster ovary (CHO)-K1 cells to hydroxychavicol induced chromosomal aberrations and increased micronucleus frequencies.

(viii) *Catechu* (Acacia catechu)

Catechu extract (< 250 µg/plate) and catechin were not mutagenic to *S. typhimurium* TA98, TA100, TA1535 or TA1538.

Exposure of human lymphocytes to catechu (200 µg/mL) for 6 days did not induce a statistically significant increase in the number of micronuclei. However, sister chromatid exchange in bone-marrow cells was significantly elevated in a dose-dependent manner following intraperitoneal administration of catechu extract (3 mg/kg bw) to male Swiss albino mice.

(ix) *Urine from chewers*

Urine isolated from controls and chewers of *masheri* ($n = 23$) and betel quid with tobacco in addition to *masheri* ($n = 34$) induced little or weak mutation in *S. typhimurium* TA98 and TA100. In the presence of metabolic activation and nitrite, the mutagenicity of urine samples collected from controls and chewers showed greater mutagenicity in *S. typhimurium* TA98 but not in TA100 compared with urine samples from control subjects (Govekar & Bhisey, 1993).

Cultured CHO cells were exposed to urine concentrates (10 µL/mL) collected from 20 tobacco and areca-nut chewers (without smoking or alcohol drinking) for 3 h. Marked elevation of chromosomal aberrations and sister chromatid exchange was noted compared with exposure to urine concentrates from control subjects, even without metabolic activation (Trivedi *et al.*, 1995).

(b) *Oncogenes and tumour-suppressor genes*

Treatment of oral mucosal fibroblasts with areca-nut extract (200 µg/mL) or arecoline (10 µg/mL) for 1 h induced an approximately threefold increase in c-*jun* mRNA levels. This increase was transient and c-*jun* mRNA returned rapidly to control levels thereafter (Ho *et al.*, 2000). However, areca-nut extract and arecoline did not induce c-*fos* mRNA expression. Furthermore, preincubation of cells with either *N*-acetyl-cysteine, a GSH precursor, or BSO, a specific inhibitor of GSH biosynthesis, had a minimal effect on arecoline-induced c-*jun* expression, suggesting that this effect is independent of GSH status (Ho *et al.*, 2000).

Lin *et al.* (2000b) established a cell line, HCDB-1, from tumours induced by the application of 7,12-dimethylbenz[*a*]anthracene (DMBA)/betel-quid extract from Taiwan, China, to hamster buccal pouch. Mutational analysis of *TP53* revealed a C→T transition at codon 141 (Ala→Val) in these cells. The HCDB-1 cells were tumorigenic in nude mice.

The *APC* gene of cultured cells from oral submucous fibrosis patients (8/8) had a CGA→GGA missense mutation at codon 498 (Arg→Gly) and 7/8 cell cultures from these patients had an adenine deletion at nucleotide 1494 that created a stop codon (TGA) at codon 504, while all (8/8) normal human gingival fibroblast cultures expressed the wild-type APC protein (Liao *et al.*, 2001).

(c) *Polymorphisms in carcinogen metabolizing genes*

No studies on genetic polymorphisms in experimental systems were available to the Working Group.

(d) *Markers of tumour promotion*

The promoting effects of betel quid and lime–piper additives (*Piper betle* flower and slaked lime paste) in betel quid on epidermal hyperplasia were investigated in CD-1 mouse skin. Aqueous extracts of these materials were condensed to powder and then kept as a 200-mg/mL stock solution in water/ethanol (5:3 v/v). They were applied twice daily for 4 days to the dorsal skin of female CD-1 mice, which were killed 18 h after the last dose. At concentrations of 50, 100 and 150 mg/mL, both extracts caused a significant induction of hyperplasia. The extract of the lime–piper additives at concentrations of 25, 50 and 75 mg/mL caused an increase in the activity of epidermal ornithine decarboxylase (ODC) by 1.4, 1.6 and 1.6 compared with the control, and an increase in the production of $H_2O_2$ of 2.4-, 3.9- and 3.8-fold, respectively. In addition, the activity of myeloperoxidase (MPO) was increased by 1.4-, 2.7- and 2.3-fold, respectively. Application of both extracts at 50, 100 and 150 mg/mL caused induction of protein kinase C-α (PKC-α) and NF-κB, with the lime–piper additives showing the strongest effect. The results show that betel quid has potential tumour-promoting activity, that the lime–piper additives probably play a major role in enhancing the effects of betel quid-induced skin hyperplasia and inflammation, and that only lime–piper additives induced the ODC activity. These promoting effects on mouse skin were associated with the induction of the expression of PKC and NF-κB (Lee *et al.*, 2002).

(e) *Preventive effects*

Padma *et al.* (1989b) found that *Piper betle* leaf extract dose-dependently decreased the mutagenicity of tobacco-specific nitrosamines, NNN and NNK, to *S. typhimurium* TA100 in the presence of metabolic activation. It also decreased the mutagenicity of *N*-methyl-*N*-nitrosourea towards TA100 and TA1535 (Nagabhushan *et al.*, 1989).

*Piper betle* leaf extract (250 mg/kg, twice) almost completely prevented the NNN- and NNK (250 mg/kg bw)-induced formation of micronuclei in the bone marrow of Swiss albino mice *in vivo* (Padma *et al.*, 1989a). This could be partly attributed to the content of eugenol and hydroxychavicol in *Piper betle* leaf (Amonkar *et al.*, 1989).

Administration of hydroxychavicol (100 mg/kg bw) decreased NNN- and NNK (500 mg/kg bw)-induced formation of micronucleated cells in the bone marrow of Swiss mice *in vivo* (Amonkar *et al.*, 1989). Furthermore, hydroxychavicol (6–96 µg/plate) and eugenol (56–222 µg/plate) inhibited DMBA (5 µg/plate)-induced mutation in *S. typhimurium* TA98 in the presence of exogenous metabolic activation systems (Amonkar *et al.*, 1986).

In addition, catechu extract (25–20 µg/plate) and catechin (12–100 µg/plate) inhibited the benzo[*a*]pyrene- and DMBA-induced mutation in *S. typhimurium* TA98. In another assay, catechu extract (2–10 mg/mL) and catechin (0.5–6 mg/mL) inhibited $N$-methyl-$N$-nitrosourea-induced mutation in *S. typhimurium* TA1535 (Nagabhushan *et al.*, 1988). Catechu (30–200 µg/plate) and catechin (15–100 µg/plate) inhibited the mutagenic effects of cigarette-smoke condensate (150 µg/plate), tobacco (100 µg/plate) and *masheri* (100 µg/plate) extract in *S. typhimurium* TA98 in the presence of an exogenous metabolic activation system (Nagabhushan & Bhide, 1988).

Acetone/ether extract of Purnark (a mixture of turmeric, betel leaf and catechu; 100 and 200 µg/mL) was shown to give 40–60% protection against benzo[*a*]pyrene (5 and 10 µg/mL)-induced formation of sister chromatid exchange and micronuclei in human lymphocytes after 3 days of exposure (Ghaisas & Bhide, 1994).

In the presence of mouse or rat liver microsomal fractions, [$^3$H]benzo[*a*]pyrene showed efficient binding to calf thymus DNA within 30 min of incubation at 37 °C ($n$ = 10). Hydroxychavicol (25 µM) [3.7 µg/mL] prevented [$^3$H]benzo[*a*]pyrene binding to DNA by 97%, whereas eugenol (25 µM) [4 µg/mL] and catechin (25 µM) [7.3 µg/mL] inhibited this binding by 84% and 82%, respectively (Lahiri & Bhide, 1993) [only a single dose was tested]. Chang, M.C. *et al.* (2002a) reported the reactive oxygen species scavenging effect of hydroxychavicol. Effective hydroxychavicol concentrations toward $H_2O_2$, superoxide radicals and hydroxyl radicals are > 10 µM [1.5 µg/mL], > 0.02 µM [0.003 µg/mL] and > 1.6 µM [0.25 µg/mL], respectively.

Nair, U.J. *et al.* (1987) detected the production of superoxide radicals and $H_2O_2$ by catechu at pH higher than 9.5. The production of superoxide was enhanced by $Fe^{2+}$, $Fe^{3+}$ and $Cu^{2+}$, but inhibited by $Mn^{2+}$. When incubated with calf thymus DNA under alkaline conditions, catechu and catechin also promoted the formation of 8-OHdG, especially in the presence of $Fe^{2+}$ and $Fe^{3+}$. It was suggested that decreasing the lime content of betel quid prevented its toxicity. Aqueous catechu extract (5–60 µg/mL) inhibited the γ-radiation-induced lipid peroxidation of rat liver microsome and was an effective scavenger of 2,2′-diphenyl-1-picrylhydrazyl radicals (Naik *et al.*, 2003).

## 4.5 Mechanistic considerations

**Betel-quid and areca-nut chewing without tobacco**

Evidence for possible human exposure to carcinogenic compounds following the use of areca nut and other betel-quid ingredients, such as lime, catechu, betel leaf and arecoline — the principal alkaloid of areca nut — was considered. Data on toxicity, genotoxicity, mutation in cancer-related genes, immunological effects and gene–environment interactions were evaluated. [The Working Group noted that tobacco chewing and smoking probably modulate the effects of betel-quid use because of the presence of numerous carcinogens in tobacco and tobacco smoke. Therefore, the discussion in this section is restricted to the use of betel quid and areca nut without tobacco.]

The areca-nut-derived nitrosamines MNPN, a rodent carcinogen, NGC and NGL have been detected in the saliva of betel-quid chewers. In-vitro nitrosation experiments using nitrite and arecoline yielded MNPA in addition to MNPN and NGL. In-vitro nitrosation of betel quid with nitrite and thiocyanate (both are present in human saliva) yielded NGL. By use of a modified NPRO test, the formation of NPRO in the oral cavity has been demonstrated to occur during chewing of betel quid to which proline was added. Bacterial plaque also plays a role in the formation of nitroso compounds in the oral cavity. MNPN forms the DNA adducts 7-methylguanine and $O^6$-methylguanine (a pro-mutagenic DNA adduct) as well as (2-cyanoethyl)guanines in treated animals (Prokopczyk et al., 1987, 1988; see the monograph on some areca-nut-derived $N$-nitrosamines, Section 4.4.2 of this volume). Such DNA adducts could trigger the tumorigenic process in the oral cavity of betel-quid chewers. There is some evidence that betel-leaf extract can inhibit $O^6$-methylguanine–DNA methyltransferase (MGMT), an enzyme responsible for removal of $O^6$-alkylated guanine residues from DNA.

The formation of reactive oxygen species has been demonstrated in the oral cavity of betel-quid chewers. In-vitro studies suggest that the superoxide anion is generated because of auto-oxidation of polyphenols found in areca nut and catechu, which is enhanced by the alkaline pH of lime. Superoxide anion is converted to $H_2O_2$, which reacts in the presence of transition metals, such as copper and iron, to generate hydroxy radicals. Copper and iron are present in microgram per gram amounts in areca nut, *pan masala*, catechu and slaked lime. This generation of hydroxyl radicals may be a critical event in carcinogenesis. In-vitro studies have demonstrated that areca nut and catechu in the presence of lime can induce oxidation of deoxyguanosine in DNA to yield 8-OHdG, which could trigger the tumorigenic process in the oral cavity. In addition, reactive oxygen species can induce DNA strand breaks.

Depletion of GSH (a cellular anti-oxidant) and reduction of the activity of GST — a detoxifying enzyme for carcinogenic electrophiles — have been demonstrated in cultured human oral keratinocytes and fibroblasts, and in the liver of mice treated with areca-nut extract and arecoline. GSH depletion and decrease in GST activity can lead to increased cellular and DNA damage, which is known to induce several response signals implicated in carcinogenesis.

Micronuclei and other markers of DNA damage have been demonstrated in exfoliated cells obtained from chewers of betel quid and users of *pan masala*. Animal studies and in-vitro test systems support the suggestion that extracts of areca nut and *pan masala* can exert genotoxic effects.

Arecoline caused the inhibition of both humoral and cell-mediated immune responses in mice. Areca-nut extract produced adverse effects on the proliferation of phytohaemagglutinin-stimulated human lymphocytes *in vitro*, suggesting that there may be impaired immune surveillance in areca-nut chewers.

Arecoline modulates matrix metalloproteinases and their tissue inhibitors, as well as the activity of lysyl oxidase, which leads to the accumulation of collagen in oral mucosal fibroblasts. Areca-nut polyphenols inhibit collagenases and increase the cross-linkage of collagen, reducing its degradation. These events may underly the generation of oral submucous fibrosis, which could be further enhanced by the presence of copper ions.

Continuous local irritation and trauma caused by betel quid and *pan masala* can generate chronic inflammation, oxidative stress and cytokine production. In-vitro studies have demonstrated the adhesive nature of areca-nut particles to cultured oral mucosal cells, leading to morphological changes and membrane damage. Oxidative stress and the generation of reactive oxygen species can drive affected cells to proliferation, senescence or cell death. Chronic occurrence of these events can lead to hyperplastic/dysplastic lesions in the oral cavity and could drive some of these preneoplastic lesions to malignancy.

In summary, multiple features of the carcinogenic process have been observed to occur *in vitro* and *in situ* in the oral cavity of betel-quid chewers, and in experimental animals treated with the betel-quid ingredients areca nut, arecoline, catechu and slaked lime.

## 5. Summary of Data Reported and Evaluation

### 5.1 Exposure data

Areca nut is one of the most widely used psychoactive substances with several hundred million users worldwide, predominantly in southern Asia. Areca nut can be chewed alone or in a variety of ways that differ by region.

The habit of chewing betel quid, containing fresh, dried or cured areca nut, catechu, slaked lime and flavouring ingredients wrapped in betel leaf, is widespread in India, Pakistan, Bangladesh and Sri Lanka and in migrant populations coming from these regions. Tobacco is often added. Many people in these regions chew areca nut, with a somewhat higher usage among women. Since the 1980s, the use of industrially manufactured products, often containing tobacco, has increased, especially among children and adolescents.

In Taiwan, China, the unripe areca nut is chewed with slaked lime and betel inflorescence, sometimes wrapped in betel leaf. Tobacco is not added. About 10% of the population, including adolescents, chew areca nut, with highest usage among men (90% of users) and in certain rural ethnic groups.

In parts of southern China (Hainan Island, Xiangtan), areca nut is chewed after treatment with maltose and slaked lime and is wrapped in betel leaf. Tobacco is never added. About one third of the population, both men and women, use areca nut.

In other South-East Asian countries such as Myanmar, Thailand, The Lao People's Republic, Cambodia and the Philippines, the betel quid contains areca nut, slaked lime, catechu and betel leaf. Tobacco is often added. In some of these countries, especially Thailand and Cambodia, the habit is only common among elderly women and usage is declining.

In Papua New Guinea, unripe or uncured ripe areca nut is chewed, sometimes with betel leaf, betel inflorescence or wild ginger. A stick is dipped in slaked lime and applied to the mouth. Tobacco is never added. Over 80% of coastal inhabitants and more than 20% of highland inhabitants chew areca nut. Male and female usage is similar.

In the South Pacific island of Palau, the unripe areca nut is chewed, mixed with slaked lime, betel leaf and, frequently, tobacco. Some 80% of the population chews areca nut, and male and female usage is similar.

Betel-quid or areca-nut chewing results in exposure to areca nut alkaloids, $N$-nitroso-compounds formed from these compounds during chewing, polyphenols, trace elements and, in some cases, to tobacco.

## 5.2    Human carcinogenicity data

In the previous *IARC Monographs* that considered betel-quid and areca-nut chewing (Volume 37 and Supplement 7), the evidence for the carcinogenicity to humans of betel quid with tobacco was evaluated as sufficient; the evidence for betel quid without tobacco was evaluated as inadequate. Many more studies now provide evidence for the carcinogenicity of betel quid without tobacco for oral cancer and for betel quid with tobacco for cancers of the oral cavity, pharynx and oesophagus.

### Oral cancer

Several case–control studies and two cohort studies reported increased risks for oral cancer for betel-quid chewing with tobacco. The statistical significance of the risk persisted after stratification for smoking and alcohol use; a strong dose–response relationship for frequency and duration of chewing was observed.

The risk for chewers of betel quid without tobacco was statistically significant in one study each from India, Pakistan and Taiwan, China, after stratifying for betel-quid chewing with tobacco, tobacco smoking and alcohol use. Several additional studies showed significant risks after stratifying or adjusting for potential confounding variables, including smoking, alcohol and human papillomavirus. A dose–response relationship for betel-quid chewing without tobacco was available in one study and was statistically significant. Suppportive evidence comes from studies that reported significant dose–response relationships for the combined categories of betel-quid chewing with and without tobacco.

### Pharynx

Four studies reported results on the association of chewing betel quid with tobacco and cancer of the pharynx. In three studies that provided results stratified for smoking, the risks were significant for chewing betel quid with tobacco. One of the studies also stratified for alcohol; two studies provided significant dose–response relationships for the frequency and duration of chewing betel quid with tobacco.

### Oesophagus

The risk for cancer of the oesophagus was significantly increased among chewers of betel quid in five case–control studies, four from India and one from Taiwan, China. This evidence comes from studies investigating populations that chew betel quid with and without tobacco. Significantly increased risks persisted in two studies that provided results stratified for smoking and alcohol intake. One additional study stratified for smoking only. The dose–response relationship was significant in three studies, two from India and one from Taiwan, China. The study from Taiwan, China, adjusted for smoking and alcohol.

### Other cancers

Two case–control studies and one cohort study reported an association between chewing betel quid (with and without tobacco) and hepatocellular carcinoma, either stratifying or adjusting for hepatitis B and/or hepatitis C virus positivity. Similar results were seen in one case–control study for cholangiocarcinoma.

A few case–control studies were reported for cancers of the larynx, stomach, lung and cervix. The results for cancers of the stomach and cervix were suggestive of an association with chewing betel quid.

### Precancerous lesions and conditions

In case–control, cross-sectional and cohort studies, chewing betel quid was strongly associated with leukoplakia. One intervention study showed decreased risk for leukoplakia in the intervention cohort. In several studies, oral submucous fibrosis was reported to occur among chewers of areca nut only, chewers of betel quid without tobacco and chewers of betel quid with tobacco, and the observed relative risk was usually extremely high. Follow-up studies showed high risks for malignant transformation of leukoplakia and oral submucous fibrosis.

### 5.3    Animal carcinogenicity data

### Betel quid without tobacco

Betel-quid extract given by gavage produced lung adenocarcinomas in male mice. Subcutaneous injection produced fibrosarcomas at the injection site in male mice.

Cheek-pouch application of betel quid did not produce tumours in three studies in hamsters. In a fourth study, it produced carcinomas locally and in the stomach. Local application on the cheek pouch did not produce tumours in male or female baboons.

The tumour-promoting effect of betel quid was demonstrated in two studies in hamsters.

### Betel quid with tobacco

Extract of betel quid combined with tobacco extract and given by gavage produced lung adenocarcinomas in male mice. Skin application produced a local squamous-cell papilloma and squamous-cell carcinomas in mice. Subcutaneous injection produced unspecified local tumours in male mice. Cheek-pouch application produced local and stomach carcinomas in hamsters, but no tumours in male or female baboons.

### Areca nut

Areca-nut extracts given by gavage produced carcinomas of the lung, liver and stomach, benign liver tumours and salivary gland tumours of an unknown nature in male mice. In another study, lung adenocarcinomas were produced.

Areca nut given in the diet produced squamous-cell carcinomas of the stomach and unspecified malignant uterine tumours in one study and oesophageal papillomas and a carcinoma in another study in male and female mice. In male hamsters, malignant lymphomas were observed. In male and female rats, no tumours were observed.

In male and female mice, oral application of areca nut produced papillomas and carcinomas in the oesophagus. In another study, skin application did not produce tumours.

Subcutaneous injection of areca-nut extract produced fibrosarcomas at the injection site in male and female mice. In another study in male mice with three types of areca-nut extract, two of the extracts produced local fibrosarcomas, liver haemangiomas, hepatomas and lung carcinomas. In a third study, local fibrosarcomas were produced in male and female rats.

Intraperitoneal injection of areca-nut extract did not produce tumours in male mice.

Cheek-pouch application of areca-nut extract produced local squamous-cell carcinomas in hamsters. In another study in females, it produced a local papilloma and a local squamous-cell carcinoma and, in a third study, local and stomach carcinomas were produced. In three other studies, no tumours were seen.

The tumour-promoting effect of areca nut was demonstrated in one study in mice, one study in rats and three studies in hamsters.

### Areca nut with tobacco

Skin application of areca-nut extract with tobacco extract produced local papillomas and squamous-cell carcinomas in male and female mice.

In three studies, cheek-pouch application of areca-nut and tobacco extract in hamsters produced local squamous-cell carcinomas in males, stomach tumours in males, and local and stomach carcinomas, respectively. No tumours were seen in two other studies.

### Areca nut with slaked lime

In one study, areca nut with slaked lime in the diet produced papillomas in the oral cavity and the forestomach, and carcinomas in various major organs in male and female rats. In another study, no tumours were produced.

### Areca nut with tobacco and slaked lime

Cheek-pouch application of areca nut with slaked lime and tobacco produced local and stomach carcinomas in hamsters.

### Areca nut with betel leaf

Areca-nut extract with betel-leaf extract given by gavage produced lung adenocarcinomas in male mice. It did not produce tumours when given subcutaneously to male mice or applied to the cheek pouch of male and female hamsters.

### Betel leaf

Betel-leaf extract given by gavage in two studies or intraperitoneally to male mice, in the diet to male and female rats or by cheek-pouch application to hamsters in two studies did not produce tumours.

Betel leaf also showed some antitumorigenic activity in three studies in mice, in one study in rats and in three studies in hamsters.

### *Pan masala*

*Pan masala* in the diet produced benign and malignant tumours in various organs, most frequently adenocarcinoma of the lung, in male and female mice. *Pan masala* extract did not produce tumours when administered by gavage to male and female mice, or when applied orally to rats in another study.

The tumour-promoting effect of *pan masala* was demonstrated in one study in mice. The number of studies investigating this substance in animals is limited.

### Arecoline

Arecoline given by gavage produced lung adenocarcinomas, stomach squamous-cell carcinomas and liver haemangiomas in male mice. It did not produce tumours when given by gavage to female mice or in the drinking-water to male and female hamsters, when injected subcutaneously into male mice or when administered intraperitoneally to male mice.

No tumours were produced by local intraoral painting in rats.

No initiating effect of arecoline was demonstrated in one study in male hamsters.

### Arecoline with slaked lime

Cheek-pouch application of arecoline following application of slaked lime produced an oesophageal papilloma in female hamsters. In two studies in male and female hamsters, no tumours were seen after administration in the diet or in drinking-water.

### Slaked lime

Slaked lime did not produce tumours in male or female mice when given by gavage, in male or female hamsters when given in the drinking-water or diet or in three cheek-pouch application studies in hamsters.

No promoting effect for slaked lime was shown in male and female hamsters.

**Arecaidine alone**

Local application of arecaidine to the cheek pouch did not produce tumours in male hamsters.

The tumour-promotion effect of arecaidine was demonstrated in one study in hamsters.

## 5.4 Other relevant data

Areca nut is chewed for its psychostimulating effects, such as relaxation, improved concentration and enhanced satisfaction after eating. A majority of users reported the development of tolerance to these effects. Withdrawal symptoms on trying to quit the habit were mood swings, anxiety, irritability, reduced concentration, sleep disturbance and craving. These findings are regarded to be consistent with the existence of a dependence syndrome among regular users. In rare cases, areca nut psychosis has been reported to occur in heavy users following abrupt cessation of the habit.

**Human studies**

Powdered areca nut placed in the oral cavity of human volunteers gives rise to the rapid appearance of arecoline in blood plasma, indicating systemic absorption of this alkaloid. Peak concentrations of arecoline in blood plasma have been measured in human subjects 5–10 h after application of a dermal dose.

Eugenol and dihydroxychavicol, metabolites of safrole, are found in the urine of betel-quid chewers.

The areca-nut-derived nitrosamines, *N*-nitrosoguvacoline and 3-(methylnitroso)-propionitrile, have been detected in saliva and are most probably produced *in situ* during betel-quid chewing. This nitrosation reaction can be mimicked *in vitro*. In addition, the volatile nitrosamines, *N*-nitrosodimethylamine and *N*-nitrosodiethylamine, and the tobacco-specific nitrosamines, *N*-nitrosonornicotine, 4-(methylnitrosamino)-1-(3-pyridyl)-1-butanone and *N'*-nitrosoanabasine, are present in the saliva of chewers of betel quid with tobacco. Endogenous nitrosation has been demonstrated in chewers of betel quid mixed with proline, by measuring *N*-nitrosoproline in saliva and urine.

Formation of reactive oxygen species in the oral cavity during betel-quid chewing has been demonstrated. In-vitro studies have shown that the generation of reactive oxygen species is due to auto-oxidation of the polyphenols in areca nut and catechu. This reaction is enhanced by alkaline pH (from the slaked lime) and by the presence of the transition metals, copper and iron.

Areca-nut chewing has significant effects on the hard and soft tissues of the oral cavity. Although some studies have described a protective effect of areca-nut chewing on dental caries, the habit causes severe tooth wear and may also enhance gingivitis. Areca-nut polyphenols increase cross-linkage of collagen and inhibit the activity of collagenase.

Arecoline modulates the activity of matrix metalloproteinases, their tissue inhibitors and lysyl oxidase, which leads to the accumulation of collagen in the fibroblasts of the oral mucosa. This may result in the development of submucous fibrosis. The significant amounts of soluble copper released into the oral cavity by areca-nut chewing may further contribute to the development of this condition.

Betel-quid chewing by pregnant women has been associated with adverse pregnancy outcomes including reduction in birth weight, pre-term delivery, stillbirth and fetal malformation.

The alkaloids in areca nut have antimuscarinic effects. Areca-nut chewing increases the blood plasma concentrations of adrenaline and noradrenaline. Arecoline and betel-quid use increase occipital $\alpha$ activity and generalized $\beta$ activity in electroencephalograms. Betel-nut chewing has antidepressant effects and increases heart rate and blood flow through carotid arteries.

Areca-nut chewing is said to soothe digestion and enhances the production and secretion of saliva.

Betel-quid chewing aggravates asthma by reducing the forced expiratory volume. Arecoline can cause constriction of bronchial smooth muscle tissue *in vitro* and bronchoconstriction in betel-quid users with asthma.

Although short-term hypoglycaemic effects have been reported, areca nut can clearly cause chronic hyperglycaemia. The alkaloids in areca nut block the receptor of $\gamma$-aminobutyric acid, which increases the release of glucagon. Areca-nut use has been shown to be an independent risk factor for type-2 diabetes.

Areca-nut chewing increases skin temperature, pulse rate and — in novice users — blood pressure.

Elevated micronucleus formation and chromosome breaks have been reported in oral exfoliated cells in chewers of betel quid with or without tobacco. Micronucleus formation has been observed in precancerous lesions in the oral cavity of chewers.

Elevated sister chromatid exchange and micronucleus formation have been demonstrated in cultured peripheral lymphocytes collected from chewers of *pan masala* and areca nut with and without tobacco and slaked lime.

*TP53* mutations were infrequent or absent in oral premalignant lesions and squamous-cell carcinomas in subjects chewing betel quid without tobacco, but accumulation of p53 protein was observed. *TP53* or *ras* mutations, p53 or ras protein accumulation and a number of other gene/protein alterations were observed in premalignant lesions and squamous-cell carcinomas of chewers of betel quid with tobacco.

No clear gene–environment interaction could be established for polymorphisms in carcinogen metabolic enzymes because of the presence of concurrent confounding habits of tobacco chewing or smoking or alcohol consumption in cases.

Elevated COX2 protein levels have been detected in 'moderate human submucous fibrosis' tissue by immunohistochemistry.

## Animal studies

In rats, the major metabolic pathway of arecoline is via de-esterification and production via conjugated mercapturic acid. In-vitro data suggest that arecoline is metabolized by carboxylesterase (EC 3.1.1.1) in mouse liver and kidney.

Male Swiss albino mice fed areca-nut powder or arecoline showed enhanced levels of the hepatic cytochromes P450 and $b_5$ and decreased levels of hepatic glutathione. When given orally to these mice, betel-leaf extract enhanced hepatic superoxide dismutase activity, increased vitamin A and C concentrations in the liver and inhibited catalase activity.

*Pan masala* reduced testis weight in mice and enhanced the frequency of morphological abnormalities in mouse sperm. Areca-nut extracts were embryotoxic when given to pregnant mice during early gestation, and teratogenic when administered into the yolk sac of chick embryos. Extracts of *Piper betle* stalks disturbed the estrus cycle in female rats and reduced fertility in males. In mice, arecoline was genotoxic to early spermatids and it increased the frequency of abnormal sperm.

The diabetogenic effects of areca nut were produced in mice fed ground areca nut and were observed in subsequent generations not fed betel quid.

Arecoline caused inhibition of both humoral and cell-mediated immune responses in mice.

At higher doses, betel-quid extracts reduce the activity of hepatic glutathione peroxidase and glutathione $S$-transferase.

In rats, *pan masala* impaired liver function and decreased relative weights of gonads and brain. Areca nut and areca-nut ingredients influenced the rate of RNA and DNA synthesis in various tissues of treated mice. Effects on gastrointestinal tract function and control of the cardiovascular system have been described for areca nut and its ingredients in a number of experimental models, both *in vivo* and *in vitro*. In general, the effects observed correspond to those seen in regular users of areca nut and betel quid.

## In-vitro studies

Glutathione depletion and reduction of glutathione $S$-transferase activity have been demonstrated in cultured human oral keratinocytes and in fibroblasts treated with arecoline.

Areca-nut extract enhanced COX2 expression and prostaglandin $E_2$ production in cultured human gingival keratinocytes and human buccal mucosa fibroblasts.

Phytohaemagglutinin-stimulated proliferation of human lymphocytes *in vitro* was inhibited by areca-nut extract.

Extracts (water, water/ethanol, dimethyl sulfoxide) of *pan masala* were weakly mutagenic in bacteria, but induced chromosomal aberrations, sister chromatid exchange and micronucleus formation in Chinese hamster ovary cells in the absence of metabolic activation. Sister chromatid exchange and sperm abnormalities were induced by these extracts in mice *in vivo*.

Extracts of betel quid with or without tobacco were mutagenic in bacteria, but only extracts with tobacco induced mutations in Chinese hamster V79 cells. Betel-quid extracts without tobacco were weak inducers of sister chromatid exchange in Chinese hamster ovary-K1 cells *in vitro* and did not give rise to micronucleus formation in mouse bone marrow.

Aqueous extracts of areca nut produced gene conversion in yeast, DNA strand breaks in mouse kidney cells, and gene mutation, chromosomal aberrations, sister chromatid exchange and micronucleus formation in Chinese hamster ovary cells *in vitro*. These extracts also induced chromosomal aberrations and cell transformation in mouse C3H 10T1/12 cells. Areca-nut extracts induced DNA strand breaks and DNA–protein cross-links in cultured human primary buccal epithelial cells, DNA strand breaks in human oral mucosal fibroblasts and unscheduled DNA synthesis in Hep2 human laryngeal carcinoma cells and in primary human gingival keratinocytes. Sister chromatid exchange and micro-nucleus formation were seen in bone-marrow cells of mice treated with these extracts *in vivo*. Micronuclei were also induced in cheek-pouch epithelial cells of hamsters treated *in vivo*, with or without slaked lime, and in fibroblasts of healthy subjects and ataxia telangiectasia patients. All these effects of areca-nut extracts were seen without metabolic activation.

Arecoline and other areca-nut alkaloids gave positive responses in most bacterial mutagenicity assays, and induced chromosomal aberrations, micronucleus formation and sister chromatid exchange in mammalian cells, both *in vitro* and *in vivo*.

Data on the genotoxicity of aqueous extracts of *Piper betle* L. inflorescence and of betel leaf are limited, and generally negative. Inflorescence was reported to induce DNA strand breaks in cultured human oral mucosa fibroblasts in one study.

Safrole and eugenol did not induce mutation in bacteria, whereas hydroxychavicol gave inconsistent results. However, the latter compound did induce chromosomal aberrations and micronucleus formation in Chinese hamster ovary cells.

Catechu was not mutagenic in bacteria.

## 5.5 Evaluation

There is *sufficient evidence* in humans for the carcinogenicity of betel quid with tobacco. Betel quid with tobacco causes oral cancer and cancer of the pharynx and oesophagus.

There is *sufficient evidence* in humans for the carcinogenicity of betel quid without tobacco. Betel quid without tobacco causes oral cancer.

There is *sufficient evidence* in experimental animals for the carcinogenicity of betel quid without tobacco.

There is *sufficient evidence* in experimental animals for the carcinogenicity of betel quid with tobacco.

There is *sufficient evidence* in experimental animals for the carcinogenicity of areca nut.

There is *sufficient evidence* in experimental animals for the carcinogenicity of areca nut with tobacco.

There is *limited evidence* in experimental animals for the carcinogenicity of arecoline.

There is *inadequate evidence* in experimental animals for the carcinogenicity of arecaidine.

There is *evidence suggesting lack of carcinogenicicy* in experimental animals for betel leaf.

There is *evidence suggesting lack of carcinogenicicy* in experimental animals for slaked lime.

**Overall evaluation**

Betel quid with tobacco is *carcinogenic to humans (Group 1)*.
Betel quid without tobacco is *carcinogenic to humans (Group 1)*.
Areca nut is *carcinogenic to humans (Group 1)*.

In reaching the latter conclusion, the Working Group noted that a common component of all betel-quid preparations is the areca nut. This evaluation is based on strong evidence that areca nut causes oral submucous fibrosis, a precancerous condition in humans, and sufficient evidence of carcinogenicity in experimental animals. In addition, there is strong supporting evidence for this conclusion.

# 6. References

Adhikary, P., Banerji, J., Chowdhury, D., Das, A.K., Deb, C.C., Mukherjee, S.R. & Chatterjee, A. (1989) Antifertility effect of *Piper betle* Linn. extract on ovary and testis of albino rats. *Indian J. exp. Biol.*, **27**, 868–870

Adhikary, P., Banerji, J., Choudhuri, D., Das, A.K., Deb, C.C., Mukherjee, S.R. & Chatterjee, A. (1990a) Effect of oral administration of stalk of leaves of *Piper betle* Linn on oestrous cycle and its antifertility activity in rats. *Indian J. phys. all. Sci.*, **44**, 116–123

Adhikary, P., Banerji, J., Choudhuri, D., Das, A.K. Deb, C.C., Mukherjee, S.R. & Chatterjee, A. (1990b) Effect of *Piper betle* Linn (stalk) extract on male rat fertility. *Indian J. Pharmacol.*, **22**, 145–149

Adhvaryu, S.G., Bhatt, R.G., Dayal, P.K., Trivedi, A.H., Dave, B.J., Vyas, R.C. & Jani, K.H. (1986) SCE frequencies in lymphocytes of tobacco/betel nut chewers and patients with oral submucous fibrosis. *Br. J. Cancer*, **53**, 141–143

Adhvaryu, S.G., Dave, B.J. & Trivedi, A.H. (1991) Cytogenetic surveillance of tobacco-areca nut (mava) chewers, including patients with oral cancers and premalignant conditions. *Mutat. Res.*, **261**, 41–49

Agarwal, V. & Arora, M.M. (1964) Oropharyngeal cancer in Bhopal. *J. Indian med. Assoc.*, **42**, 519–521

Agarwal, S., Mathur, M., Srivastava, A. & Ralhan, R. (1999) MDM2/p53 co-expression in oral premalignant and malignant lesions: Potential prognostic implications. *Oral Oncol.*, **35**, 209–216

Ahluwalia, H.S. & Duguid, J.B. (1966) Malignant tumours in Malaya. *Br. J. Cancer*, **20**, 12–15

Ahmed, W., Qureshi, H., Alam, S.E. & Zuberi, S.J. (1993) Association of upper gastrointestinal lesions with addictions. *J. Pak. med. Assoc.*, **43**, 176–177

Alfthan, G., Aro, A. & Gey, K.F. (1997) Plasma homocysteine and cardiovascular disease mortality. *Lancet*, **349**, 397

Amarasena, N., Ekanayake, A.N.I., Herath, L. & Miyazaki, H. (2003) Association between smoking, betel chewing and gingival bleeding in rural Sri Lanka. *J. clin. Periodontol.*, **30**, 403–408

Amonkar, A.J., Nagabhushan, M., D'Souza, A.V. & Bhide, S.V. (1986) Hydroxychavicol: A new phenolic antimutagen from betel leaf. *Food chem. Toxicol.*, **24**, 1321–1324

Amonkar, A.J., Padma, P.R. & Bhide, S.V. (1989) Protective effect of hydroxychavicol, a phenolic component of betel leaf, against the tobacco-specific carcinogens. *Mutat. Res.*, **210**, 249–253

Anantha, N., Nandakumar, A., Vishwanath, N., Venkatesh, T., Pallad, Y.G., Manjunath, P., Kumar, D.R., Murthy, S.G.S., Shivashankariah & Dayananda C.S. (1995) Efficacy of an anti-tobacco community education program in India. *Cancer Causes Control*, **6**, 119–129

Ånerud, Å., Löe, H. & Boysen, H. (1991) The natural history and clinical course of calculus formation in man. *J. clin. Periodontol.*, **18**, 160–170

Anisimov, V.N. (1978) Pharmacological study of cholinergic mechanisms of compensatory ovarian hypertrophy in rats. *Endokrinologie*, **71**, 149–153

Anon. (2003) Betelnut: Mama'on [http://ns.gov.gu/pugua.html]

Arbeille, P., Bosc, M., Vaillant, M.C. & Tranquart, F. (1992) Nicotine-induced changes in the cerebral circulation in ovine fetuses. *Am. J. Perinatol.*, **9**, 270–274

Arjungi, K.N. (1976) Areca nut: A review. *Arzneim.-Forsch. (Drug Res)*, **26**, 951–957

Asma, S. (1997) Smokeless tobacco: Betel quid chewing among adult women in Lao People's Democratic Republic. *Tobacco Control*, **6**, 157–158

Asthana, S., Greig, N.H., Holloway, H.W., Raffaele, K.C., Berardi, A., Schapiro, M.B., Rapoport, S.I. & Soncrant, T.T. (1996) Clinical pharmacokinetics of arecoline in subjects with Alzheimer's disease. *Clin. Pharmacol. Ther.*, **60**, 276–282

Atkinson, L., Chester, I.C., Smyth, F.G. & ten Seldam R.E.J. (1964) Oral cancer in New Guinea: A study in demography and etiology. *Cancer*, **17**, 1289–1298

Atkinson, L., Purohit, R., Reay-Young, P. & Scott, G.C. (1982) Cancer reporting in Papua New Guinea: 1958–70 & 1971–78. *Natl Cancer Inst. Monogr.*, **62**, 65–71

Atwal, G.S., Warnakulasuriya, K.A.A.S. & Gelbier, S. (1996) Betel-quid chewing habits among a sample of South Asians. *J. dent. Res.*, **75**, 1151

Awang, M.N. (1986) Estimation of arecoline contents in commercial areca (betel) nuts and its relation to oral precancerous lesions. *Singapore med. J.*, **27**, 317–320

Awang, M.N. (1987) Quantitative analysis of areca catechu (betel) nut flavanols (tannins) in relation to oral submucous fibrosis. *Dent. J. Malaysia*, **9**, 29–32

Awang, M.N. (1988) Fate of betel nut chemical constituents following nut treatment prior to chewing and its relation to oral precancerous and cancerous lesion. *Dent. J. Malaysia*, **10**, 33–37

Axéll, T., Zain, R.B., Siwamoghstam, P., Tantinran, D. & Thampipit, J. (1990) Prevalence of oral soft tissue lesions in out-patients at two Malaysian and Thai dental schools. *Community dent. oral Epidemiol.*, **18**, 95–99

Azuine, M.A. & Bhide, S.V. (1992) Protective single/combined treatment with betel leaf and turmeric against methyl (acetoxymethyl) nitrosamine-induced hamster oral carcinogenesis. *Int. J. Cancer*, **51**, 412–415

Azuine, M.A., Amonkar, A.J. & Bhide, S.V. (1991) Chemopreventive efficacy of betel leaf extract and its constituents on 7,12-dimethylbenz(a)anthracene induced carcinogenesis and their effect on drug detoxification system in mouse skin. *Indian J. exp. Biol.*, **29**, 346–351

Babu, S., Bhat, R.V., Kumar, P.U., Sesikaran, B., Rao, K.V., Aruna, P. & Reddy, P.R.R. (1996) A comparative clinico-pathological study of oral submucous fibrosis in habitual chewers of pan masala and betel quid. *J. Toxicol. clin. Toxicol.*, **34**, 317–322

Bagchi, M., Balmoori, J., Bagchi, D., Stohs, S.J., Chakrabarti, J. & Das, D.K. (2002) Role of reactive oxygen species in the development of cytotoxicity with various forms of chewing tobacco and pan masala. *Toxicology*, **179**, 247–255

Bagwe, A.N., Ganu, U.K., Gokhale, S.V. & Bhisey, R.A. (1990) Evaluation of the mutagenicity of 'pan masala', a chewing substitute widely used in India. *Mutat. Res.*, **241**, 349–354

Balaram, P., Pillai, M.R. & Abraham, T. (1987) Immunology of premalignant and malignant conditions of the oral cavity. II. Circulating immune complexes. *J. oral Pathol.*, **16**, 389–391

Balaram, P., Nalinakumari, K.R., Abraham, E., Balan, A., Hareendran, N.K., Bernard, H.U. & Chan, S.-Y. (1995) Human papillomaviruses in 91 oral cancers from Indian betel quid chewers — High prevalence and multiplicity of infections. *Int. J. Cancer*, **61**, 450–454

Balaram, P., Sridhar, H., Rajkumar, T., Vaccarella, S., Herrero, R., Nandakumar, A., Ravichandran, K., Ramadas, K., Sankaranarayanan, R., Gajalakshmi, V., Munoz, N. & Franceschi, S. (2002) Oral cancer in southern India: The influence of smoking, drinking, paan chewing and oral hygiene. *Int. J. Cancer*, **98**, 440–445

Balendra, W. (1949) Symposium on oral diseases in tropical countries. I. The effect of betel chewing on the dental and oral tissues and its possible relationship to buccal carcinoma. *Br. dent. J.*, **87**, 83–87

Balendra, W. (1965) The incidence of oral carcinoma in Ceylon. *Br. J. oral Surg.*, **3**, 101–105

Baral, R.N., Patnaik, S. & Das, B.R. (1998) Co-overexpression of p53 and c-myc proteins linked with advanced stages of betel- and tobacco-related oral squamous cell carcinomas from eastern India. *Eur. J. oral Sci.*, **106**, 907–913

Bedi, R. (1996) Betel-quid and tobacco chewing among the United Kingdom's Bangladeshi community. *Br. J. Cancer*, **74** (Suppl. 29), S73–S77

Bedi, R. & Gilthorpe, M.S. (1995) Betel-quid and tobacco chewing among the Bangladeshi community in areas of multiple deprivation. In: Bedi, R. & Jones, P., eds, *Betel-quid and Tobacco Chewing among the Bangladeshi Community in the United Kingdom, Usage and Health Issues*, London, Centre for Transcultural Oral Health, pp. 37–52

Behari, M., Sharma, A.K., Changkakoti, S., Sharma, N. & Pandey, R.M. (2000) Case–control study of Meige's syndrome. Result of a pilot study. *Neuroepidemiology*, **19**, 275–280

Benjamin, A.L. (2001) Community screening for diabetes in the National Capital District, Papua New Guinea: Is betelnut chewing a risk factor for diabetes? *Papua New Guinea med. J.*, **44**, 101–107

Bentall, W.C. (1908) Cancer in Travancore, South India. A summary of 1700 cases. *Br. med. J.*, ii, 1428–1431

Bhargava, K., Smith, L.W., Mani, N.J., Silverman, S., Jr, Malaowalla, A.M. & Bilimoria, K.F. (1975) A follow-up study of oral cancer and precancerous lesions in 57 518 industrial workers of Gujarat, India. *Indian J. Cancer*, **12**, 124–129

Bhide, S.V., Shivapurkar, N.M., Gothoskar, S.V. & Ranadive, K.J. (1979) Carcinogenicity of betel quid ingredients: Feeding mice with aqueous extract and the polyphenol fraction of betel nut. *Br. J. Cancer*, **40**, 922–926

Bhide, S.V., Gothoskar, S.V. & Shivapurkar, N.M. (1984) Arecoline tumorigenicity in Swiss strain mice on normal and vitamin B deficient diet. *J. Cancer Res. clin. Oncol.*, **107**, 169–171

Bhide, S.V., Nair, U.J., Nair, J., Spiegelhalder, B. & Preussmann, R. (1986) *N*-Nitrosamines in the saliva of tobacco chewers or masheri users. *Food chem. Toxicol.*, **24**, 293–297

Bhide, S.V., Zariwala, M.B., Amonkar, A.J. & Azuine, M.A. (1991) Chemopreventive efficacy of a betel leaf extract against benzo[a]pyrene-induced forestomach tumors in mice. *J. Ethnopharmacol.*, **34**, 207–213

Bhisey, R.A., Ramchandani, A.G., D'Souza, A.V., Borges, A.M. & Notani, P.N. (1999) Long-term carcinogenicity of pan masala in Swiss mice. *Int. J. Cancer*, **83**, 679–684

Bhurgri Y. (2001) History of cancer registration in Pakistan. *Asian Pacific J. Cancer Prev.*, **2** (IACR Suppl.), 51–54

Bolton, J.L., Valerio, L.G., Jr & Thompson, J.A. (1992) The enzymatic formation and chemical reactivity of quinone methides correlate with alkylphenol-induced toxicity in rat hepatocytes. *Chem. Res. Toxicol.*, **5**, 816–822

Boonyaphiphat, P., Thongsuksai, P., Sriplung, H. & Puttawibul, P. (2002) Lifestyle habits and genetic susceptibility and the risk of esophageal cancer in the Thai population. *Cancer Lett.*, **186**, 193–199

Borle, R.M. & Gupta, D.S. (1987) Fungal contamination of arecanut. *Indian J. Pathol. Microbiol.*, **30**, 357–360

Boucher, B.J. & Mannan, N. (2002) Metabolic effects of the consumption of Areca catechu. *Addict. Biol.*, **7**, 103–110

Boucher, B.J., Ewen, S.W.B. & Stowers, J.M. (1994) Betel nut (*Areca catechu*) consumption and the induction of glucose intolerance in adult CD1 mice and in their F1 and F2 offspring. *Diabetologia*, **37**, 49–55

Boucher, B.J., Mannan, N., Noonan, K., Hales, C.N. & Evans, S.J.W. (1995) Glucose intolerance and impairment of insulin secretion in relation to vitamin D deficiency in East London Asians. *Diabetologia*, **38**, 1239–1245

Boyland, E. & Nery, R. (1969) Mercapturic acid formation during the metabolism of arecoline and arecaidine in the rat. *Biochem. J.*, **113**, 123–130

Bravo, L. (1998) Polyphenols: Chemistry, dietary sources, metabolism, and nutritional significance. *Nutr. Rev.*, **56**, 317–333

Buch, S.C., Notani, P.N. & Bhisey, R.A. (2002) Polymorphism at *GSTM1*, *GSTM3* and *GSTT1* gene loci and susceptibility to oral cancer in an Indian population. *Carcinogenesis*, **23**, 803–807

Budhy, T.I., Soenarto, S.D., Yaacob, H.B. & Ngeow, W.C. (2001) Changing incidence of oral and maxillofacial tumours in East Java, Indonesia, 1987–1992. Part 2: Malignant tumours. *Br. J. oral maxillofac. Surg.*, **39**, 460–464

Burt, A.D. (1993) C.L. Oakley Lecture 1993. Cellular and molecular aspects of hepatic fibrosis. *J. Pathol.*, **170**, 105–114

Burton-Bradley, B.G. (1977) Papua and New Guinea transcultural psychiatry: Some implications of betel chewing. In: Burton-Bradley, B.G., ed., *Some Aspects of South Pacific Ethnopsychiatry*, New Caledonia, South Pacific Commission, pp. 29–36

Burton-Bradley, B.G. (1978) Betel chewing in retrospect. *Papua New Guinea med. J.*, **21**, 236–241

Byun, S.-J., Kim, H.-S., Jeon, S.-M., Park, Y.B. & Choi, M.S. (2001) Supplementation of *Areca catechu* L. extracts alters triglyceride absorption and cholesterol metabolism in rats. *Ann. Nutr. Metab.*, **45**, 279–284

Caggiula, A.R., McAllister, C.G., Epstein, L.H., Antelman, S.M., Knopf, S., Saylor, S. & Perkins, K.A. (1992) Nicotine suppresses the proliferative response of peripheral blood lymphocytes in rats. *Drug Dev. Res.*, **26**, 473–479

Calmels, S., Ohshima, H. & Bartsch, H. (1988) Nitrosamine formation by denitrifying and non-denitrifying bacteria: Implication of nitrite reductase and nitrate reductase in nitrosation catalysis. *J. gen. Microbiol.*, **134**, 221–226

Canniff, J.P. & Harvey, W. (1981) The aetiology of oral submucous fibrosis: The stimulation of collagen synthesis by extracts of areca nut. *Int. J. oral Surg.*, **10** (Suppl. 1), 163–167

Canniff, J.P., Harvey, W. & Harris, M. (1986) Oral submucous fibrosis: Its pathogenesis and management. *Br. dent. J.*, **160**, 429–434

Carley, K.W., Puttaiah, R., Alvarez, J.O., Heimburger, D.C. & Anantha, N. (1994) Diet and oral premalignancy in female south Indian tobacco and betel chewers: A case–control study. *Nutr. Cancer*, **22**, 73–84

Carossa, S., Pera, P., Doglio, P., Lombardo, S., Colagrande, P., Brussino, L., Rolla, G. & Bucca, C. (2001) Oral nitric oxide during plaque deposition. *Eur. J. clin. Invest.*, **31**, 876–879

Cawte, J. (1985) Psychoactive substances in the South seas: Betel, kava, and pituri. *Aust. N.Z. J. Psychiat.*, **19**, 83–87

Chakrabarti, R.N., Dutta, K., Ghosh, K. & Sikdar, S. (1990) Uterine cervical dysplasia with reference to the betel quid chewing habit. *Eur. J. Gynaecol. Oncol.*, **11**, 57–59

Chakradeo, P.P., Nair, J. & Bhide, S.V. (1994) Endogenous formation of N-nitrosoproline and other N-nitrosamino acids in tobacco users. *Cancer Lett.*, **86**, 187–194

Chakravarti, N., Mathur, M., Bahadur, S., Shukla, N.K., Rochette-Egly, C. & Ralhan, R. (2001) Expression of RARα and RARβ in human oral potentially malignant and neoplastic lesions. *Int. J. Cancer*, **91**, 27–31

Chakravarti, N., Mathur, M., Bahadur, S., Kumar Shukla, N. & Ralhan, R. (2003) Retinoic acid receptor-alpha as a prognostic indicator in oral squamous cell carcinoma. *Int. J. Cancer*, **103**, 544–549

Chan, J.M., Rimm, E.B., Colditz, G.A., Stampfer, M.J. & Willett, W.C. (1994) Obesity, fat distribution, and weight gain as risk factors for clinical diabetes in men. *Diabetes Care*, **17**, 961–969

Chandra, A. (1962) Different habits and their relation with cancer cheek. *Chittaranjan Cancer Hosp. Calcutta natl. Cancer Res. Centre Bull.*, 33–36

Chang, K.-M. (1964) Betel nut chewing and mouth cancer in Taiwan. First report: Survey of disposition of mouth cancer in Taiwan. *J. Formosan med. Assoc.*, **63**, 437–448

Chang, K.-W., Chang, C.-S., Lai, K.-S., Chou, M.-J. & Choo, K.-B. (1989) High prevalence of human papilloma virus infection and possible association with betel quid chewing and smoking in oral epidermoid carcinomas in Taiwan. *J. med. Virol.*, **28**, 57–61

Chang, Y.-S., Lin, T.-J., Tsai, C.-N., Shu, C.-H., Tsai, M.-S., Choo, K.-B. & Liu, S.-T. (1992) Detection of mutations in the p53 gene in human head and neck carcinomas by single strand conformation polymorphism analysis. *Cancer Lett.*, **67**, 167–174

Chang, M.-C., Kuo, M.Y.-P., Hahn, L.-J., Hsieh, C.-C., Lin, S.-K. & Jeng, J.-H. (1998) Areca nut extract inhibits the growth, attachment, and matrix protein synthesis of cultured human gingival fibroblasts. *J. Periodontol.*, **69**, 1092–1097

Chang, Y.C., Tai, K.W., Cheng, M.H., Chou, L.S.S. & Chou, M.Y. (1998) Cytotoxic and non-genotoxic effects of arecoline on human buccal fibroblasts *in vitro*. *J. oral Pathol. Med.*, **27**, 68–71

Chang, M.C., Ho, Y.S., Lee, P.H., Chan, C.P., Lee, J.J., Hahn, L.J., Wang, Y.J. & Jeng, J.H. (2001) Areca nut extract and arecoline induced the cell cycle arrest but not apoptosis of cultured oral KB epithelial cells: Association of glutathione, reactive oxygen species and mitochondrial membrane potential. *Carcinogenesis*, **22**, 1527–1535

Chang, Y.-C., Hu, C.-C., Tseng, T.-H., Tai, K.-W., Lii, C.-K. & Chou, M.-Y. (2001a) Synergistic effects of nicotine on arecoline-induced cytotoxicity in human buccal mucosal fibroblasts. *J. oral Pathol. Med.*, **30**, 458–464

Chang, Y.-C., Lii, C.-K., Tai, K.-W. & Chou, M.-Y. (2001b) Adverse effects of arecoline and nicotine on human periodontal ligament fibroblasts in vitro. *J. clin. Periodontol.*, **28**, 277–282

Chang, K.-C., Su, I.-J., Tsai, S.-T., Shieh, D.-B. & Jin, T.-T. (2002) Pathological features of betel quid-related oral epithelial lesions in Taiwan with special emphasis on the tumor progression and human papillomavirus association. *Oncology*, **63**, 362–369

Chang, K.-W., Kao, S.-Y., Tzeng, R.-J., Liu, C.-J., Cheng, A.-J., Yang, S.-C., Wong, Y.-K. & Lin, S.-C. (2002) Multiple molecular alterations of *FHIT* in betel-associated oral carcinoma. *J. Pathol.*, **196**, 300–306

Chang, M.C., Uang, B.J., Wu, H.L., Lee, J.J., Hahn, L.J. & Jeng, J.H. (2002a) Inducing the cell cycle arrest and apoptosis of oral KB carcinoma cells by hydroxychavicol: Roles of glutathione and reactive oxygen species. *Br. J. Pharmacol.*, **135**, 619–630

Chang, M.C., Ho, Y.S., Lee, J.J., Kok, S.H., Hahn, L.J. & Jeng, J.H. (2002b) Prevention of the areca nut extract-induced unscheduled DNA synthesis of gingival keratinocytes by vitamin C and thiol compounds. *Oral Oncol.*, **38**, 258–265

Chang, M.J.W., Ko, C.Y., Lin, R.F. & Hsieh, L.L. (2002) Biological monitoring of environment exposure to safrole and the Taiwanese betel quid chewing. *Arch. environ. Contam. Toxicol.*, **43**, 432–437

Chang, Y.-C., Yang, S.-F., Tai, K.-W., Chou, M.-Y. & Hsieh, Y.-S. (2002a) Increased tissue inhibitor of metalloproteinase-1 expression and inhibition of gelatinase A activity in buccal mucosal fibroblasts by arecoline as possible mechanisms for oral submucous fibrosis. *Oral Oncol.*, **38**, 195–200

Chang, Y.-C., Tsai, C.-H., Tai, K.-W., Yang, S.-H., Chou, M.-Y. & Lii, C.-K. (2002b) Elevated vimentin expression in buccal mucosal fibroblasts by arecoline *in vitro* as a possible pathogenesis for oral submucous fibrosis. *Oral Oncol.*, **38**, 425–430

Chatterjee, A. & Deb, S. (1999) Genotoxic effect of arecoline given either by peritoneal or oral route in murine bone marrow cells and the influence of *N*-acetylcysteine. *Cancer Lett.*, **139**, 23–31

Chauhan, R. (2000) *The Sale of Pan and Smokeless Tobacco Products (Betel Quid, Gutka) within Greater London and Pattern of Consumption amongst a Minority Asian Community Residing in London*, MSc Thesis, London, University of London

Chempakan, B. (1993) Hypoglycaemic activity of arecoline in betel nut *Areca catechu* L. *Indian J. exp. Biol.*, **31**, 474–475

Chen, J.W. & Shaw, J.H. (1996) A study on betel quid chewing behavior among Kaohsiung residents aged 15 years and above. *J. oral Pathol. Med.*, **25**, 140–143

Cheng, Y.-A. & Tsai, C.-C. (1999) Nicotine- and arecoline-induced interleukin-1 secretion and intercellular adhesion molecular-1 expression in human oral epidermoid carcinoma cells in vitro. *Arch. oral Biol.*, **44**, 843–851

Chen, H.-C., Chang, Y.-S. & Lee, T.-C. (1984) The mutagenicity of nitrite-treated aqueous extract of *Piper betle* L. *Proc. natl Sci. Counc. Repub. China B*, **8**, 4–10

Chen, S.J., Wu, B.N., Yeh, J.L., Lo, Y.C., Chen, I.S. & Chen, I.J. (1995) C-fiber evoked autonomic cardiovascular effects after injection of *Piper betle* inflorescence extracts. *J. Ethnopharmacol.*, **45**, 183–188

Chen, C.-L., Chi, C.-W., Chang, K.-W. & Liu, T.-Y. (1999) Safrole-like DNA adducts in oral tissue from oral cancer patients with a betel quid chewing history. *Carcinogenesis*, **20**, 2331–2334

Chen, C.-L., Chi, C.-W. & Liu, T.-Y. (2000) Enhanced hydroxychavicol-induced cytotoxic effects in glutathione-depleted HepG2 cells. *Cancer Lett.*, **155**, 29–35

Chen, K.T., Chen, C.J., Fagot-Campagna, A. & Narayan, K.M. (2001) Tobacco, betel quid, alcohol, and illicit drug use among 13- to 35-year-olds in I-Lan, rural Taiwan: Prevalence and risk factors. *Am. J. Public Health*, **91**, 1130–1134

Chen, C.-L., Chi, C.-W. & Liu, T.-Y. (2002) Hydroxyl radical formation and oxidative DNA damage induced by areca quid in vivo. *J. Toxicol. environ. Health*, **A65**, 327–336

Chen, P.C., Kuo, C., Pan, C.C. & Chou, M.Y. (2002) Risk of oral cancer associated with human papillomavirus infection, betel quid chewing, and cigarette smoking in Taiwan — An integrated molecular and epidemiological study of 58 cases. *J. Oral Pathol. Med.*, **31**, 317–322

Cheng, Y.-A., Shiue, L.-F., Yu, H.-S., Hsieh, T.-Y. & Tsai, C.-C. (2000) Interleukin-8 secretion by cultured oral epidermoid carcinoma cells induced with nicotine and/or arecoline treatments. *Kaoshiung J. med. Sci.*, **16**, 126–133

Cheong, Y.H. (1984) The fading links between tradition and oral health in Singapore. *Int. dent. J.*, **34**, 253–256

Chiang, C.-P., Huang, J.-S., Wang, J.-T., Liu, B.-Y., Kuo, Y.-S., Hahn, L.-J. & Kuo, M.Y.-P. (1999) Expression of p53 protein correlates with decreased survival in patients with areca quid chewing and smoking-associated oral squamous cell carcinomas in Taiwan. *J. oral Pathol. Med.*, **28**, 72–76

Chiang, C.-P., Lang, M.-J., Liu, B.-Y., Wang, J.-T., Leu, J.-S., Hahn, L.-J. & Kuo, M.Y.-P. (2000a) Expression of p53 protein in oral submucous fibrosis, oral epithelial hyperkeratosis, and oral epithelial dysplasia. *J. Formos. med. Assoc.*, **99**, 229–234

Chiang, C.P., Lang, M.J., Liu, B.Y., Wang, J.T., Leu, J.S., Hahn, L.J. & Kuo, M.Y.P. (2000b) Expression of proliferating cell nuclear antigen (PCNA) in oral submucous fibrosis, oral epithelial hyperkeratosis and oral epithelial dysplasia in Taiwan. *Oral Oncol.*, **36**, 353–359

Chiang, C.P., Hsieh, R.P., Chen, T.H.H., Chang, Y.F., Liu, B.Y., Wang, J.T., Sun, A. & Kuo, M.Y.P. (2002a) High incidence of autoantibodies in Taiwanese patients with oral submucous fibrosis. *J. oral Pathol. Med.*, **31**, 402–409

Chiang, C.P., Wu, H.Y., Liu, B.Y., Wang, J.T. & Kuo, M.Y.P. (2002b) Quantitiative analysis of immunocompetent cells in oral submucous fibrosis in Taiwan. *Oral Oncol.*, **38**, 56–63

Chiba, I., Muthumala, M., Yamazaki, Y., Uz Zaman, A., Iizuka, T., Amemiya, A., Shibata, T., Kashiwazaki, H., Sugiura, C. & Fukuda, H. (1998) Characteristics of mutations in the *p53* gene of oral squamous-cell carcinomas associated with betel-quid chewing in Sri Lanka. *Int. J. Cancer*, **77**, 839–842

Chin, C.T. & Lee, K.W. (1970) The effects of betel-nut chewing on the buccal mucosa of 296 Indians and Malays in West Malaysia. A clinical study. *Br. J. Cancer*, **24**, 427–432

Chiu, C.-J., Chang, M.-L., Chiang, C.-P., Hahn, L.-J., Hsieh, L.-L. & Chen, C.-J. (2002) Interaction of collagen-related genes and susceptibility to betel quid-induced oral submucous fibrosis. *Cancer Epidemiol. Biomarkers Prev.*, **11**, 646–653

Chong, M.-Y., Chan, K.-W. & Cheng, A.T.A. (1999) Substance use disorders among adolescents in Taiwan: Prevalence, sociodemographic correlates and psychiatric co-morbidity. *Psych. Med.*, **29**, 1387–1396

Choonoo, A.G. (1967) *Indentured Indian Immigration into Natal 1860–1911 with Particular Reference to its Role in the Development of the Natal Sugar Industry*, MA Thesis, Durban, University of Natal, p. 27

Choudhary, D. & Kale, R.K. (2002) Antioxidant and non-toxic properties of *Piper betle* leaf extract: *In vitro* and *in vivo* studies. *Phytother. Res.*, **16**, 461–466

Chu, N.-S. (1993) Cardiovascular responses to betel chewing. *J. Formos. med. Assoc.*, **92**, 835–837

Chu, N.-S. (1994) Effects of betel chewing on electroencephalographic activity: Spectral analysis and topographic mapping. *J. Formos. med. Assoc.*, **93**, 167–169

Chu, N.S. (1995a) Sympathetic response to betel chewing. *J. psychoact. Drugs*, **27**, 183–186

Chu, N.S. (1995b) Effect of betel chewing on RR interval variation. *J. Formos. med. Assoc.*, **94**, 106–110

Chu, N.-S. (2001) Effects of betel chewing on the central and autonomic nervous systems. *J. biomed. Sci.*, **8**, 229–236

Chu, N.-S. (2002) Neurological aspects of areca and betel chewing. *Addict. Biol.*, **7**, 111–114

Cooke, R.A. (1969) Verrucous carcinoma of the oral mucosa in Papua-New Guinea. *Cancer*, **24**, 397–402

Council of Agriculture, ROC (2003) Available at [http://stat.cora.gov.tw/dba_as/english/as_root.htm] under *4. Agricultural Production, Quantity of Major Agricultural Production, Crops, d. Fruits*

Council of the European Communities (2001) Directive 2001/37/EC of the European Parliament and of the Council of 5 June 2001 on the approximation of the laws, regulations and administrative provisions of the Member States concerning the manufacture, presentation and sale of tobacco products. *Off. J. Eur. Communities*, **L194**, 26–34

Council of the Pharmaceutical Society of Great Britain (1911) *The British Pharmaceutical Codex, 1911*, London, The Pharmaceutical Press; available at [http://www.ibiblio.org/herbmed/eclectic/bpc/1911/main.html]

Cox, S.C. & Walker, D.M. (1996) Epithelial growth fraction and expression of p53 tumour suppressor gene in oral submucous fibrosis. *Aust. dent. J.*, **41**, 91–96

Croucher, R. & Islam, S. (2002) Socio-economic aspects of areca nut use. *Addict. Biol.*, **7**, 139–146

Daftary, D.K., Bhonsle, R.B., Murti, R.B., Pindborg, J.J. & Mehta, F.S. (1980) An oral lichen planus-like lesion in Indian betel-tobacco chewers. *Scand. J. dent. Res.*, **88**, 244–249

Dar, A. & Khatoon, S. (2000) Behavioral and biochemical studies of dichloromethane fraction from the *Areca catechu* nut. *Pharmacol. Biochem. Behav.*, **65**, 1–6

Dave, B.J., Trivedi, A.H. & Adhvaryu, S.G. (1991) Cytogenetic studies reveal increased genomic damage among 'pan masala' consumers. *Mutagenesis*, **6**, 159–163

Dave, B.J., Trivedi, A.H. & Adhvaryu, S.G. (1992a) Role of areca nut consumption in the cause of oral cancers: A cytogenetic assessment. *Cancer*, **70**, 1017–1023

Dave, B.J., Trivedi, A.H. & Adhvaryu, S.G. (1992b) In vitro genotoxic effects of areca nut extract and arecoline. *Cancer Res. clin. Oncol.*, **118**, 283–288

Davis, G.G. (1915) Buyo cheek cancer with special reference to etiology. *J. Am. med. Assoc.*, **64**, 711–718

Dayal, P.K., Mani, N.J. & Bhargava, K. (1978) Prevalence of oral cancer and precancerous lesions in 'pan'/'supari' chewers. *Indian J. publ. Health*, **22**, 234–245

De Costa, C. & Griew, A.R. (1982) Effects of betel chewing on pregnancy outcome. *Aust. N.Z. J. Obstet. Gynaecol.*, **22**, 22–24

Deahl, M. (1989) Betel nut-induced extrapyramidal syndrome: An unusual drug interaction. *Mov. Disord.*, **4**, 330–333

Deb, S. & Chatterjee, A. (1998) Influence of buthionine sulfoximine and reduced glutathione on arecoline-induced chromosomal damage and sister chromatid exchange in mouse bone marrow cells *in vivo*. *Mutagenesis*, **13**, 243–248

Deng, J.-F., Ger, J., Tsai, W.-J., Kao, W.-F. & Yang, C.-C. (2001) Acute toxicities of betel nut: Rare but probably overlooked events. *J. Toxicol. clin. Toxicol.*, **39**, 355–360

Desai, S.S., Ghaisas, S.D., Jakhi, S.D. & Bhide, S.V. (1996) Cytogenetic damage in exfoliated oral mucosal cells and circulating lymphocytes of patients suffering from precancerous oral lesions. *Cancer Lett.*, **109**, 9–14

Dikshit, R.P. & Kanhere, S. (2000) Tobacco habits and risk of lung, oropharyngeal and oral cavity cancer: A population-based case–control study in Bhopal, India. *Int. J. Epidemiol.*, **29**, 609–614

Dockrat, I. & Shear, M. (1969) Oral submucous fibrosis in Natal. In: Cahn, L., ed., *Fourth Proceedings of the International Academy of Oral Pathology*, New York, Gordon & Breach, pp. 57–63

Donaldson, L.J. & Clayton, D.G. (1984) Occurrence of cancer in Asians and non-Asians. *J. Epidemiol. Commmunity Health*, **38**, 203–207

Dunham, L.J. & Herrold, K.M. (1962) Failure to produce tumors in the hamster cheek-pouch by exposure to ingredients of betel quid; Histopathologic changes in the pouch and other organs by exposure to known carcinogens. *J. natl Cancer Inst.*, **29**, 1047–1067

Dunham, L.J., Muir, C.S. & Hamner, J.E., III (1966) Epithelial atypia in hamster cheek-pouches treated repeatedly with calcium hydroxide. *Br. J. Cancer*, **20**, 588–593

Dunham, L.J., Sheets, R.H. & Morton, J.F. (1974) Proliferative lesions in cheek-pouch and esophagus of hamsters treated with plants from Curaçao, Netherland Antilles. *J. natl Cancer Inst.*, **53**, 1259–1269

Dunham, L.J., Snell, K.C. & Stewart, H.L. (1975) Argyrophilic carcinoids in two Syrian hamsters *(Mesocricetus auratus)*. *J. natl Cancer Inst.*, **54**, 507–513

Dunn, B.P. & Stich, H.F. (1986) $^{32}$P-Postlabelling analysis of aromatic DNA adducts in human oral mucosal cells. *Carcinogenesis*, **7**, 1115–1120

Eisen, M. J. (1946) Betel chewing among natives of the Southwest Pacific Islands: Lack of carcinogenic action. *Cancer Res.*, **6**, 139–141

Ernst, H., Ohshima H., Bartsch, H., Mohr, U. & Reichart, P. (1987) Tumorigenicity study in Syrian hamsters fed areca nut together with nitrite. *Carcinogenesis*, **8**, 1843–1845

Fabunmi, R.P., Sukhova, G.K., Sugiyama, S. & Libby, P. (1998) Expression of tissue inhibitor of metalloproteinases-3 in human atheroma and regulation in lesion-associated cells: A potential protective mechanism in plaque stability. *Circ. Res.*, **83**, 270–278

FAO (2003) FAO *Statistical Databases: Agriculture*, available at [http://apps.fao.org/page/collections?subset=agriculture], under Crops Primary

Farago, C. (1963a) Review of 110 cases of cancer of oral cavity in Papua and New Guinea. *Br. med. J.*, **i**, 1264–1266

Farago, C. (1963b) Report of 1160 registered tumor cases in Papua and New Guinea. *Cancer*, **16**, 670–680

Farrand, P., Rowe, R.M., Johnston, A. & Murdoch, H. (2001) Prevalence, age of onset and demographic relationships of different areca nut habits amongst children in Tower Hamlets, London. *Br. dent. J.*, **190**, 150–154

Fells, A. (1908) Cancer of the mouth in southern India, with an analysis of 209 operations. *Br. med. J.*, **ii**, 1357–1358

Ferlay, J., Bray, F., Pisani, P. & Parkin, D.M. (2001) *Globocan 2000: Cancer Incidence, Mortality and Prevalence Worldwide, Version 1.0. IARC CancerBase No. 5*, Lyon, IARCPress

Forlen, H.P., Hornstein, O. & Stüttgen, G. (1965) Betel quid and leukoplakia. *Arch. klin. exp. Dermatol.*, **221**, 463–480 (in German)

Frewer, L.J. (1990) The effect of betel nut on human performance. *Papua New Guinea med. J.*, **33**, 143–145

Furatado, C.X. (1933) The limits of the genus *Areca Linn* and its section. *Fedde's Repertor. Spec. Navar. Regn. Veget.*, **33**, 217–239

Gajalakshmi, C.K. & Shanta, V. (1996) Lifestyle and risk of stomach cancer: A hospital-based case–control study. *Int. J. Epidemiol.*, **25**, 1146–1153

Gajalakshmi, V., Hung, R.J., Mathew, A., Varghese, C., Brennan, P. & Boffetta, P. (2003) Tobacco smoking and chewing, alcohol drinking and lung cancer risk among men in southern India. *Int. J. Cancer*, **107**, 441–447

Galis, Z.S., Sukhova, G.K., Lark, M.W. & Libby, P. (1994) Increased expression of matrix metalloproteinases and matrix degrading activity in vulnerable regions of atherosclerotic plaques. *J. clin. Invest.*, **94**, 2493–2503

Gan, C. (1998) Tobacco usage among rural Bajaus in Sabah, Malaysia. *Southeast Asian J. trop. Med. Public Health*, **29**, 643–648

Gandagule, V.N. & Agarwal, S. (1969) Oral and pharyngeal cancer in Madhya Pradesh. *J. Indian med. Assoc.*, **53**, 582–585

Gao, Y.J., Yin, X.M. & Wu, H.J. (2001) [Relationship between vertical root fracture and the habits of chewing betel nut.] *Hunan Yi Ke Da Xue Xue Bao*, **26**, 161–162 (in Chinese)

Geng, Y., Savage, S.M., Johnson, L.J. Seagrave, J. & Sopori, M.L. (1995) Effects of nicotine on immune response: I. Chronic exposure to nicotine impairs antigen receptor-mediated signal transduction in lymphocytes. *Toxicol. appl. Pharmacol.*, **135**, 268–278

Geng, Y. Savage, S.M., Razani-Boroujerdi, S. & Sopori, M.L. (1996) Effects of nicotine on the immune response: II. Chronic nicotine treatment induces T cell anergy. *J. Immunol.*, **156**, 2384–2390

George, A., Varghese, C., Sankaranarayanan, R. & Nair, M.K. (1994) Use of tobacco and alcoholic beverages by children and teenagers in a low-income coastal community in South India. *J. Cancer Educ.*, **9**, 111–113

Gerry, R.G., Smith, S.T. & Calton, M.L. (1952) The oral characteristics of Guamanians including the effects of betel chewing on the oral tissues. Part I. Part II. Diseases of the oral mucous membranes and dental supporting tissues in Guamanians. Part III. *Oral Surg.*, **5**, 762–781, 884–894, 1004–1011

Ghaisas, S.D. & Bhide, S.V. (1994) In vitro studies on chemoprotective effect of Purnark against benzo(a)pyrene-induced chromosomal damage in human lymphocytes. *Cell Biol. int.*, **18**, 21–27

Gilani, A.H., Aziz, N., Khurran, I.M., Rao, Z.A. & Ali, N.K. (2000) The presence of cholinomimetic and calcium channel antagonist constituents in *Piper betle* Linn. *Phytother. Res.*, **14**, 436–442

Giri, A.K., Banerjee, T.S., Talukder, G. & Sharma, A. (1987) Induction of sister chromatid exchange and dominant lethal mutation by 'Katha' (catechu) in male mice. *Cancer Lett.*, **36**, 189–196

Gopalan, C., Rama Sastri, B.V., Balasubramanian, S.C., Narasinga Rao, B.S., Deosthale, Y.G. & Pant, K.C. (1989) *Nutritive Value of Indian Foods*, Hyderabad, Indian Council of Medical Research, National Institute of Nutrition

Gothoskar, S.V. & Pai, S.R. (1986) A study on parotid gland tumor induced in Swiss mice by tanin containing fraction of betelnut. *Indian J. exp. Biol.*, **24**, 229–231

Goto, H., Tanaka, N., Tanigawa, K., Shimada, Y., Itoh, T. & Terasawa, K. (1997) Endothelium dependent vasodilator effect of extract prepared from seeds of Areca catechu on isolated rat aorta. *Phytother. Res.*, **11**, 457–459

Govekar, R.B. & Bhisey, R.A. (1993) Mutagenic activity in urine samples from female tobacco habitues. *Cancer Lett.*, **69**, 75–80

Gupta, D.S., Gupta, M. & Oswal, R.H. (1985) Estimation of major immunoglobulin profile in oral submucous fibrosis by radial immunodiffusion. *Int. J. oral Surg.*, **14**, 533–537

Gupta, P.C. (1984) A study of dose–response relationship between tobacco habits and oral leukoplakia. *Br. J. Cancer*, **50**, 527–531

Gupta, P.C. (1996) Survey of sociodemographic characteristics of tobacco use among 99 598 individuals in Bombay, India using handheld computers. *Tob. Control*, **5**, 114–120

Gupta, P.C. (1999) Mouth cancer in India: A new epidemic? *J. Indian med. Assoc.*, **97**, 370–373

Gupta, P.C. & Ray, C.S. (2002) Tobacco and youth in the South East Asian region. *Indian J. Cancer*, **39**, 5–34

Gupta, P.C. & Warnakulasuriya, S. (2002) Global epidemiology of areca nut usage. *Addict. Biol.*, **7**, 77–83

Gupta, P.C., Mehta, F.S., Daftary, D.K., Pindborg, J.J., Bhonsle, R.B., Jalnawalla, P.N., Sinor, P.N., Pitkar, V.K., Murti, P.R., Irani, R.R., Shah, H.T., Kadam, P.M., Iyer, K.S.S., Iyer, H.M., Hegde, A.K., Chandrashekar, G.K., Shroff, B.C., Sahiar, B.E. & Mehta, M.N. (1980) Incidence rates of oral cancer and natural history of oral precancerous lesions in a 10-year follow-up study of Indian villagers. *Community Dent. Oral Epidemiol.*, **8**, 283–333

Gupta, P.C., Aghi, M.B., Bhonsle, R.B., Murti, P.R., Mehta, F.S., Mehta, C.R. & Pindborg, J.J. (1986) An intervention study of tobacco chewing and smoking habits for primary prevention of oral cancer among 12 212 Indian villagers. In: Zaridze, D.G. & Peto, R., eds, *Tobacco: A Major International Health Hazard* (IARC Scientific Publications No. 74), Lyon, IARC*Press*, pp. 307–318

Gupta, P.C., Bhonsle, R.B., Murti, P.R., Daftary, D.K., Mehta, F.S. & Pindborg, J.J. (1989) An epidemiologic assessment of cancer risk in oral precancerous lesions in India with special reference to nodular leukoplakia. *Cancer*, **63**, 2247–2252

Gupta, P.C., Murti, P.R., Bhonsle, R.B., Mehta, F.S. & Pindborg, J.J. (1995) Effect of cessation of tobacco use on the incidence of oral mucosal lesions in a 10-year follow-up study of 12,212 users. *Oral Dis.*, **1**, 54–58

Gupta, P.C., Bhonsle, R.B. & Murti, P.R. (1997) Oral mucosal lesions related to betel-quid chewing — An epidemiologic assessment from a 10-year follow-up study of 12,212 individuals in Ernakulam district, Kerala, India. *Dent. J. Malaysia*, **18**, 38–42

Gupta, P.C., Sinor, P.N., Bhonsle, R.B., Pawar, V.S. & Mehta, H.C. (1998) Oral submucous fibrosis in India: A new epidemic? *Natl med. J. India*, **11**, 113–116

Hada, S., Kakiuchi, N., Hattori, M. & Namba, T. (1989) Identification of antibacterial principles against *Streptococcus mutans* and inhibitory principles against glucosyltransferase from the seed of *Areca catechu* L. *Phytother. Res.*, **3**, 140–144

Hafström, O. Milerad, J. & Sundell, H.W. (2002) Prenatal nicotine exposure blunts the cardiorespiratory response to hypoxia in lambs. *Am. J. respir. crit. Care Med.*, **166**, 1544–1549

Hamner, J.E., III (1972) Betel quid inducement of epithelial atypia in the buccal mucosa of baboons. *Cancer*, **30**, 1001–1005

Haque, M.F., Harris, M., Meghji, S. & Speight, P.M. (1997) An immunohistochemical study of oral submucous fibrosis. *J. oral Pathol. Med.*, **26**, 75–82

Harvey, W., Scutt, A., Meghji, S. & Canniff, J.P. (1986) Stimulation of human buccal mucosa fibroblasts in vitro by betel-nut alkaloids. *Arch. oral Biol.*, **31**, 45–49

Hashibe, M., Sankaranarayanan, R., Thomas, G., Kuruvilla, B., Mathew, B., Somanathan, T., Parkin, D.M. & Zhang, Z.F. (2000a) Alcohol drinking, body mass index and the risk of oral leukoplakia in an Indian population. *Int. J. Cancer*, **88**, 129–134

Hashibe, M., Mathew, B., Kuruvilla, B., Thomas, G., Sankaranarayanan, R., Parkin, D.M. & Zhang, Z.F. (2000b) Chewing tobacco, alcohol and the risk of erythroplakia. *Cancer Epidemiol. Biomarkers Prev.*, **9**, 639–645

Hashibe, M., Sankaranarayanan, R., Thomas, G., Kuruvilla, B., Mathew, B., Somanathan, T., Parkin, D.M. & Zhang, Z.F. (2002) Body mass index, tobacco chewing, alcohol drinking, and the risk of oral submucous fibrosis in Kerala, India. *Cancer Causes Control*, **13**, 55–64

Hashibe, M., Jacob, B.J., Thomas, G., Ramadas, K., Mathew, B., Sankaranarayanan, R. & Zhang, Z.F. (2003) Socioeconomic status, lifestyle factors and oral premalignant lesions. *Oral Oncol.*, **39**, 664–671

Hayes, P.A. (1985) Oral submucous fibrosis in a 4-year-old girl. *Oral Surg. oral Med. oral Pathol.*, **59**, 475–478

Hayes, M.J., Khemani, L., Bax, M. & Alkalay, D. (1989) Quantitative determination of arecoline in plasma by gas chromatography chemical ionization mass spectrometry. *Biomed. environ. mass Spectrom.*, **18**, 1005–1009

Hazare, V.K., Goel, R.R. & Gupta, P.C. (1998) Oral submucous fibrosis, areca nut and pan masala use: A case–control study. *Natl med. J. India*, **11**, 299

Health Canada (1995) *Herbs Used as Non-medicinal Ingredients in Nonprescription Drugs for Human Use*; available at [www.hc-sc.gc.ca/hpfb-dgpsa/tpd-dpt/herbnmi_c/html]

Heinzel, P.A., Balaram, P. & Bernard, H.U. (1996) Mutations and polymorphisms in the *p53*, *p21* and *p16* genes in oral carcinomas of Indian betel quid chewers. *Int. J. Cancer*, **68**, 420–423

Henderson, B.E. & Aiken, G.H. (1979) Cancer in Papua-New Guinea. *Natl. Cancer Inst. Monogr.* **53**, 67–72

Higdon, J.V. & Frei, B. (2003) Tea catechins and polyphenols: Health effects, metabolism, and antioxidant functions. *Crit. Rev. Food Sci. Nutr.*, **43**, 89–143

Hirayama, T. (1966) An epidemiological study of oral and pharyngeal cancer in central and South-East Asia. *Bull. World Health Organization*, **34**, 41–69

Ho, C.S., Gee, M.J., Tsai, C.C., Lo, C.I. & Hwang, M.N. (2000a) Factors related to betel chewing among junior high school students in Taiwan. *Community Dent. oral Epidemiol.*, **28**, 150–154

Ho, C.S., Gee, M.J., Tsai, C.C., Lo, C.I. & Hwang, M.N. (2000b) The prevalence of betel chewing among the students of the different senior high schools in southern Taiwan. *Kaohsiung. J. Med. Sci.*, **16**, 32–38

Ho, T.-J., Chiang, C.-P., Hong, C.-Y., Kok, S.-H., Kuo, Y.-S. & Kuo, M.Y.-P. (2000) Induction of the c-*jun* protooncogene expression by areca nut extract and arecoline on oral mucosal fibroblasts. *Oral Oncol.*, **36**, 432–436

Ho, P.S., Ko, Y.C., Yang, Y.C., Shieh, T.Y. & Tsai, C.C. (2002) The incidence of oropharyngeal cancer in Taiwan: An endemic betel quid chewing area. *J. oral Pathol. Med.*, **31**, 213–219

Hogan, J. (2000) Tobacco products require redefining. *Br. dent. J.*, **188**, 61

Holdsworth, D.K., Jones, R.A. & Self, R. (1998) Volatile alkaloids from *Areca catechu*. *Phytochemistry*, **48**, 581–582

Howden, G.F. (1984) The cariostatic effect of betel nut chewing. *Papua New Guinea med. J.*, **27**, 123–131

Hsieh, L.-L., Wang, P.-F., Chen, I.-H., Liao, C.-T., Wang, H.-M., Chen, M.-C., Chang, J.T.-C. & Cheng, A.-J. (2001) Characteristics of mutations in the *p53* gene in oral squamous cell carcinoma associated with betel quid chewing and cigarette smoking in Taiwanese. *Carcinogenesis*, **22**, 1497–1503

Hsieh, L.-L., Chien, H.-T., Chen, I.-H., Liao, C.-T., Wang, H.-M., Jung, S.-M., Wang, P.-F., Chang, J.T.-C., Chen, M.-C. & Cheng, A.-J. (2003) The *XRCC1* 339Gln polymorphism and the frequency of *p53* mtuations in Taiwanese oral squamous cell carcinomas. *Cancer Epidemiol. Biomarkers Prev.*, **12**, 439–443

Hsu, H.-J, Chang, K.-L., Uang, Y.-H. & Shieh, T.-Y. (2001) The effects of arecoline on the release of cytokines using cultured peripheral blood mononuclear cells from patients with oral mucous diseases. *Kaohsiung J. med. Sci.*, **17**, 175–182

Huang, J.L. & McLeish, M.J. (1989) High-performance liquid chromatographic determination of the alkaloids in betel nut. *J. Chromatogr.*, **475**, 447–450

Huang, J.-S., Ho. T.-J., Chiang, C.-P., Kok, S.-H., Kuo, Y.-S. & Kuo, M.Y.-P. (2001) MDM2 expression in areca quid chewing-associated oral squamous cell carcinomas in Taiwan. *J. oral Pathol. Med.*, **30**, 53–58

Hung, C.-R. & Cheng, J.-T. (1994) Betel quid chewing damaged gastric mucosa: Protective effects of cimetidine and sodium bicarbonate. *Chin. J. Physiol.*, **37**, 213–218

Hung, D.-Z. & Deng, J.-F. (1998) Acute myocardial infarction temporally related to betel nut chewing. *Vet. hum. Toxicol.*, **40**, 25–28

Hung, H.-C., Chuang, J., Chien, Y.-C., Chern, H.-D., Chiang, C.-P., Kuo, Y.-S., Hildesheim, A. & Chen, C.-J. (1997) Genetic polymorphisms of CYP2E1, GSTM1, and GSTT1; environmental factors and risk of oral cancer. *Cancer Epidemiol. Biomarkers Prev.*, **6**, 901–905

Hung, S.-L., Chen, Y.-L., Wan, H.-C., Liu, T.-Y., Chen, Y.-T. & Ling, L.-J. (2000) Effects of areca nut extracts on the function of human neutrophils *in vitro. J. periodont. Res.*, **35**, 186–193

Huq, S.F. (1965) Some aspect of site distribution of cancer in East Pakistan. *J. Pak. med. Assoc.*, **15**, 237–245

Hwang, L.S., Wang, C.K., Sheu, M.J. & Kao, L.S. (1992) Phenolic compounds of *Piper betle* flower as flavoring and neuronal activity modulating agents. In: Ho, C.T., Lee, C.Y. & Huang, M.T., eds, *Phenolic Compounds in Food and their Effects on Health*, Vol. 1, *Analysis, Occurrence and Chemistry*, Washington DC, American Chemical Society, pp. 200–213

IARC (1976) *IARC Monographs on the Evaluation of the Carcinogenic Risk of Chemicals to Humans*, Vol. 10, *Some Naturally Occurring Substances*, Lyon, IARCPress

IARC (1985a) *IARC Monographs on the Evaluation of the Carcinogenic Risk of Chemicals to Humans*, Vol. 37, *Tobacco Habits Other than Smoking; Betel-Quid and Areca-nut Chewing; and Some Related Nitrosamines*, Lyon, IARCPress

IARC (1985b) *IARC Monographs on the Evaluation of the Carcinogenic Risk of Chemicals to Humans*, Vol. 36, *Allyl Compounds, Aldehydes, Epoxides and Peroxides*, Lyon, IARCPress, pp. 75–97

IARC (1986) *IARC Monographs on the Evaluation of the Carcinogenic Risk of Chemicals to Humans*, Vol. 40, *Some Naturally Occurring and Synthetic Food Components, Furocoumarins and Ultraviolet Radiation*, Lyon, IARCPress, pp. 123–159, 161–206

IARC (1987) *IARC Monographs on the Evaluation of the Carcinogenic Risks to Humans*, Suppl. 7, *Overall Evaluations of Carcinogenicity: An Updating of IARC Monographs Volumes 1 to 42*, Lyon, IARCPress, p. 63

IARC (2002) *IARC Monographs on the Evaluation of Carcinogenic Risks to Humans*, Vol. 82, *Some Traditional Herbal Medicines, Some Mycotoxins, Naphthalene and Styrene*, Lyon, IARCPress, pp. 171–274

IARC (2004) *IARC Monographs on the Evaluation of Carcinogenic Risks to Humans*, Vol. 83, *Tobacco Smoke and Involuntary Smoking*, Lyon, IARCPress

ICMR (Indian Council of Medical Research) (2001) *Consolidated Report of the Population Based Cancer Registries: Incidence and Distribution of Cancer: 1990–96*, National Cancer Registry Programme, New Delhi, pp 34–37

Ikeda, N., Handa, Y., Khim, S.P. Durward, C., Axéll, T., Mizuno, T., Fukano, H. & Kawai, T. (1995) Prevalence study of oral mucosal lesions in a selected Cambodian population. *Community dent. oral Epidemiol.*, **23**, 49–54

Inokuchi, J.-I., Okabe, H., Yamauchi, T., Nagamatsu, A., Nonaka, G.-I. & Nishioka, I. (1986) Antihypertensive substance in seeds of *Areca catechu* L. *Life Sci.*, **38**, 1375–1382

Iverson, S.L., Hu, L.Q., Vukomanovic, V. & Bolton, J.L. (1995) The influence of the *p*-alkyl substituent on the isomerization of *o*-quinones to *p*-quinone methides: Potential bioactivation mechanism for catechols. *Chem. Res. Toxicol.*, **8**, 537–544

Jafarey, N.A., Mahmood, Z. & Zaidi, S.H.M. (1977) Habits and dietary pattern of cases of carcinoma of the oral cavity and oropharynx. *J. Pak. med. Assoc.*, **27**, 340–343

Jaiswal, N., Jaiswal, R.K. & Malik, K.U. (1991) Muscarinic receptor-mediated prostacyclin and cGMP synthesis in cultured vascular cells. *Mol. Pharmacol.*, **40**, 101–106

Jaju, R.J., Patel, R.K., Bakshi, S.R., Trivedi, A.H., Dave, B.J. & Adhvaryu, S.G. (1992) Chromosome damaging effects of pan masala. *Cancer Lett.*, **65**, 221–226

Jamrozik, K. (1985) Regional variation of oral cancer in Papua New Guinea. *Papua New Guinea med. J.*, **28**, 9–13

Jayalakshmi, A. & Mathew, A.G. (1982) Chemical composition and processing. In: Bavappa, K.V.A., Nair, M.K. & Kumar, T.P., eds, *The Arecanut Palm*, Kerala, Central Plantation Crops Research Institute, pp. 225–244

Jayant, K., Balakrishnan, V., Sanghvi, L.D. & Jussawalla, D.J. (1977) Quantification of the role of smoking and chewing tobacco in oral, pharyngeal, and oesophageal cancers. *Br. J. Cancer*, **35**, 232–235

Jeng, J.H., Kuo, M.L., Hahn, L.J. & Kuo, M.Y.P. (1994a) Genotoxic and non-genotoxic effects of betel quid ingredients on oral mucosal fibroblasts *in vitro*. *J. dent. Res.*, **73**, 1043–1049

Jeng, J.H., Hahn, L.J., Lu, F.J., Wang, Y.J. & Kuo, M.Y.P. (1994b) Eugenol triggers different pathobiological effects on human oral mucosal fibroblasts. *J. dent. Res.*, **73**, 1050–1055

Jeng, J.H., Lan, W.H., Hahn, L.J., Hsieh, C.C. & Kuo, M.Y.P. (1996) Inhibition of the migration, attachment, spreading, growth and collagen synthesis of human gingival fibroblasts by arecoline, a major areca alkaloid, in vitro. *J. oral Pathol. Med.*, **25**, 371–375

Jeng, J.H., Tsai, C.L., Hahn, L.J., Yang, P.J., Kuo, S. & Kuo, M.Y.P. (1999a) Arecoline cytotoxicity on human oral mucosal fibroblasts related to cellular thiol and esterase activities. *Food. chem. Toxicol.*, **37**, 751–756

Jeng, J.-H., Hahn, L.-J., Lin, B.-R., Hsieh, C.-C., Chan, C.-P. & Chang, M.-C. (1999b) Effects of areca nut, inflorescence Piper betle extracts and arecoline on cytotoxicity, total and unscheduled DNA synthesis in cultured gingival keratinocytes. *J. oral Pathol. Med.*, **28**, 64–71

Jeng, J.H., Ho, Y.S., Chan, C.P., Wang, Y.J., Hahn, L.J., Lei, D., Hsu, C.C. & Chang, M.C. (2000) Areca nut extract up-regulates prostaglandin production, cyclooxygenase-2 mRNA and protein expression of human oral keratinocytes. *Carcinogenesis*, **21**, 1365–1370

Jeng, J.-H., Chen, S.-Y., Liao, C.-H., Tung, Y.-Y., Lin, B.-R., Hahn, L.-J. & Chang, M.-C. (2002) Modulation of platelet aggregation by areca nut and betel leaf ingredients: Role of reactive oxygen species and cyclooxygenase. *Free Rad. Biol. Med.*, **32**, 860–871

Jeng, J.-H., Wang, Y.-J., Chiang, B.-L., Lee, P.-H., Chan, C.-P., Ho, Y.-S., Wang, T.-M., Lee, J.-J., Hahn, L.-J. & Chang, M.-C. (2003) Roles of keratinocyte inflammation in oral cancer: Regulating the prostaglandin $E_2$, interleukin-6 and TNF-$\alpha$ production of oral epithelial cells by areca nut extract and arecoline. *Carcinogenesis*, **24**, 1301–1315

Jensen, G.D. & Polloi, A.H. (1988) The very old of Palau: Health and mental state. *Age Ageing*, **17**, 220–226

Jeon, S.-M., Kim, H.-S., Lee, T.-G., Ryu, S.-H., Suh, P.-G., Byun, S.-J., Park, Y.B. & Choi, M.-S. (2000) Lower absorption of cholesteryl oleate in rats supplemented with *Areca catechu* L. extract. *Ann. Nutr. Metab.*, **44**, 170–176

Jin, Y.T., Tsai, S.T., Wong, T.Y., Chen, F.F. & Chen, R.M. (1996) Studies on promoting activity of Taiwan betel quid ingredients in hamster buccal pouch carcinogenesis. *Eur. J. Cancer*, **32B**, 343–346

Johnson, J.D., Houchens, D.P., Kluwe, W.M., Craig, D.K. & Fisher, G.L. (1990) Effects of mainstream and environmental tobacco smoke on the immune system in animals and humans, a review. *Crit. Rev. Toxicol.*, **20**, 369–395

Johnston, G.A.R., Krogsgaard-Larsen, P. & Stephanson, A. (1975) Betel nut constituents as inhibitors of $\gamma$-aminobutyric acid uptake. *Nature*, **258**, 627–628

Joseph, K.C. & Sitaram, N. (1990) Topographical sleep EEG response to arecoline. *Psychiatry Res.*, **35**, 91–94

Jussawalla, D.J. & Deshpande, V.A. (1971) Evaluation of cancer risk in tobacco chewers and smokers: An epidemiologic assessment. *Cancer*, **28**, 244–252

Kai, H., Ikeda, H., Yasukawa, H., Kai, M., Seki, Y., Kuwahara, F., Ueno, T., Sugi, K. & Imaizumi, T. (1998) Peripheral blood levels of matrix metalloproteases-2 and -9 are elevated in patients with acute coronary syndromes. *J. Am. Coll. Cardiol.*, **32**, 368–372

Kalra, R., Singh, S.P., Savage, S.M., Finch, G.L. & Sopori, M.L. (2000) Effects of cigarette smoke on immune response: Chronic exposure to cigarette smoke impairs antigen-mediated signaling in T cells and depletes IP3-sensitive $Ca^{2+}$ stores. *J. Pharmacol. exp. Ther.*, **293**, 166–171

Kandarkar, S.V. & Sirsat, S.M. (1977) Changes in vitamin A conditioned hamster cheek pouch epithelium on exposure to commercial shell lime (calcium hydroxide) and tobacco. I. Optical histopathology. *J. oral Pathol.*, **6**, 191–202

Kao, S.-Y., Tu, H.-F., Chang, K.-W., Chang, C.-S., Yang, C.-C. & Lin, S.-C. (2002a) The retinoic acid receptor-β (RAR-β) mRNA expression in the oral squamous cell carcinoma associated with betel quid use. *J. oral Pathol. Med.*, **31**, 220–226

Kao, S.-Y., Wu, C.-H., Lin, S.-C., Yap, S.-K., Chang, C.-S., Wong, Y.-K., Chi, L.-Y. & Liu, T.-Y. (2002b) Genetic polymorphism of cytochrome P4501A1 and susceptibility to oral squamous cell carcinoma and oral precancer lesions associated with smoking/betel use. *J. oral Pathol. Med.*, **31**, 505–511

Kapadia, G.J., Chung, E.B., Ghosh, B., Shukla, Y.N., Basak, S.P., Morton, J.F. & Pradhan, S.N. (1978) Carcinogenicity of some folk medicinal herbs in rats. *J. natl Cancer Inst.*, **60**, 683–686

Kaur, J. & Ralhan, R. (1995) Differential expression of 70-kDa heat shock-protein in human oral tumorigenesis. *Int. J. Cancer*, **63**, 774–779

Kaur, J., Srivastava, A. & Ralhan, R. (1994) Overexpression of p53 protein in betel- and tobacco-related human oral dysplasia and squamous-cell carcinoma in India. *Int. J. Cancer*, **58**, 340–345

Kaur, J., Srivastava, A. & Ralhan, R. (1998a) Prognostic significance of p53 protein overexpression in betel- and tobacco-related oral oncogenesis. *Int. J. Cancer*, **79**, 370–375

Kaur, J., Srivastava, A. & Ralhan, R. (1998b) Expression of 70-kDa heat shock protein in oral lesions: Marker of biological stress or pathogenicity. *Oral Oncol.*, **34**, 496–501

Kayal, J.J., Trivedi, A.H., Dave, B.J., Nair, J., Nair, U.J., Bhide, S.V., Goswami, U.C. & Adhvaryu, S.G. (1993) Incidence of micronuclei in oral mucosa of users of tobacco products singly or in various combinations. *Mutagenesis*, **8**, 31–33

Kerdpon, D. & Sriplung, H. (2001) Factors related to advanced stage oral squamous cell carcinoma in southern Thailand. *Oral Oncol.*, **37**, 216–221

Kerdpon, D., Sriplung, H. & Kietthubthew, S. (2001) Expression of p53 in oral squamous cell carcinoma and its association with risk habits in southern Thailand. *Oral Oncol.*, **37**, 553–557

Kevekordes, S., Mersch-Sundermann, V., Burghaus, C.M., Spielberger, J., Schmeiser, H.H., Arlt, V.M. & Dunkelberg, H. (1999) SOS induction of selected naturally occurring substances in *Escherichia coli* (SOS chromotest). *Mutat. Res.*, **445**, 81–91

Kevekordes, S., Spielberger, J., Burghaus, C.M., Birkenkamp, P., Zietz, B., Paufler, P., Diez, M., Bolten, C. & Dunkelberg, H. (2001) Micronucleus formation in human lymphocytes and in the metabolically competent human hepatoma cell line Hep-G2: Results with 15 naturally occurring substances. *Anticancer Res.*, **21**, 461–470

Khan, F.A., Robinson, P.G., Warnakulasuriya, K.A.A.S., Newton, J.T., Gelbier, S. & Gibbons, D.E. (2000) Predictors of tobacco and alcohol consumption and their prevalence to oral cancer control amongst people from minority ethnic communities in the South Thames health region, England. *J. oral Pathol. Med.*, **29**, 214–219

Khanna, N.N., Pant, G.C., Tripathi, F.M., Sanyal, B. & Gupta, S. (1975) Some observations on the etiology of oral cancer. *Indian J. Cancer*, **12**, 77–83

Khanolkar, V.R. (1944) Oral cancer in Bombay, India. A review of 1,000 consecutive cases. *Cancer Res.*, **4**, 313–319

Khanolkar, V.R. (1959) Oral cancer in India. *Acta Unio int. contra Cancrum*, **15**, 67–77

Khrime, R.D., Mehra, Y.N., Mann, S.B.S., Mehta, S.K. & Chakraborti, R.N. (1991) Effect of instant preparation of betel nut (*pan masala*) on the oral mucosa of albino rats. *Indian J. med. Res.*, **94**, 119–124

Kietthubthew, S., Sriplung, H. & Au, W.W. (2001) Genetic and environmental interactions on oral cancer in southern Thailand. *Environ. mol. Mutag.*, **37**, 111–116

Kiyingi, K.S. (1991) Betel-nut chewing may aggravate asthma. *Papua New Guinea med. J.*, **34**, 117–121

Kiyingi, K.S. & Saweri, A. (1994) Betelnut chewing causes bronchoconstriction in some asthma patients. *Papua New Guinea med. J.*, **37**, 90–99

Knudsen, B., Knudsen, B. & Saleem, M. (1985) [Dental diseases and betel chewing among Maldivian school children.] *Dan. Dent. J. (Tandlagebladed)*, **89**, 264–267 (in Danish)

Ko, Y.C., Chiang, T.A., Chang, S.J. & Hsieh, S.F. (1992) Prevalence of betel quid chewing habit in Taiwan and related sociodemographic factors. *J. oral Pathol. Med.*, **21**, 261–264

Ko, Y.C., Huang, Y.L., Lee, C.H., Chen, M.J., Lin, L.M. & Tsai, C.C. (1995) Betel quid chewing, cigarette smoking and alcohol consumption related to oral cancer in Taiwan. *J. oral Pathol. Med.*, **24**, 450–453

Kok, S.-H., Lee, J.-J., Hsu, H.-C., Chiang, C.-P., Kuo, Y.-S. & Kuo, M.Y.-P. (2002) Mutations of the *adenomatous polyposis coli* gene in areca quid and tobacco-associated oral squamous cell carcinomas in Taiwan. *J. oral. Pathol. Med.*, **31**, 395–401

Krol, E.S. & Bolton, J.L. (1997) Oxidation of 4-alkylphenols and catechols by tyrosinase: *ortho*-Substituents alter the mechanism of quinoid formation. *Chem.-biol. Interactions*, **104**, 11–27

Kuek, L.B.K., Chin, T.W. & Fong, K.W. (1990) Lip and intraoral tumours: A local perspective. *Ann. Acad. Med. Singapore*, **19**, 178–181

Kumar, M., Kannan, A. & Upreti, R.K. (2000) Effect of betel/areca nut (*Areca catechu*) extracts on intestinal epithelial cell lining. *Vet. hum. Toxicol.*, **42**, 257–260

Kuo, M.Y.P., Jeng, J.H., Chiang, C.P. & Hahn, L.J. (1994) Mutations of Ki-*ras* oncogene codon 12 in betel quid chewing-related human oral squamous cell carcinoma in Taiwan. *J. oral Pathol. Med.*, **23**, 70–74

Kuo, M.Y.P., Chen, H.M., Hahn, L.J., Hsieh, C.C. & Chiang, C.P. (1995a) Collagen biosynthesis in human oral submucous fibrosis fibroblast cultures. *J. dent. Res.*, **74**, 1783–1788

Kuo, M.Y.P., Chang, H.H., Hahn, L.J., Wang, J.T. & Chiang, C.P. (1995b) Elevated ras p21 expression in oral premalignant lesions and squamous cell carcinoma in Taiwan. *J. oral Pathol. Med.*, **24**, 255–260

Kuo, M.Y.-P., Huang, J.-S., Hsu, H.-C., Chiang, C.-P., Kok, S.-H., Kyo, Y.-S. & Hong, C.-Y. (1999a) Infrequent p53 mutations in patients with areca quid chewing-associated oral squamous cell carcinomas in Taiwan. *J. oral Pathol. Med.*, **28**, 221–225

Kuo, M.Y.-P., Lin, C.-Y., Hahn, L.-J., Cheng, S.-J. & Chiang, C.-P. (1999b) Expression of cyclin D1 is correlated with poor prognosis in patients with areca quid chewing-associated oral squamous cell carcinomas in Taiwan. *J. oral Pathol. Med.*, **28**, 165–169

Kuo, M.Y.-P., Huang, J.-S., Kok, S.-H., Kuo, Y.-S. & Chiang, C.-P. (2002a) Prognostic role of p21$^{WAF1}$ expression in areca quid chewing and smoking-associated oral squamous cell carcinoma in Taiwan. *J. oral Pathol. Med.*, **31**, 16–22

Kuo, M.Y.-P., Hsu, H.-Y., Kok, S.-H., Kuo, R.-C., Yang, H., Hahn, L.-J. & Chiang, C.-P. (2002b) Prognostic role of p27$^{Kip1}$ expression in oral squamous cell carcinoma in Taiwan. *Oral Oncol.*, **38**, 172–178

Kuo, P.-H., Yang, H.-J., Soong, W.-T. & Chen, W.J. (2002) Substance use among adolescents in Taiwan: Associated personality traits, incompetence, and behavioral/emotional problems. *Drug. Alcohol Depend.*, **67**, 27–39

Kuruppuarachchi, K.A.L.A. & Williams, S.S. (2003) Betel use and schizophrenia. *Br. J. Psychiatry*, **182**, 455

Kuttan, N.A.A., Rosin, M.P., Ambika, K., Priddy, R.W., Bhakthan, N.M.G. & Zhang, L. (1995) High prevalence of expression of p53 oncoprotein in oral carcinomas from India associated with betel and tobacco chewing. *Eur. J. Cancer*, **31B**, 169–173

Kwan, H.-W. (1976) A statistical study on oral carcinomas in Taiwan with emphasis on the relationship with betel nut chewing: A preliminary report. *J. Formosa med. Assoc.*, **75**, 497–505

Lahiri, M. & Bhide, S.V. (1993) Effect of four plant phenols, β-carotene and α-tocopherol on 3(H)-benzopyrene-DNA interaction in vitro in the presence of rat and mouse liver postmitochondrial fraction. *Cancer Lett.*, **73**, 35–39

Lay, K.M., Sein, K., Myint, A., Ko Ko, S. & Pindborg, J.J. (1982) Epidemiologic study of 6000 villagers of oral precancerous lesions in Bilugyun: Preliminary report. *Community dent. oral Epidemiol.*, **10**, 152–155

Lee, C.H., Lin, R.H., Liu, S.H. & Lin-Shiau, S.Y. (1996) Mutual interactions among ingredients of betel quid in inducing genotoxicity on Chinese hamster ovary cells. *Mutat. Res.*, **367**, 99–104

Lee, H.-C., Yin, P.-H., Yu, T.-N., Chang, Y.-D., Hsu, W.-C., Kao, S.-Y., Chi, C.-W., Liu, T.-Y. & Wei, Y.-H. (2001) Accumulation of mitochondrial DNA deletions in human oral tissues—Effects of betel quid chewing and oral cancer. *Mutat. Res.*, **493**, 67–74

Lee, J.-M., Lee, Y.-C., Yang, S.-Y., Yang, P.-W., Luh, S.-P., Lee, C.-J., Chen, C.-J. & Wu, M.-T. (2001) Genetic polymorphisms of *XRCC1* and risk of the esophageal cancer. *Int. J. Cancer*, **95**, 240–246

Lee, M.-J., Hsu, J.-D., Lin, C.-L., Lin, M.-H., Yuan, S.-C. & Wang, C.-J. (2002) Induction of epidermal proliferation and expression of PKC and NF-κB by betel quid extracts in mouse: The role of lime-piper additives in betel quid. *Chem.-biol. Interactions*, **140**, 35–48

Lee, C.H., Ko, Y.C., Huang, H.L., Chao, Y.Y., Tsai, C.C., Shieh, T.Y. & Lin, L.M. (2003) The precancer risk of betel quid chewing, tobacco use and alcohol consumption in oral leukoplakia and oral submucous fibrosis in southern Taiwan. *Br. J. Cancer*, **88**, 366–372

Lee-Chen, S.-F., Chen, C.-L., Ho, L.-Y., Hsu, P.-C., Chang, J.-T., Sun, C.-M., Chi, C.-W. & Liu, T.-Y. (1996) Role of oxidative DNA damage in hydroxychavicol-induced genotoxicity. *Mutagenesis*, **11**, 519–523

Lei, D., Chan, C.-P., Wang, Y.-J., Wang, T.-M., Lin, B.-R., Huang, C.-H., Lee, J.-J., Chen, H.-M., Jeng, J.-H. & Chang, M.-C. (2003) Antioxidative and antiplatelet effects of aqueous inflorescence *piper betle* extract. *J. agric. Food Chem.*, **51**, 2083–2088

Len Meng, M. (1969) [Betel chewing.]. *Rev. Stomatol.*, **70**, 417–430 (in French)

Liao, P.-H., Lee, T.-L., Yang, L.-C., Yang, S.-H., Chen, S.-L. & Chou, M.-Y. (2001) Adenomatous polyposis coli gene mutation and decreased wild-type p53 protein expression in oral submucous fibrosis: A preliminary investigation. *Oral Surg. oral Med. oral Pathol. oral Radiol. Endod.*, **92**, 202–207

Lichtensteiger, W. & Schlumpf, M. (1985) Prenatal nicotine affects fetal testosterone and sexual dimorphism of saccharin preference. *Pharmacol. Biochem. Behav.*, **23**, 439–444

Lin, L.M., Chen, Y.K., Lai, D.R. & Huang, Y.L. (1996) Minimal arecaidine concentrations showing a promotion effect during DMBA-induced hamster cheek pouch carcinogenesis. *J. oral Pathol. Med.*, **25**, 65–68

Lin, L.M., Chen, Y.K., Lai, D.R., Huang, Y.L. & Chen, H.R. (1997) Cancer-promoting effect of Taiwan betel quid in hamster buccal pouch carcinogenesis. *Oral Dis.*, **3**, 232–235

Lin, S.-C., Chang, K.-W., Chang, C.-S., Liu, T.-Y., Tzeng, Y.-S., Yang, F.-S. & Wong, Y.-K. (2000a) Alterations of *p16/MTS1* gene in oral squamous cell carcinomas from Taiwanese. *J. oral Pathol. Med.*, **29**, 159–166

Lin, S.-C., Chang, K.-W., Chang, C.-S., Yu, S.-Y., Chao, S.-Y. & Wong, Y.-K. (2000b) Establishment and characterization of a cell line (HCDB-1) derived from a hamster buccal pouch carcinoma induced by DMBA and Taiwanese betel quid extract. *Proc. natl Sci. Counc. Repub. China*, **B24**, 129–135

Lin, S.-C., Chen, Y.-J., Kao, S.-Y., Hsu, M.-T., Lin, C.-H., Yang, S.-C., Liu, T.-Y. & Chang, K.-W. (2002) Chromosomal changes in betel-associated oral squamous cell carcinomas and their relationship to clinical parameters. *Oral Oncol.*, **38**, 266–273

Lin, S.-H., Lin, Y.-F., Cheema-Dhadli, S., Davids, M.R. & Halperin, M.L. (2002) Hypercalcaemia and metabolic alkalosis with betel nut chewing: Emphasis on its integrative pathophysiology. *Nephrol. Dial. Transplant.*, **17**, 708–714

Lin, S.-K., Chang, Y.-J., Ryu, S.-J. & Chu, N.-S. (2002) Cerebral hemodynamic responses to betel chewing: A Doppler study. *Clin. Neuropharmacol.*, **25**, 244–250

Ling, L.-J., Hung, S.-L., Tseng, S.-C., Chen, Y.-T., Chi, L.-Y., Wu, K.-M. & Lai, Y.-L. (2001) Association between betel quid chewing, periodontal status and periodontal pathogens. *Oral Microbiol. Immunol.*, **16**, 364–369

Liu, C.J., Chen, C.L., Chang, K.W., Chu, C.H. & Liu, T.Y. (2000) Safrole in betel quid may be a risk factor for hepatocellular carcinoma: Case report. *CMAJ*, **162**, 359–360

Liu, T.-Y., Chen, C.-L. & Chi, C.-W. (1996) Oxidative damage to DNA induced by areca nut extract. *Mutat. Res.*, **367**, 25–31

Liu, Y., Egyhazi, S., Hansson, J., Bhide, S.V., Kulkarni, P.S. & Grafström, R.C. (1997) $O^6$-Methylguanine–DNA methyltransferase activity in human buccal mucosal tissue and cell cultures. Complex mixtures related to habitual use of tobacco and betel quid inhibit the activity in vitro. *Carcinogenesis*, **18**, 1889–1895

Lodge, D., Johnston, G.A.R., Curtis, D.R. & Brand, S.J. (1977) Effects of Areca nut constituents arecaidine and guvacine on the action of GABA in the cat central nervous system. *Brain Res.*, **136**, 513–522

Lord, G.A., Lim, C.K., Warnakulasuriya, S. & Peters, T.J. (2002) Chemical and analytical aspects of areca nut. *Addict. Biol.*, **7**, 99–102

Lu, C.T., Lan, S.J., Hsieh, C.C., Yang, M.J., Ko, Y.C., Tsai, C.C. & Yen, Y.Y. (1993) Prevalence and characteristics of areca nut chewers among junior high school students in Changhua county, Taiwan. *Community Dent. oral Epidemiol.*, **21**, 370–373

Lu, C.T., Yen, Y.Y., Ho, C.S., Ko, Y.C., Tsai, C.C., Hsieh, C.C. & Lan, S.J. (1996) A case–control study of oral cancer in Changhua County, Taiwan. *J. oral Pathol. Med.*, **25**, 245–248

Ma, R.H., Tsai, C.C. & Shieh, T.Y. (1995) Increased lysyl oxidase activity in fibroblasts cultured from oral submucous fibrosis associated with betel nut chewing in Taiwan. *J. oral Pathol. Med.*, **24**, 407–412

MacDonald, D.G. (1986) Effects of arecaidine application to hamster cheek pouch. *J. oral Med.*, **41**, 269–270

MacDonald, D.G. (1987) Effects of arecaidine application to hamster cheek pouch. *J. oral Med.*, **42**, 61–62

MacLennan, R., Paissat, D., Ring, A. & Thomas, S. (1985) Possible aetiology of oral cancer in Papua New Guinea. *Papua New Guinea med. J.*, **28**, 3–8

Mahale, A. & Saranath, D. (2000) Microsatellite alterations on chromosome 9 in chewing tobacco-induced oral squamous cell carcinomas from India. *Oral Oncol.*, **36**, 199–206

Maher, R., Lee, A.J., Warnakulasuriya, K.A.A.S., Lewis, J.A. & Johnson, N.W. (1994) Role of areca nut in the causation of oral submucous fibrosis: A case–control study in Pakistan. *J. oral Pathol. Med.*, **23**, 65–69

Mahmood, Z., Jafarey, N.A., Samiuddin, M., Rais, A.K., Malik, S. & Qureshi, S.A. (1974) Dietary and other habits of the people of Karachi. *J. Pak. med. Assoc.*, **24**, 222–229

Mannan, N., Boucher, B.J. & Evans, S.J.W. (2000) Increased waist size and weight in relation to consumption of *Areca catechu* (betel-nut); a risk factor for increased glycaemia in Asians in East London. *Br. J. Nutr.*, **83**, 267–275

Marmot, M.G., Adelstein, A.M. & Bulusu, L. (1984) *Immigrant Mortality in England and Wales 1970-78* (Office of Population Censuses and Surveys. Studies on Medical and Population Subjects No. 47), London, Her Majesty's Stationery Office

Marsden, A.T.H. (1960) Betel cancer in Malaya. *Med. J. Malaya*, **14**, 162–165

Martin, W.M.C., Sengupta, S.K., Murthy, D.P. & Barua, D.L. (1992) The spectrum of cancer in Papua New Guinea. *Cancer*, **70**, 2942–2950

Martino, G.V., Tappaz, M.L., Braghi, S., Dozio, N., Canal, N., Pozza, G., Bottazzo, G.F., Grimaldi, M.E. & Bosi, E. (1991) Autoantibodies to glutamic acid decarboxylase (GAD) detected by an immuno-trapping enzyme activity assay: Relation to insulin-dependent diabetes mellitus and islet cell antibodies. *J. Autoimmun.*, **4**, 915–923

McAllister-Sistilli, C.G., Caggiula, A.R., Knopf, S., Rose, C.A., Miller, A.L. & Donny, E.C. (1998) The effects of nicotine on the immune system. *Psychoneuroendocrinology*, **23**, 175–187

McGurk, M. & Craig, G.T. (1984) Oral submucous fibrosis; two cases of malignant transformation in Asian immigrants to the United Kingdom. *Br. J. oral max. facial Surg.*, **22**, 56–64

Meghji, S., Scutt, A., Harvey, W. & Canniff, J.P. (1987) An in-vitro comparison of human fibroblasts from normal and oral submucous fibrosis tissue. *Arch. oral Biol.*, **32**, 213–215

Mehta, F.S., Sanjana, M.K., Shroff, B.C. & Doctor, R.H. (1961) Incidence of leukoplakia among 'pan' (betel leaf) chewers and 'bidi' smokers: A study of a sample survey. *Indian J. med. Res.*, **49**, 393–399

Mehta, F.S., Daftary, D.K., Shroff, B.C. & Sanghvi, L.D. (1969) Clinical and histologic study of oral leukoplakia in relation to habits. *Oral Pathol.,* **28**, 372–388

Mehta, F.S., Pindborg, J.J., Hamner, J.E., Gupta, P.C., Daftary, D.K., Sahiar, B.E., Shroff, B.C., Sanghvi, L.D., Bhonsle, R.B., Choksi, S.K., Dandekar, V.V., Mehta, Y.N., Pitkar, V.K., Sinor, P.N., Shah, N.C., Turner, P.S. & Upadhyay, S.A. (1971) *Report on Investigations of Oral Cancer and Precancerous Conditions in Indian Rural populations. 1966–1969,* Copenhagen, Munksgaard, pp. 48, 68, 89, 107, 120

Mehta, F.S., Shroff, B.C., Gupta, P.C. & Daftary, D.K. (1972a) Oral leukoplakia in relation to tobacco habits. A ten-year follow-up study of Bombay policemen. *Oral Surg. oral Med. oral Pathol.,* **34**, 426–433

Mehta, F.S., Gupta, P.C., Daftary, D.K., Pindborg, J.J. & Choksi, S.K. (1972b) An epidemiologic study of oral cancer and precancerous conditions among 101 761 villagers in Maharashtra, India. *Int. J. Cancer,* **10**, 134–141

Mendelson, R.W. & Ellis, A.G. (1924) Cancer as a public health problem in Siam. *J. trop. Med. Hyg.,* **27**, 274–278

Merchant, A., Husain, S.S.M., Hosain, M., Fikree, F.F., Pitiphat, W., Siddiqui, A.R., Hayder, S.J., Haider, S.M., Ikram, M., Chuang, S.K. & Saeed, S.A. (2000) Paan without tobacco: An independent risk factor for oral cancer. *Int. J. Cancer,* **86**, 128–131

Ministry of Health (1998) *National Oral Health Survey, Sri Lanka, 1994/1995,* Colombo, Ministry of Health

de Miranda, C.M., van Wyk, C.W., van der Bijl, P. & Basson, N.J. (1996) The effect of areca nut on salivary and selected oral microorganisms. *Int. dent. J.,* **46**, 350–356

Miyazawa, T. (2000) Absorption, metabolism and antioxidative effects of tea catechin in humans. *Biofactors,* **13**, 55–59

Molinengo, L., Cassone, M.C. & Orsetti, M. (1986) Action of arecoline on the levels of acetylcholine, norepinephrine and dopamine in the mouse central nervous system. *Pharmacol. Biochem. Behav.,* **24**, 1801–1803

Möller, I.J., Pindborg, J.J. & Effendi, I. (1977) The relation between betel chewing and dental caries. *Scand. J. dent. Res.,* **85**, 64–70

Monheit, A.G., Van Vunakis, H., Key, T.C. & Resnik, R. (1983) Maternal and fetal cardiovascular effects of nicotine infusion in pregnant sheep. *Am. J. Obstet. Gynecol.,* **145**, 290–296

Mori, H., Matsubara, N., Ushimaru, Y. & Hirono, I. (1979) Carcinogenicity examination of betel nuts and piper betel leaves. *Experientia,* **35**, 384–385

Mougne, C., MacLennan, R. & Atsana, S. (1982) Smoking, chewing and drinking in Ban Pong, Northern Thailand. *Soc. Sci. Med.,* **16**, 99–106

Muir, C.S. & Kirk, R. (1960) Betel, tobacco, and cancer of the mouth. *Br. J. Cancer,* **14**, 597–608

Muir, C.S. (1962) Cancer of the buccal cavity and nasopharynx in Singapore. *Br. J. Cancer,* **14**, 597–608

Mujumdar, A.M., Kapadi, A.H. & Pendse, G.S. (1979) Chemistry and pharmacology of betel nut *Areca catechu* Linn. *J. plant. Crops,* **7**, 69–92

Mujumdar, A.M., Kapadi, A.H. & Pendse, G.S. (1982) Pharmacological properties. In: Bavappa, K.V.A., ed., *The Areca Nut Palm, Central Plant Crop Research Institute Publication,* pp. 245–261

Mukherjee, A. & Giri, A.K. (1991) Sister chromatid exchange induced by 'pan masala' (a betel quid ingredient) in male mice *in vivo. Food chem. Toxicol.,* **29**, 401–403

Mukherjee, A., Chakrabarti, J., Chakrabarti, A., Banerjee, T. & Sarma, A. (1991) Effect of 'Pan masala' on the germ cells of male mice. *Cancer Lett.*, **58**, 161–165

Munirajan, A.K., Tutsumi-Ishii, Y., Mohanprasad, B.K.C., Hirano, Y., Munakata, N., Shanmugam, G. & Tsuchida, N. (1996) *p53* Gene mutations in oral carcinomas from India. *Int. J. Cancer*, **66**, 297–300

Munirajan, A.K., Mohanprasad, B.K., Shanmugam, G. & Tsuchida, N. (1998) Detection of a rare point mutation at codon 59 and relatively high incidence of H-*ras* mutation in Indian oral cancer. *Int. J. Oncol.*, **13**, 971–974

Murti, P.R., Bhonsle, R.B., Pindborg, J.J., Daftary, D.K., Gupta, P.C. & Mehta, F.S. (1985) Malignant transformation rate in oral submucous fibrosis over a 17-year period. *Community dent. oral Epidemiol.*, **13**, 340–341

Murti, P.R., Gupta, P.C., Bhonsle, R.B., Daftary, D.K., Mehta, F.S. & Pindborg, J.J. (1990) Effect on the incidence of oral submucous fibrosis of intervention in the areca nut chewing habit. *J. oral Pathol. Med.*, **19**, 99–100

Murti, P.R., Bhonsle, R.B., Gupta, P.C., Daftary, D.K., Pindborg, J.J. & Mehta, F.S. (1995) Etiology of oral submucous fibrosis with special reference to the role of areca nut chewing. *J. oral Pathol. Med.*, **24**, 145–152

Murti, P.R., Warnakulasuriya, K.A.A.S., Johnson, N.W., Bhonsle, R.B., Gupta, P.C., Daftary, D.K. & Mehta, F.S. (1998) p53 Expression in oral precancer as a marker for malignant potential. *J. oral Pathol. Med.*, **27**, 191–196

Nagabhushan, M. & Bhide, S.V. (1988) Anti-mutagenicity of catechin against environmental mutagens. *Mutagenesis*, **3**, 293–296

Nagabhushan, M., Amonkar, A.J., D'Souza, A.V. & Bhide, S.V. (1987) Nonmutagenicity of betel leaf and its antimutagenic action against environmental mutagens. *Neoplasma*, **34**, 159–167

Nagabhushan, M., Amonkar, A.J., Nair, U.J., Santhanam, U., Ammigan, N., D'Souza, A.V. & Bhide, S.V. (1988) Catechin as an antimutagen: Its mode of action. *J. Cancer Res. clin. Oncol.*, **114**, 177–182

Nagabhushan, M., Amonkar, A.J., Nair, U.J., D'Souza, A.V. & Bhide, S.V. (1989) Hydroxychavicol: A new anti-nitrosating phenolic compound from betel leaf. *Mutagenesis*, **4**, 200–204

Nagpal, J.K., Patnaik, S. & Das, B.R. (2002a) Prevalence of high-risk human papilloma virus types and its association with p53 codon 72 polymorphism in tobacco addicted oral squamous cell carcinoma (OSCC) patients of eastern India. *Int. J. Cancer*, **97**, 649–653

Nagpal, J.K., Mishra, R. & Das, B.R. (2002b) Activation of Stat-3 as one of the early events in tobacco chewing-mediated oral carcinogenesis. *Cancer*, **94**, 2393–2400

Naik, G.H., Priyadarsini, K.I., Satav, J.G., Banavalikar, M.M., Sohoni, D.P., Biyani, M.K. & Mohan, H. (2003) Comparative antioxidant activity of individual herbal components used in Ayurvedic medicine. *Phytochemistry*, **63**, 97–104

Nair, U. & Bartsch, H. (2001) Metabolic polymorphisms as susceptibility markers for lung and oral cavity cancer. In: Miller, A.B., Bartsch, H., Boffetta, P., Dragsted, L. & Vainio, H., eds, *Biomarkers in Cancer Chemoprevention* (IARC Scientific Publications 154), Lyon, *IARC*Press, pp. 271–290

Nair, J., Ohshima, H., Friesen, M., Croisy, A., Bhide, S.V. & Bartsch, H. (1985) Tobacco-specific and betel nut-specific *N*-nitroso compounds: Occurrence in saliva and urine of betel quid chewers and formation *in vitro* by nitrosation of betel quid. *Carcinogenesis*, **6**, 295–303

Nair, J., Ohshima, H., Pignatelli, B., Friesen, M., Malaveille, C, Calmels, S. & Bartsch, H. (1986) Modifiers of endogenous carcinogen formation: Studies on in vivo nitrosation in tobacco users. In: Hoffman, D. & Harris, C.C., eds, *Mechanisms in Tobacco Carcinogenisis* (Banbury Report 23), Cold Spring Harbor, NY, CSH Press, pp. 45–61

Nair, J., Nair, U.J., Ohshima, H., Bhide, S.V., & Bartsch, H. (1987) Endogenous nitrosation in the oral cavity of chewers while chewing betel quid with or without tobacco. In: Bartsch, H., O'Neill, I.K. & Schulte-Hermann, R., eds, *The Relevence of N-Nitroso Compounds in Human Cancer: Exposure and Mechanisms* (IARC Scientific Publications 84), Lyon, *IARC*Press, pp. 465–469

Nair, U.J., Floyd, R.A., Nair, J., Bussachini, V., Friesen, M. & Bartsch, H. (1987) Formation of reactive oxygen species and of 8-hydroxydeoxyguanosine in DNA in vitro with betel quid ingredients. *Chem.-biol. Interactions*, **63**, 157–169

Nair, U.J., Friesen, M., Richard, I., MacLennan, R., Thomas, S. & Bartsch, H. (1990) Effect of lime composition on the formation of reactive oxygen species from areca nut extract *in vitro*. *Carcinogenesis*, **11**, 2145–2148

Nair, U., Obe, G., Nair, J., Maru, G.B., Bhide, S.V., Pieper, R. & Bartsch, H. (1991) Evaluation of frequency of micronucleated oral mucosal cells as a marker for genotoxic damage in chewers of betel quid with or without tobacco. *Mutat. Res.*, **261**, 163–168

Nair, U.J., Obe, G., Friesen, M., Goldberg, M.T. & Bartsch, H. (1992) Role of lime in the generation of reactive oxygen species from betel-quid ingredients. *Environ. Health Perspect.*, **98**, 203–205

Nair, U.J., Nair, J., Friesen, M.D., Bartsch, H. & Ohshima, H. (1995) *ortho-* and *meta-*Tyrosine formation from phenylalanine in human saliva as a marker of hydroxyl radical generation during betel quid chewing. *Carcinogenesis*, **16**, 1195–1198

Nair, J., Ohshima, H., Nair, U.J. & Bartsch, H. (1996) Endogenous formation of nitrosamines and oxidative DNA-damaging agents in tobacco users. *Crit. Rev.Toxicol.*, **26**, 149–161

Nair, U.J., Nair, J., Mathew, B. & Bartsch, H. (1999) Glutathione *S*-transferase M1 and T1 null genotypes as risk factors for oral leukoplakia in ethnic Indian betel quid/tobacco chewers. *Carcinogenesis*, **20**, 743–748

Nandakumar, A., Thimmasetty, K.T., Sreeramareddy, N.M., Venugopal, T.C., Rajanna, Vinutha, A.T., Srinivas & Bhargava, M.K. (1990) A population-based case–control investigation on cancers of the oral cavity in Bangalore, India. *Br. J. Cancer*, **62**, 847–851

National Centre for Transcultural Oral Health (2001) *Educational Programme for Trading Standards and Customs and Excise Officers*, London, Resolutions, p. 17

Nery, R. (1971) The metabolic interconversion of arecoline and arecoline 1-oxide in the rat. *Biochem. J.*, **122**, 503–508

Ng, K.H., Siar, C.H., Ramanathan, K. & Murugasu, P. (1986) A study on the prevalence of oral habits in 100 cases of squamous cell carcinoma in Malaysia. *Ann. Dent.*, **45**, 7–10

Nieschulz, O. & Schmersahl, P. (1968) [On the pharmacology of active materials from betel. 2. Transformation of arecoline to arecaidine.] *Arzneim.-Forsch.*, **18**, 222–225 (in German)

Nigam, P. & Srivastava, A.B. (1990) Betel chewing and dental decay. *Fed. Oper. Dent.*, **1**, 36–38

Nikolic, D., Fan, P.W., Bolton, J.L. & van Breemen, R.B. (1999) Screening for xenobiotic electrophilic metabolites using pulsed ultrafiltration–mass spectrometry. *Comb. Chem. high Throughput Screen.*, **2**, 165–175

Norton, S.A. (1998) Betel: Consumption and consequences. *J. Am. Acad. Dermatol.*, **38**, 81–88

Notani, P.N. & Sanghvi, L.D. (1976) Role of diet in the cancers of the oral cavity. *Indian J. Cancer*, **13**, 156–160

Obeid, O.A., Mannan, N., Perry, G., Iles, R.A. & Boucher, B.J. (1998) Homocysteine and folate in healthy East London Bangladeshis. *Lancet*, **352**, 1829–1830

Ohshima, H. & Bartsch, H. (1981) Quantitative estimation of endogenous nitrosation in humans by monitoring *N*-nitrosoproline excreted in the urine. *Cancer Res.*, **41**, 3658–3662

Ohshima, H., Friesen, M. & Bartsch, H. (1989) Identification in rats of N-nitrosonipecotic acid as a major urinary metabolite of the areca-nut alkaloid-derived nitrosamines, N-nitrosoguvacoline and N-nitrosoguvacine. *Cancer Lett.*, **44**, 211–216

Oliver, A.J. & Radden, B.G. (1992) Oral submucous fibrosis. Case report and review of the literature. *Austr. Dent. J.*, **37**, 31–34

Orr, I.M. (1933) Oral cancers in betel nut chewers in Travancore: Its aetiology, pathology, and treatment. *Lancet*, **ii**, 575–580

Osman, S., Warnakulasuriya, S., Cooper, D. & Gelbier, S. (1997) Betel quid chewing and tobacco habits among Asian schoolchildren in Bedfordshire. *J. dent. Res.*, **76**, 1054

Padma, P.R., Lalitha, V.S., Amonkar, A.J. & Bhide, S.V. (1989a) Anticarcinogenic effect of betel leaf extract against tobacco carcinogens. *Cancer Lett.*, **45**, 195–202

Padma, P.R., Amonkar, A.J. & Bhide, S.V. (1989b) Antimutagenic effects of betel leaf extract against the mutagenicity of two tobacco-specific *N*-nitrosamines. *Mutagenesis*, **4**, 154–156

Padmavathy, G. & Reddy, D.J. (1960) Aetiological factors of carcinoma of the mouth and pharynx in Guntur. *J. Indian med. Assoc.*, **34**, 84–88

Pai, S.R., Shirke, A.J. & Gothoskar, S.V. (1981) Long-term feeding study in C17 mice administered saccharin coated betel nut and 1,4-dinitrosopiperazine in combination. *Carcinogenesis*, **2**, 175–177

Pai, C.-Y., Hsieh, L.-L., Tsai, C.-W., Chiou, F.-S., Yang, C.-H. & Hsu, B.-D. (2002) Allelic alterations at the STR markers in the buccal tissue cells of oral cancer patients and the oral epithelial cells of healthy betel quid-chewers: An evaluation of forensic applicability. *Forensic Sci. int.*, **129**, 158–167

Panda, S. & Kar, A. (1998) Dual role of betel leaf extract on thyroid function in male mice. *Pharmacol. Res.*, **38**, 493–496

Pande, P., Mathur, M., Shukla, N.K. & Ralhan, R. (1998) pRb and p16 Protein alterations in human oral tumorigenesis. *Oral Oncol.*, **34**, 396–403

Pande, P., Soni, S., Chakravarti, N., Mathur, M., Shukla, N.K., Ralhan R. (2001) Prognostic impact of Ets-1 overexpression in betel and tobacco related oral cancer. *Cancer Detect. Prev.*, **25**, 496–501

Pande, P., Soni, S., Kaur, J., Agarwal, S., Mathur, M., Shukla, N.K., Ralhan, R. (2002) Prognostic factors in betel and tobacco related oral cancer. *Oral Oncol.*, **38**, 491–499

Pandey, G.K., Raut, D.K., Hazra, S., Vajpayee, A., Pandey, A. & Chatterjee, P. (2001) Patterns of tobacco use amongst school teachers. *Indian J. public Health*, **45**, 82–87

Panigrahi, G.B. & Rao, A.R. (1984) Induction of in vivo sister chromatid exchanges by arecaidine, a betel nut alkaloid, in mouse bone-marrow cells. *Cancer Lett.*, **23**, 189–192

Panigrahi, G.B. & Rao, A.R. (1986) Study of the genotoxicity of the total aqueous extract of betel nut and its tannin. *Carcinogenesis*, **7**, 37–39

Park, Y.B., Jeon, S.-M., Byun, S.-J., Kim, H.-S. & Choi, M.-S. (2002) Absorption of intestinal free cholesterol is lowered by supplementation of *Areca catechu* L. extracts in rats. *Life Sci.*, **70**, 1849–1859

Parkin, D.M., Srivatanakul, P., Khlat, M., Chenvidhya, D., Chotiwan, P., Insiripong, S., L'Abbe, K.A. & Wild, C.P. (1991) Liver cancer in Thailand. I. A case–control study of cholangiocarcinoma. *Int. J. Cancer*, **48**, 323–328

Parkin, D.M., Whelan, S.L., Ferlay, J., Teppo, L. & Thomas, D.B. (2003) *Cancer Incidence in Five Continents, Vol. VIII* (IARC Scientific Publication No. 155), Lyon, IARC*Press*

Patel, R.S. & Rajorhia, G.S. (1979) Antioxidative role of curry (*Murraya Koenigi*) and betel (*Piper betel*) leaves in ghee. *J. Food Sci. Technol.*, **16**, 158–160

Patel, R.K., Jaju, R.J., Bakshi, S.R., Trivedi, A.H., Dave, B.J. & Adhvaryu, S.G. (1994a) Pan masala — A genotoxic menace. *Mutat. Res.*, **320**, 245–249

Patel, R.K., Trivedi, A.H., Jaju, R.J., Adhvaryu, S.G. & Balar, D.B. (1994b) Ethanol potentiates the clastogenicity of pan masala — An *in vitro* experience. *Carcinogenesis*, **15**, 2017–2021

Patnaik, S., Nayak, B.K. & Das, B.R., (1999) Genetic alterations of P53 in oral tumors. In: Varma, A.K., ed., *Oral Oncology*, Vol. VI, *Proceedings of the 6th International Congress on Oral Cancer*, New Delhi, Macmillan, pp. 87–92

Patterson, T.A. & Kosh, J.W. (1993) Elucidation of the rapid *in vivo* metabolism of arecoline. *Gen. Pharmacol.*, **24**, 641–647

Paul, K., Moitra, P.K., Maity, C.R. & Ghosal, S.K. (1996) Teratogenicity of crude area nut extract in chick embryos. *Indian J. phys. all. Sci.*, **50**, 182–187

Paul, K., Moitra, P.K. & Ghosal, S.K. (1997) Developmental toxicity of crude *areca* nut extract in chick embryos. *Trans. zool. Soc. India*, **1**, 14–17

Paul, K., Moitra, P.K., Mukherjee, I., Maity, C. & Ghosal, S.K. (1999) Teratogenicity of arecoline hydrobromide on developing chick embryos: A preliminary report. *Bull. environ. Contam. Toxicol.*, **62**, 356–362

Paymaster, J.C. (1956) Cancer of the buccal mucosa. A clinical study of 650 cases in Indian patients. *Cancer*, **9**, 431–435

Paymaster, J.C. (1962) Some observations on oral and pharyngeal carcinomas in the State of Bombay. *Cancer*, **15**, 578–583

Paymaster, J.C. & Gangadharan, P. (1970) Cancer in the Parsi community of Bombay. *Int. J. Cancer*, **5**, 426–431

Pearson, N.K. (1994) *Oral Health Status and Dental Treatment Needs of an Adult Bangladeshi Population Resident in Tower Hamlets*, MSc Thesis, London, University of London

Pearson, N., Croucher, R., Marcenes, W. & O'Farrell, M. (1999) Dental service use and the implications for oral cancer screening in a sample of Bangladeshi adult medical care users living in Tower Hamlets, UK. *Br. Dent. J.*, **186**, 517–521

Pearson, N., Croucher, R., Marcenes, W. & O'Farrell, M. (2001) Prevalence of oral lesions among a sample of Bangladeshi medical users aged 40 years and over living in Tower Hamlets, UK. *Int. dent. J.*, **51**, 30–34

Petro, T.M., Peterson, D.S & Fung, Y.K. (1992) Nicotine enhances interleukin production of rat splenic T lymphocytes. *Immunopharmacol. Immunotoxicol.*, **14**, 463–475

Phukan, R.K., Ali, M.S., Chetia, C.K. & Mahanta, J. (2001) Betel nut and tobacco chewing: Potential risk factors of cancer of oesophagus in Assam, India. *Br. J. Cancer*, **85**, 661–667

Pickwell, S.M., Schimelpfening, S. & Palinkas, L.A. (1994) 'Betelmania'. Betel quid chewing by Cambodian women in the United States and its potential health effects. *West. J. Med.*, **160**, 326–330

Pignatelli, B., Bereziat, J.-C., Descotes, G. & Bartsch, H. (1982) Catalysis of nitrosation *in vitro* and *in vivo* in rats by catechin and resorcinol and inhibition by chlorogenic acid. *Carcinogenesis*, **3**, 1045–1049

Pillai, M.R., Balaram, P., Abraham, T. & Nair, M.K. (1987) Lymphocyte populations in premalignant lesions and cancer of the oral cavity. *Neoplasma*, **34**, 469–479

Pillai, M.R., Balaram, P., Kannan, S., Sudha, L., Nalinakumari, K.R., Hareendran, N.K. & Nair, M.K. (1990) Interferon activation of latent natural killer cells and alterations in kinetics of target cell lysis: Clinical implications for oral precancerous lesions. *Oral Surg. oral Med. oral Pathol.*, **70**, 458–461

Pindborg, J.J. (1965) Oral precancerous conditions in South East Asia. *Int. dent. J.*, **15**, 190–199

Pindborg, J.J., Chawla, T.N., Misra, R.K., Nagpaul, R.K. & Gupta, V.K. (1965) Frequency of oral carcinoma, leukoplakia, leukokeratosis, leukoedema, submucous fibrosis, and lichen planus in 10 000 Indians in Lucknow, Uttar Pradesh, India. *J. dent. Res.*, **44**, 615

Pindborg, J.J., Kiaer, J., Gupta, P.C. & Chawla, T.N. (1967) Studies in oral leukoplakias. Prevalence of leukoplakia among 10 000 persons in Lucknow, India, with special reference to use of tobacco and betel nut. *Bull. World Health Organ.*, **37**, 109–116

Pindborg, J.J., Barmes, D. & Roed-Petersen, B. (1968) Epidemiology and histology of oral leukoplakia and leukoedema among Papuans and New Guineans. *Cancer*, **22**, 379–384

Pindborg, J.J., Mehta, F.S., Daftary, D.K., Gupta, P.C. & Bhonsle, R.B. (1972) Prevalence of oral lichen planus among 7639 Indian villagers in Kerala, South India. *Acta Derm. Venereol.*, **52**, 216–220

Pindborg, J.J., Zheng, K.-H., Kong, C.-R. & Lin, F.-X. (1984a) Pilot survey of oral mucosa in areca (betel) nut chewers on Hainan Island of the People's Republic of China. *Commun. Dent. oral Epidemiol.*, **12**, 195–196

Pindborg, J.J., Murti, P.R., Bhonsle, R.B., Gupta, P.C., Daftary, D.K. & Mehta, F.S. (1984b) Oral submucous fibrosis as a precancerous condition. *Scand. J. dent. Res.*, **92**, 224–229

Pindborg, J.J., Reichart, P.A., Smith, C.J. & van der Waal, I. (1996) In: Sobin, L.H., *Histological Typing of Cancer and Precancer of the Oral Mucosa, Second Edition, International Histological Classification of Tumours*, World Health Organization

Piyaratn, P. (1959) Relative incidence of malignant neoplasms in Thailand. *Cancer*, **12**, 693–696

Polasa, K., Babu, S., Shenolikar, I.S. (1993) Dose-dependent genotoxic effect of Pan masala and areca nut in the *Salmonella typhimurium* assay. *Food chem. Toxicol.*, **31**, 439–442

Prabhu, M.S., Patel, K., Saraswathi, G. & Srinivasan, K. (1995) Effect of orally administered betel leaf (*Piper betle* Linn.) on digestive enzymes of pancreas and intestinal mucosa and on bile production in rats. *Indian J. exp. Biol.*, **33**, 752–756

Prabhu, N.T., Warnakulasuriya, K.A.A.S., Gelbier, S. & Robinson, P.G. (2001) Betel quid chewing among Bangladeshi adolescents living in East London. *Int. J. paediatr. Dent.*, **11**, 18–24

Prokopczyk, B., Rivenson, A., Bertinato, P., Brunnemann, K.D. & Hoffmann, D. (1987) 3-(Methylnitrosamino)propionitrile: Occurrence in saliva of betel quid chewers, carcinogenicity, and DNA methylation in F344 rats. *Cancer Res.*, **47**, 467–471

Prokopczyk, B., Bertinato, P. & Hoffmann, D. (1988) Cyanoethylation of DNA in vivo by 3-(methylnitrosamino)propionitrile, an Areca-derived carcinogen. *Cancer Res.*, **48**, 6780–6784

Raghavan, V. & Baruah, H.K. (1958) Arecanut: India's popular masticatory — History, chemistry and utilization. *Econom. Bot.*, **12**, 315–325

Rahman, Z.A.A., Zain, R.B., Abang, Z., Ikeda, N., Razak, I.A., Aung, S. & Abdullah, F. (1997) A pilot study of oral mucosal lesions among Sarawak indigenous people. *Dent. J. Malaysia*, **18**, 26–29

Raisuddin, S. & Misra, J.K. (1991) Aflatoxin in betel nut and its control by use of food preservatives. *Food Addit. Contam.*, **8**, 707–712

Rajendran, R., Sugathan, C.K., Remani, P., Ankathil, R. & Vijayakumar, T. (1986) Cell mediated and humoral immune responses in oral submucous fibrosis. *Cancer*, **58**, 2628–2631

Rajkumar, T., Franceschi, S., Vaccarella, S., Gajalakshmi, V., Sharmila, A., Snijders, P.J.F., Munoz, N., Meijer, C.J.L.M. & Herrero, R. (2003) Role of paan chewing and dietary habits in cervical carcinoma in Chennai, India. *Br. J. Cancer*, **88**, 1388–1393

Ralhan, R., Agarwal, S., Nath, N., Mathur, M., Wasylyk, B. & Srivastava, A. (2001) Correlation between *p53* gene mutations and circulating antibodies in betel- and tobacco-consuming North Indian population. *Oral Oncol.*, **37**, 243–250

Ramanathan, K. & Lakshimi, S. (1976) Oral carcinoma in Peninsular Malaysia: Racial variations in the Indians, Malays, Chinese, and Caucasians. *Gann Monogr. Cancer Res.*, **18**, 27–36

Ramchandani, A.G., D'Souza, A.V., Borges, A.M. & Bhisey, R.A. (1998) Evaluation of carcinogenic/co-carcinogenic activity of a common chewing product, pan masala, in mouse skin, stomach and esophagus. *Int. J. Cancer*, **75**, 225–232

Ranadive, K.J., Gothoskar, S.V., Rao, A.R., Tezabwalla, B.U. & Ambaye, R.Y. (1976) Experimental studies on betel nut and tobacco carcinogenicity. *Int. J. Cancer*, **17**, 469–476

Ranadive, K.J., Ranadive, S.N., Shivapurkar, N.M. & Gothoskar, S.V. (1979) Betel quid chewing and oral cancer: Experimental studies on hamsters. *Int. J. Cancer*, **24**, 835–843

Ranasinghe, A., MacGeoch, C., Dyer, S., Spurr, N. & Johnson, N.W. (1993a) Some oral carcinomas from Sri Lankan betel/tobacco chewers overexpress p53 oncoprotein but lack mutations in exons 5–9. *Anticancer Res.*, **13**, 2065–2068

Ranasinghe, A.W., Warnakulasuriya, K.A.A.S. & Johnson, N.W. (1993b) Low prevalence of expression of p53 oncoprotein in oral carcinomas from Sri Lanka associated with betel and tobacco chewing. *Eur. J. Cancer*, **29B**, 147–150

Rao, A.R. (1984) Modifying influences of betel quid ingredients on B(a)P-induced carcinogenesis in the buccal pouch of hamster. *Int. J. Cancer*, **33**, 581–586

Rao, A.R. & Das, P. (1989) Evaluation of the carcinogenicity of different preparations of areca nut in mice. *Int J. Cancer*, **43**, 728–732

Rao, D.N. & Desai, P.B. (1998) Risk assessment of tobacco, alcohol and diet in cancers of base tongue and oral tongue — A case–control study. *Indian J. Cancer*, **35**, 65–72

Rao, A.R,. Sinha, A. & Selvan, R.S. (1985) Inhibitory action of *Piper betle* on the initiation of 7.12-dimethylbenz[*a*]anthracene-induced mammary carcinogenesis in rats. *Cancer Lett.*, **26**, 207–214

Ravi, D., Nalinakumari, K.R, Rajaram, R.S., Nair, M.K. & Pillai, M.R. (1996) Expression of programmed cell death, regulatory p53 and bcl-2 proteins in oral lesions. *Cancer Lett.*, **105**, 139–146

Ravi, D., Ramadas, K., Mathew, B.S., Nalinakumari, K.R., Nair, M.K. & Pillai, M.R. (1999) *De novo* programmed cell death in oral cancer. *Histopathology*, **34**, 241–249

Reddy, D.G. & Anguli, V.C. (1967) Experimental production of cancer with betel nut, tobacco and slaked lime mixture. *J. Indian med. Assoc.*, **49**, 315–318

Reddy, M.S., Naik, S.R., Bagga, O.P. & Chuttani, H.K. (1980) Effect of chronic tobacco-betel-lime 'quid' chewing on human salivary secretions. *Am. J. clin. Nutr.*, **33**, 77–80

Reichart, P.A. (1995) Oral cancer and precancer related to betel and *miang* chewing in Thailand: A review. *J. oral Pathol. Med.*, **24**, 241–243

Reichart, P. & Gehring, F. (1984) *Streptococcus mutans* and caries prevalence in Lisu and Karen of Northern Thailand. *J. dent. Res.*, **63**, 56–58

Reichart, P., Böning, W., Srisuwan, S., Theetranont, C. & Mohr, U. (1984) Ultrastructural findings in the oral mucosa of betel chewers. *J. oral Pathol.*, **13**, 166–177

Reichart, P.A., Mohr, U., Srisuwan, S., Geerlings, H., Theetranont, C. & Kangwanpong T. (1987) Precancerous and other oral mucosal lesions related to chewing, smoking and drinking habits in Thailand. *Community dent. oral Epidemiol.*, **15**, 152–160

Reichart, P.A., Schmidtberg, W. & Scheifele, C. (1996) Betel chewer's mucosa in elderly Cambodian women. *J. oral Pathol. Med.*, **25**, 367–370

Reichart, P.A., Schmidtberg, W. & Scheifele, C. (1997) Khmer dental and medical students' knowledge about the betel quid chewing habit in Cambodia. *Eur. J. dent. Educ.*, **1**, 129–132

Reichart, P.A., Khongkhunthian, P., Scheifele, C. & Lohsuwan, P. (1999) Thai dental students' knowledge of the betel quid chewing habit in Thailand. *Eur. J. dent. Educ.*, **3**, 126–132

Reichart, P.A., Schmidtberg, W., Samaranayake, L.P. & Scheifele, C. (2002) Betel quid-associated oral lesions and oral *Candida* species in a female Cambodian cohort. *J. oral Pathol. Med.*, **31**, 468–472

Remani, P., Ankathil, R., Vijayan, K.K., Haseena Beevi, V.M., Rajendran, R. & Vijayakumar, T. (1988) Circulating immune complexes as an immunological marker in premalignant and malignant lesions of the oral cavity. *Cancer Lett.*, **40**, 185–191

Ridge, C., Akanle, O. & Spyrou, N.M. (2001) Elemental composition of betel nut and associated chewing materials. *J. radioanal. nucl. Chem.*, **249**, 67–70

Ridge, C., Okanle, O. & Spyrou, N.M. (2001) Elemental composition of betel nut and associated chewing materials. *J. radioanal. nucl. Chem.*, **249**, 67–70

Rosazza, J.P.N., Huang, Z., Dostal, L., Volm, T. & Rousseau, B. (1995) Review: Biocatalytic transformations of ferulic acid: An abundant aromatic natural product. *J. ind. Microbiol.*, **15**, 457–471

Rosin, M.P. (1984) The influence of pH on the convertogenic activity of plant phenolics. *Mutat. Res.*, **135**, 109–113

Rudat, K. (1994) *Black and Minority Ethnic Groups in England: Health and Lifestyles*, London, Health Education Authority, pp. 82–83

Rupa, D.S. & Eastmond, D.A. (1997) Chromosomal alterations affecting the 1cen-1q12 region in buccal mucosal cells of betel quid chewers detected using multicolor fluorescence *in situ* hybridization. *Carcinogenesis*, **18**, 2347–2351

Saikia, M. & Vaidehi, M.P. (1983) Studies on the pathological effects of feeding betel-nut meal in albino rats. *Br. J. exp. Med.*, **64**, 515–517

Salley, J.J. (1954) Experimental carcinogenesis in the cheek pouch of the Syrian hamster. *J. dent. Res.*, **33**, 253–262

Samuel, K.C., Navani, H. & Logani, K.B. (1969) Epidemiology of oral carcinoma in eastern districts of Uttar Pradesh. *J. Indian med. Assoc.*, **53**, 179–186

Sanghvi, L.D., Rao, K.C.M. & Khanolkar, V.R. (1955) Smoking and chewing of tobacco in relation to cancer of the upper alimentary tract. *Br. med. J.*, **i**, 1111–1114

Sankaranarayanan, R., Duffy, S.W., Day, N.E., Nair, M.K. & Padmakumary, G. (1989a) A case–control investigation of cancer of the oral tongue and the floor of the mouth in Southern India. *Int. J. Cancer*, **44**, 617–621

Sankaranarayanan, R., Duffy, S.W., Padmakumary, G., Day, N.E. & Padmanabhan, T.K. (1989b) Tobacco chewing, alcohol and nasal snuff in cancer of the gingiva in Kerala, India. *Br. J. Cancer*, **60**, 638–643

Sankaranarayanan, R., Duffy, S.W., Padmakumary, G., Day, N.E. & Nair, M.K. (1990a) Risk factors for cancer of the buccal and labial mucosa in Kerala, southern India. *J. Epidemiol. Community Health*, **44**, 286–292

Sankaranarayanan, R., Duffy, S.W., Nair, M.K., Padmakumary, G. & Day, N.E. (1990b) Tobacco and alcohol as risk factors in cancer of the larynx in Kerala, India. *Int. J. Cancer*, **45**, 879–882

Sankaranarayanan, R., Duffy, S.W., Padmakumary, G., Muralidharan Nair, S., Day, N.E. & Padmanabhan, T.K. (1991) Risk factors for cancer of the oesophagus in Kerala, India. *Int. J. Cancer*, **49**, 485–489

Sankaranarayanan, R., Mathew, B., Jacob, B.J., Thomas, G., Somanathan,T., Pisani, P., Pandey, M., Ramadas, K., Najeeb, K. & Abraham, E. for the Trivandrum Oral Cancer Screening Study Group (2000) Early findings from a community-based, cluster-randomized, controlled oral cancer screening trial in Kerala, India. *Cancer*, **188**, 664–673

Saranath, D., Mukhopadhyaya, R., Rao, R.S., Fakih, A.R., Naik, S.L. & Gangal, S.G. (1985) Cell-mediated immune status in patients with squamous cell carcinoma of the oral cavity. *Cancer*, **56**, 1062–1070

Saranath, D., Bhoite, L.T., Mehta, A.R., Sanghavi, V. & Deo, M.G. (1991a) Loss of allelic heterozygosity at the harvey *ras* locus in human oral carcinomas. *Cancer Res. clin. Oncol.*, **117**, 484–488

Saranath, D., Chang, S.E., Bhoite, L.T., Panchal, R.B., Kerr, I.B., Mehta, A.R., Johnson, N.W. & Deo, M.G. (1991b) High frequency mutation in codons 12 and 61 of H-*ras* oncogene in chewing tobacco-related human oral carcinoma in India. *Br. J. Cancer*, **63**, 573–578

Saranath, D., Tandle, A.T., Teni, T.R., Dedhia, P.M., Borges, A.M., Parikh, D., Sanghavi, V. & Mehta, A.R. (1999) p53 Inactivation in chewing tobacco-induced oral cancers and leukoplakias from India. *Oral Oncol.*, **35**, 242–250

Sarkar, M., Gangopadhyay, P., Basak, B., Chakrabarty, K., Banerji, J., Adhikary, P. & Chatterjee, A. (2000) The reversible antifertility effect of *Piper betle* Linn. on Swiss albino male mice. *Contraception*, **62**, 271–274

Sarma, S.N. (1958) A study into the incidence and etiology of cancer of the larynx and adjacent parts in Assam. *Indian J. med. Res.*, **46**, 525–533

Sarma, A.B., Chakrabarti, J., Chakrabarti, A., Banerjee, T.S., Roy, D., Mukherjee, D. & Mukherjee, A. (1992) Evaluation of pan masala for toxic effects on liver and other organs. *Food chem. Toxicol.*, **30**, 161–163

Saunders, J., Showell, G.A., Snow, R.J., Baker, R., Harley, E.A. & Freedman, S.B. (1988) 2-Methyl-1,3-dioxaazaspiro[4,5]decanes as novel muscarinic cholinergic agonists. *J. med. Chem.*, **31**, 486–491

Scalbert, A., Morand, C., Manach, C. & Rémésy, C. (2002) Absorption and metabolism of polyphenols in the gut and impact on health. *Biomed. Pharmacother.*, **56**, 276–282

Schamschula, R.G., Adkins, B.L., Barmes, D.E. & Charlton, G. (1977) Betel chewing and caries experience in New Guinea. *Community dent. oral Epidemiol.*, **5**, 284–286

Schneider, E. (1986) [Betel – A popular pleasure – giving substance in South Asia.] *Pharm. Uns. Zeit*, **15**, 161–166 (in German)

Schonland, M.N. & Bradshaw, E. (1969) Upper alimentary tract cancer in Natal Indians with special reference to the betel-chewing habit. *Br. J. Cancer*, **23**, 670–682

Scrimgeour, E.M. & Jolley, D. (1983) Trends in tobacco consumption and incidences of associated neoplasms in Papua New Guinea. *Br. med. J.*, **286**, 1414–1416

Scutt, A., Meghji, S., Canniff, J.P. & Harvey, W. (1987) Stabilisation of collagen by betel nut polyphenols as a mechanism in oral submucous fibrosis. Experientia, 43, 391–393

Seedat, H.A. (1985) *Oral Submucous Fibrosis in Durban, Natal: A Study of its Epidemiology, Aetiology and Morphological Features* (PhD Thesis), Stellenbosch, University of Stellenbosch, South Africa

Seedat, H.A. & Van Wyk, C.W. (1988) Betel-nut chewing and submucous fibrosis in Durban. *S. Afr. Med. J.*, **74**, 568–571

Sein, K., Maung, K.K. & Aung, T.H. (1992) An epidemiologic study of 70 oral cancer cases at the Institute of Dental Medicine, Yangon, Myanmar, 1985–1988. *Odontostomatol. Trop.*, **15**, 5–8

Self, R., Jones, A. & Holdsworth, D.K. (1999) Gas chromatography/mass spectrometry analysis of alkaloids in betel nut (*Areca catechu*). *Eur. mass Spectrom.*, **5**, 213–219

Selvan, R.S. & Rao, A.R. (1993) Influence of arecoline on immune system: III. Suppression of B cell-mediated immune response in mice after short-term exposure. *Immunopharmacol. Immunotoxicol.*, **15**, 291–305

Selvan, R.S., Venkateswaran, K.S. & Rao, A.R. (1989) Influence of arecoline on immune system: I. Short term effects on general parameters and on the adrenal and lymphoid organs. *Immunopharmacol. Immunotoxicol.*, **11**, 347–377

Selvan, R.S., Selvakumaran, M. & Rao, A.R. (1991) Influence of arecoline on immune system: II. Suppression of thymus-dependent immune responses and parameter of non-specific resistance after short-term exposure. *Immunopharmacol. Immunotoxicol.*, **13**, 281–309

Senewiratne, B. & Uragoda, C.G. (1973) Betel chewing in Ceylon. *Am. J. trop. Med. Hyg.*, **22**, 418–422

Shah, N. & Sharma, P.P. (1998) Role of chewing and smoking habits in the etiology of oral submucous fibrosis (OSF): A case–control study. *J. oral Pathol. Med.*, **27**, 475–479

Shah, N., Kumar, R. & Shah, M.K. (1994) Immunological studies in oral submucous fibrosis. *Indian J. dent. Res.*, **5**, 81–87

Shah, B., Lewis, M.A.O. & Bedi, R. (2001) Oral submucous fibrosis in a 11-year-old Bangladeshi girl living in the United Kingdom. *Br. dent. J.*, **191**, 130–132

Shah, S.M.A., Merchant, A.T., Luby, S.P. & Chotani, R.A. (2002) Addicted schoolchildren: Prevalence and characteristics of areca nut chewers among primary school children in Karachi, Pakistan. *J. Paediatr. Child Health*, **38**, 507–510

Shahabuddin, S. Rao, A.R. & Mustafa, A.S. (1980) Effect of arecoline on the humoral and cell-mediated immune responses in mice. *Indian J. exp. Biol.*, **18**, 1493–1494

Shannon, H.E., Bymaster, F.P., Calligaro, D.O., Greenwood, B., Mitch, C.H., Sawyer, B.D., Ward, J.S., Wong, D.T., Olesen, P.H., Sheardown, M.J., Swedberg, M.D.B., Suzdak, P.D. & Sauerberg, P. (1994) Xanomeline: A novel muscarinic receptor agonist with functional selectivity for $M_1$ receptors. *J. Pharmacol. exp. Ther.*, **269**, 271–281

Shanta, V. & Krishnamurthi, S. (1959) A study of aetiological factors in oral squamous cell carcinoma. *Br. J. Cancer*, **13**, 381–388

Shanta, V. & Krishnamurthi, S. (1963) Further study in aetiology of carcinomas of the upper alimentary tract. *Br. J. Cancer*, **17**, 8–23

Sharan, R.N. & Wary, K.K. (1992) Study of unscheduled DNA synthesis following exposure of human cells to arecoline and extracts of betel nut in vitro. *Mutat. Res.*, **278**, 271–276

Sharma, B.B. (2002) *Prevention of Food Adulteration Act, 1954* (Notification No. PFA/574-2002/7, dated 23 July), Mumbai, Commissioner for Food and Drug Administration and Food (Health) Authority, Maharashtra State

Shear, M., Lemmer, J. & Dockrat, I. (1967) Oral submucous fibrosis in South African Indians: An epidemiological study. *S. Afr. J. med. Sci.*, **32**, 41–46

Shetty, K.V. & Johnson, N.W. (1999) Knowledge, attitudes and beliefs of adult South Asians living in London regarding risk factors and signs for oral cancer. *Community Dent. Health*, **16**, 227–231

Shirname, L.P., Menon, M.M., Nair, J. & Bhide, S.V. (1983) Correlation of mutagenicity and tumorigenicity of betel quid and its ingredients. *Nutr. Cancer*, **5**, 87–91

Shirname, L.P., Menon, M.M. & Bhide, S.V. (1984) Mutagenicity of betel quid and its ingredients using mammalian test systems. *Carcinogenesis*, **5**, 501–503

Shiu, M.N., Chen, T.H.H., Chang, S.H. & Hahn, L.J. (2000) Risk factors for leukoplakia and malignant transformation to oral carcinoma: A leukoplakia cohort in Taiwan. *Br. J. Cancer*, **82**, 1871–1874

Shivapurkar, N.M. & Bhide, S.V. (1979) Effect of betel-nut constituents on nucleic acid metabolism. *Indian J. exp. Biol.*, **17**, 1141–1144

Shivapurkar, N.M., Bhide, S.V. & Ranadive, K.J. (1978) Biochemical studies of betel nut constituents. *Indian J. Pharmacol.*, **10**, 191–200

Shivapurkar, N.M., Ranadive, S.N., Gothoskar, S.V., Bhide, S.V. & Ranadive, K.J. (1980) Tumorigenic effect of aqueous and polyphenolic fractions of betel nut in Swiss strain mice. *Indian J. exp. Biol.*, **18**, 1159–1161

Shivashankar, S., Dhanaraj, S., Mathew, A.G., Srinivasa Murthy, S., Vyasamurthy, M.N. & Govindarajan, V.S. (1969) Physical and chemical characteristics of processed areca nuts. *J. Food Sci. Technol.*, **41**, 113–116

Shwe, M., Chiguchi, G., Yamada, S., Nakajima, T., Maung, K.K., Takagi, M., Amagasa, T. & Tsuchida, N. (2001) p53 and MDM2 co-expression in tobacco and betel chewing-associated oral squamous cell carcinomas. *J. med. dent. Sci.*, **48**, 113–119

Sidiq, Y., Rajagopalan, K.R., & Krishnamurthy M.S. (1964) Aetiology and epidemiology of oral cavity cancers. *J. Indian med. Assoc.* **43**, 526–529

Silverman, S., Jr, Bhargava, K., Mani, N.J., Smith, L.W. & Malaowalla, A.M. (1976) Malignant transformation and natural history of oral leukoplakia in 57 518 industrial workers of Gujarat, India. *Cancer*, **38**, 1790–1795

Simarak, S., de Jong, U.W., Breslow, N., Dahl, C.J., Ruckphaopunt, K., Scheelings, P. & MacLennan, R. (1977) Cancer of the oral cavity, pharynx/larynx and lung in North Thailand: Case–control study and analysis of cigar smoke. *Br. J. Cancer*, **36**, 130–140

Singh, A.D. & von Essen, C.F. (1966) Buccal mucosa cancer in South India. Etiologic and clinical aspects. *Am. J. Roentgenol. Radium Ther. Nucl. Med.*, **96**, 6–14

Singh, A. & Rao, A.R. (1993a) Modulatory effect of areca nut on the action of MACE (*Myristica fragrans*, Houtt) on hepatic detoxification system in mice. *Food chem. Toxicol.*, **31**, 517–521

Singh, A. & Rao, A.R. (1993b) Effect of arecanut on the black mustard (*Brassica niger*, L.)-mediated detoxication enzymes and sulfhydryl content in the liver of mice. *Cancer Lett.*, **72**, 45–51

Singh, A. & Rao, A.R. (1993c) Effect of arecoline on Phase I and Phase II drug metabolizing system of enzymes, sulphydryl content and lipid peroxidation in mouse liver. *Biochem. mol. Biol. int.*, **30**, 763–772

Singh, A. & Rao, A.R. (1995a) Modulatory influence of arecanut on the mouse hepatic xenobiotic detoxication system and skin papillomagenesis. *Teratog. Carcinog. Mutag.*, **15**, 135–146

Singh, A. & Rao, A.R. (1995b) Evaluation of the modifying influence of arecanut on the garlic-modulated hepatic detoxication system enzymes, sulfyhydryl content and lipid peroxidation. *Teratog. Carcinog. Mutag.*, **15**, 127–134

Singh, A. & Rao, A.R. (1995c) Modulatory influence of arecanut on antioxidant 2(3)-*tert*-butyl-4-hydroxy anisole-induced hepatic detoxification system and antioxidant defence mechanism in mice. *Cancer Lett.*, **91**, 107–114

Singh, A., Sing, S.P. & Bamezai, R. (1996) Postnatal effect of arecoline on chlorophyllin-modulated hepatic biotransformation system enzymes in suckling neonate and lactating mice. *Teratog. Carcinog. Mutag.*, **16**, 89–96

Singh, A., Singh, S.P. & Bamezai, R. (1997) Modulatory influence of arecoline on the phytic acid-altered hepatic biotransformation system enzymes, sulfhydryl content and lipid peroxidation in a murine system. *Cancer Lett.*, **117**, 1–6

Singh, A., Singh, S.P. & Bamezai, R. (2000) Direct and translactational effect of arecoline alkaloid on the clocimum oil-modulated hepatic drug metabolizing enzymes in mice. *Food. chem. Toxicol.*, **38**, 627–635

Sinha, A. & Rao, A.R. (1985a) Embryotoxicity of betel nuts in mice. *Toxicology*, **37**, 315–326

Sinha, A. & Rao, A.R. (1985b) Induction of shape abnormality and unscheduled DNA synthesis by arecoline in the germ cells of mice. *Mutat. Res.*, **158**, 189–192

Sinha, A. & Rao, A.R. (1985c) Transplacental micronucleus inducing ability of arecoline, a betel nut alkaloid, in mice. *Mutat. Res.*, **158**, 193–194

Sinha, D.N. & Gupta, P.C. (2001) Tobacco and areca nut use in male medical students of Patna. *Natl med. J. India*, **14**, 176–178

Sinor, P.N., Gupta, P.C., Murti, P.R., Bhonsle, R.B., Daftary, D.K., Mehta, F.S. & Pindborg, J.J. (1990) A case–control study of oral submucous fibrosis with special reference to the etiologic role of areca nut. *J. oral Pathol. Med.*, **19**, 94–98

Sirsat, S.M. & Khanolkar, V.R. (1962) The effect of arecoline on the palatal and buccal mucosa of the Wistar rat. An optical and electron microscope study. *Indian J. med. Sci.*, **16**, 198–202

Slotkin, T.A. (1992) Prenatal exposure to nicotine: What can we learn from animal models? In: Zagon, I.S. & Slotkin. T.A., eds, *Maternal Substance Abuse and the Developing Nervous System*, San Diego, Academic Press, pp. 97–124

Slotkin, T.A., Greer, N., Faust, J., Cho, H. & Seidler, F.J. (1986) Effects of maternal nicotine injections on brain development in the rat: Ornithine decarboxylase activity, nucleic acids and proteins in discrete brain regions. *Brain Res. Bull.*, **17**, 41–50

Slotkin, T.A., Lappi, S.E. & Seidler, F.J. (1993) Impact of fetal nicotine exposure on development of rat brain regions: Critical sensitive periods or effects of withdrawal? *Brain Res. Bull.*, **31**, 319–328

Smismans, A., Schuit, F. & Pipeleers, D. (1997) Nutrient regulation of gamma-butyric acid release from islet beta cells. *Diabetologia*, **40**, 1411–1415

Smith, L.W., Bhargava, K., Mani, N.J., Malaowalla, A.M. & Silverman, S., Jr (1975) Oral cancer and precancerous lesions in 57,518 industrial workers of Gujarat, India. *Indian J. Cancer*, **12**, 118–123

Sopori, M.L & Kozak, W. (1998) Immunomodulatory effects of cigarette smoke. *J. Neuroimmunol.*, **83**, 148–156

Sorenson, R.L., Garry, D.G. & Brelje, T.C. (1991) Structural and functional considerations of GABA in islets of Langerhans, β-cells and nerves. *Diabetes*, **40**, 1365–1374

Srinivasan, M. & Jewell, S.D. (2001a) Quantitative estimation of PCNA, *c-myc*, EGFR and TGF-α in oral submucous fibrosis — An immunohistochemical study. *Oral Oncol.*, **37**, 461–467

Srinivasan, M. & Jewell, S.D. (2001b) Evaluation of TGF-α and EGFR expression in oral leukoplakia and oral submucous fibrosis by quantitative immunohistochemistry. *Oncology*, **61**, 284–292

Srivastava, S.P. & Sharma, S.C. (1968) Gingival cancer. *Indian J. Cancer*, **5**, 89–97

Srivatanakul, P., Parkin, D.M., Khlat, M., Chenvidhya, D., Chotiwan, P., Insiripong, S., L'Abbe, K.A. & Wild C.P. (1991) Liver cancer in Thailand. II. A case–control study of hepatocellular carcinoma. *Int. J. Cancer*, **48**, 329–332

Stanley, K. & Stjernsward, J. (1986) A survey on the control of oral cancer in India. *Indian J. Cancer*, **23**, 105–111

Stephen, S.J. & Uragoda, C.G. (1970) Some observations on oesophageal carcinoma in Ceylon including its relationship to betel chewing. *Br. J. Cancer*, **24**, 11–15

Stich, H.F. & Dunn, B.P. (1986) Relationship between cellular levels of beta-carotene and sensitivity to genotoxic agents. *Int. J. Cancer*, **38**, 713–717

Stich, H.F. & Tsang, S.S. (1989) Promoting activity of betel quid ingredients and their inhibition by retinol. *Cancer Lett.*, **45**, 71–77

Stich, H.F., Stich, W. & Parida, B.B. (1982) Elevated frequency of micronucleated cells in the buccal mucosa of individuals at high risk for oral cancer: Betel quid chewers. *Cancer Lett.*, **17**, 125–134

Stich, H.F., Ohshima, H., Pignatelli, B., Michelon, J. & Bartsch, H. (1983) Inhibitory effect of betel nut extracts on endogenous nitrosation in humans. *J. natl Cancer Inst.*, **70**, 1047–1050

Stich, H.F., Dunn, B.P., Pignatelli, B., Ohshima, H. & Bartsch, H. (1984a) Dietary phenolics and betel nut extracts as modifiers of *N*-nitrosation in rat and man. In: O'Neill, I.K., von Borstel, R.C., Miller, C.T., Long, J. & Bartsch, H., eds, N-*Nitroso Compounds: Occurrence, Biological Effects and Relevance to Human Cancer* (IARC Scientific Publications No. 57), Lyon, *IARC*Press, pp. 213–222

Stich, H.F., Rosin, M.P. & Vallejera, M.O. (1984b) Reduction with vitamin A and beta-carotene administration of proportion of micronucleated buccal mucosal cells in Asian betel nut and tobacco chewers. *Lancet*, **i**, 1204–1206

Stich, H.F., Stich, W., Rosin, M.P. & Vallejera, M.O. (1984c) Use of the micronucleus test to monitor the effect of vitamin A, beta-carotene and canthaxanthin on the buccal mucosa of betel nut/tobacco chewers. *Int. J. Cancer*, **34**, 745–750

Stich, H.F., Rosin, M.P. & Brunnemann, K.D. (1986) Oral lesions, genotoxicity and nitrosamines in betel quid chewers with no obvious increase in oral cancer risk. *Cancer Lett.*, **31**, 15–25

Stich, H.F., Rosin, M.P., Hornby, A.P., Mathew, B., Sankaranarayanan, R. & Nair, M.K. (1988) Remission of oral leukoplakias and micronuclei in tobacco/betel quid chewers treated with beta-carotene and with beta-carotene plus vitamin A. *Int. J. Cancer*, **42**, 195–199

Stich, H.F., Brunnemann, K.D., Mathew, B., Sankaranayanan, R. & Nair, M.K. (1989) Chemopreventive trials with vitamin A and β-carotene: Some unresolved issues. *Prev. Med.*, **18**, 732–739

Stich, H.F., Mathew, B., Sankaranarayanan, R. & Nair, M.K. (1991) Remission of precancerous lesions in the oral cavity of tobacco chewers and maintenance of the protective effect of β-carotene or vitamin A. *Am. J. clin. Nutr.*, **53**, 298S–304S

Strickland, S.S. & Duffield, A.E. (1997) Anthropometric status and resting metabolic rate in users of the areca nut and smokers of tobacco in rural Sarawak. *Ann. hum. Biol.*, **25**, 453–474

Strickland, S.S., Veena, G.V., Houghton, P.J., Stanford S.C. & Kurpad, A.V. (2003) Areca nut, energy metabolism and hunger in Asian men. *Ann. hum. Biol.*, **30**, 26–52

Sullivan, R.J. & Hagen, E.H. (2002) Psychotropic substance-seeking: Evolutionary pathology or adaptation? *Addiction*, **97**, 389–400

Summers, R.M., Williams, S.A. & Curzon, M.E.J. (1994) The use of tobacco and betel quid ('pan') among Bangladeshi women in West Yorkshire. *Community Dent. Health*, **11**, 12–16

Sun, C.A., Wu, D.M., Lin, C.C., Lu, S.N., You, S.L., Wang, L.Y., Wu, M.H. & Chen, C.J. (2003) Incidence and cofactors of hepatitis C virus-related hepatocellular carcinoma: A prospective study of 12 008 men in Taiwan. *Am. J. Epidemiol.*, **157**, 674–682

Sundqvist, K. & Grafström, R.C. (1992) Effects of areca nut on growth, differentiation and formation of DNA damage in cultured human buccal epithelial cells. *Int. J. Cancer*, **52**, 305–310

Sundqvist, K., Liu, Y., Nair, J., Bartsch, H., Arvidson, K. & Grafström, R.C. (1989) Cytotoxic and genotoxic effects of areca nut-related compounds in cultured human buccal epithelial cells. *Cancer Res.*, **49**, 5294–5298

Suri, K., Goldman, H.M. & Wells, H. (1971) Carcinogenic effect of a dimethyl sulphoxide extract of betel nut on the mucosa of the hamster buccal pouch. *Nature*, **230**, 383–384

Swerdlow, A.J., Marmot, M.G., Grulich, A.E. & Head, J. (1995) Cancer mortality in Indian and British ethnic immigrants from the Indian subcontinent to England and Wales. *Br. J. Cancer*, **72**, 1312–1319

Syiem, D., Syngai, G., Khup, P.Z., Khongwir, B.S., Kharbuli, B. & Kayang, H. (2002) Hypoglycemic effects of *Potentilla fulgens* L. in normal and alloxan-induced diabetic mice. *J. Ethnopharmacol.*, **83**, 55–61

Talonu, N.T. (1989) Observation on betel-nut use, habituation, addiction and carcinogenesis in Papua New Guineans. *Papua New Guinea med. J.*, **32**, 195–197

Tan, B.S., Rosman, A., Ng, K.H. & Ahmad, N. (2000) Profile of the betel/tobacco quid chewers in six Malaysian estates. *Annal. Dent. Univ. Malaya*, **7**, 1–5

Tanaka, T., Mori, H., Fujii, M., Takahashi, M. & Hirono, I. (1983) Carcinogenicity examination of betel quid. II. Effect of vitamin A deficiency on rats fed semipurified diet containing betel nut and calcium hydroxide. *Nutr. Cancer*, **4**, 260–266

Tanaka, T., Kuniyasu, T., Shima, H., Sugie, S., Mori, H., Takahashi, M. & Hirono, I. (1986) Carcinogenicity of betel quid. III. Enhancement of 4-nitroquinoline-1-oxide- and N-2-fluorenylacetamide-induced carcinogenesis in rats by subsequent administration of betel nut. *J. natl Cancer Inst.*, **77**, 777–781

Tandle, A.T., Sanghvi, V. & Saranath, D. (2001) Determination of *p53* genotypes in oral cancer patients from India. *Br. J. Cancer*, **84**, 739–742

Tang, J.G., Jian, X.F., Gao, M.L., Ling, T.Y. & Zhang, K.H. (1997) Epidemiological survey of oral submucous fibrosis in Xiangtan City, Hunan Province, China. *Community Dent. Oral Epidemiol.*, **25**, 177–180

Tang, J.G., Jian, X.F., Gao, M.L., Ling, T.Y. & Zhang, K.H. (1997) Epidemiological survey of oral submucous fibrosis in Xiangtan City, Hunan Province, China. *Community dent. oral Epidemiol.*, **25**, 177–178

Taylor, F., Al-Jarad, N., John, L.M.E., Conroy, D.M. & Barnes, N.C. (1992) Betel-nut chewing and asthma. *Lancet*, **339**, 1134–1136

Thomas, S.J. & MacLennan, R. (1992) Slaked lime and betel nut cancer in Papua New Guinea. *Lancet*, **340**, 577–578

Thomas, S., Brennan, J., Martel, G., Frazer, I., Montesano, R., Sidransky, D. & Hollstein, M. (1994) Mutations in the conserved regions of *p53* are infrequent in betel-associated oral cancers from Papua-New Guinea. *Cancer Res.*, **54**, 3588–3593

Thomas, G., Hashibe, M., Jacob, B.J., Ramadas, K., Mathew, B., Sankaranarayanan, R. & Zhang, Z.F. (2003) Risk factors for multiple oral premalignant lesions. *Int. J. Cancer*, **107**, 285–291

Thompson, D.C., Thompson, J.A., Sugumaran, M. & Moldéus, P. (1993) Biological and toxicological consequences of quinone methide formation. *Chem.-biol. Interactions*, **86**, 129–162

Thongsuksai, P. & Boonyaphiphat, P. (2001) Lack of association between p53 expression and betel nut chewing in oral cancers from Thailand. *Oral Oncol.*, **37**, 276–281

Timms, P.M., Srikanthan, V.A., Lindsay, M., Maxwell, P., Wright, A. & Dunn, F.G. (1998) Plasma tissue inhibitor of metalloproteinase-1 is elevated in hypertension (Abstract). *Am. J. Hypertens.*, **11**, 1A

Timms, P.M., Mannan, N., Hitman, G.A., Noonan, K., Mills, P.G., Syndercombe-Court, Y.D., Aganna, E., Price, C.P. & Boucher, B.J. (2002a) Circulating MMP9, vitamin D and variation in the TIMP-1 response with VDR genotype: Mechanisms for inflammatory damage in chronic disorders? *Q. J. Med.*, **95**, 787–796

Timms, P.M., Wright, A., Maxwell, P., Campbell, S., Dawnay, A.B. & Srikanthan, V. (2002b) Plasma tissue inhibitor of metalloproteinase-1 levels are elevated in essential hypertension and related to left ventricular hypertrophy. *Am. J. Hypertens.*, **15**, 269–272

Tolentino, A.D., Jr, Erese, B.C. & Soriano, O.L. (1963) Malignant and pre-malignant lesions of the oral cavity. *Philippine J. Cancer*, **5**, 406–416

Topcu, Z., Chiba, I., Fujieda, M., Shibata, T., Ariyoshi, N., Yamazaki, H., Sevgican, F., Muthumala, M., Kobayashi, H. & Kamataki, T. (2002) *CYP2A6* gene deletion reduces oral cancer risk in betel quid chewers in Sri Lanka. *Carcinogenesis*, **23**, 595–598

Trendelenburg, P. (1912) Physiologische und pharmakologische Untersuchungen an der isolierten Bronchialmuskulatur. *Arch. exp. Pathol. Pharm.*, **69**, 79

Trivedy, C.R. (2001) The legislative issues related to the sale and consumption of areca (betel) nut products in the UK: Current status and objectives for the future. *J. Indian Med. Assoc.*, **1**, 10–16

Trivedi, A.H., Dave, B.J. & Adhvaryu, S.C. (1993) Genotoxic effects of nicotine in combination with arecoline on CHO cells. *Cancer Lett.*, **74**, 105–110

Trivedi, A.H., Roy, S.K., Patel, R.K., Adhvaryu, S.G. & Balar, D.B. (1995) Urine of tobacco/areca nut chewers causes genomic damage in Chinese hamster ovary cells. *Carcinogenesis*, **16**, 205–208

Trivedy, C., Baldwin, D., Warnakulasuriya, S., Johnson, N. & Peters, T. (1997) Copper content in *Areca catechu* (betel nut) products and oral submucous fibrosis. *Lancet*, **349**, 1447

Trivedy, C., Warnakulasuriya, K.A.A.S., Tavassoli, M., Steingrimsdottir, H., Penhallow, J., Maher, R. & Johnson, N.W. (1998) p53 Aberrations in oral submucous fibrosis and oral squamous cell carcinoma detected by immunocytochemistry and PCR-SSCP. *J. oral Pathol. Med.*, **27**, 72–77

Trivedy, C., Warnakulasuriya, S. & Peters, T.J. (1999a) Areca nuts can have deleterious effects. *Br. med. J.*, **318**, 1287

Trivedy, C., Warnakulasuriya, S., Hazarey, V.K. & Johnson, N.W. (1999b) The role of copper in the aetiopathogenesis of oral submucous fibrosis. In: Varma, A.K., ed., *Oral Oncology*, Vol. VI, *Proceedings of the 6th International Congress on Oral Cancer*, New Delhi, Macmillan Press, pp. 7–10

Trivedy, C., Warnakulasuriya, K.A.A.S., Hazarey, V.K., Tavassoli, M., Sommer, P. & Johnson, N.W. (1999c) The upregulation of lysyl oxidase in oral submucous fibrosis and squamous cell carcinoma. *J. oral Pathol. Med.*, **28**, 246–251

Trivedy, C.R., Warnakulasuriya, K.A.A.S., Peters, T.J., Senkus, R., Hazarey, V.K. & Johnson, N.W. (2000) Raised tissue copper levels in oral submucous fibrosis. *J. oral Pathol. Med.*, **29**, 241–248

Trivedy, C., Meghji, S., Warnakulasuriya, K.A.A.S., Johnson, N.W. & Harris, M. (2001) Copper stimulates human oral fibroblasts *in vitro*: A role in the pathogenesis of oral submucous fibrosis. *J. oral Pathol. Med.*, **30**, 465–470

Tsai, C.C., Ma, R.H. & Shieh, T.Y. (1999) Deficiency in collagen and fibronectin phagocytosis by human buccal mucosa fibroblasts *in vitro* as a possible mechanism for oral submucous fibrosis. *J. oral Pathol. Med.*, **28**, 59–63

Tsai, J.F., Chuang, L.Y., Jeng, J.E., Ho, M.S., Hsieh, M.Y., Lin, Z.Y. & Wang, L.Y. (2001) Betel quid chewing as a risk factor for hepatocellular carcinoma: A case–control study. *Br. J. Cancer*, **84**, 709–713

Tsai, C.-H., Chou, M.-Y. & Chang, Y.-C. (2003) The upregulation of cyclooxygenase-2 expression in human buccal mucosal fibroblasts by arecoline: A possible role in the pathogenesis of oral submucous fibrosis. *J. oral Pathol. Med.*, **32**, 146–153

Van der Bijl, P. & Van Wyk C.W. (1995) Estimation of areca nut consumption among South African Indians. *J. int. dent. Assoc.*, **66**, 52–54

Van der Bijl, P., Stockenström, S., Vismer, H.F. & van Wyk, C.W. (1996) Incidence of fungi and aflatoxins in imported areca nut samples. *S. Afr. J. Sci.*, **92**, 154–156

Verma, R.C., Chansoriya, M. & Kaul, K.K. (1983) Effect of tobacco chewing by mothers on fetal outcome. *Indian Pediatr.*, **20**, 105–111

Vineis, P., d'Errico, A., Malats, N. & Boffetta, P. (1999) Overall evaluation and research perspectives. In: Vineis, P., Malats, N., Lang, M., d'Errico, A., Caporaso, J., Cuzick, J. & Boffetta, P., eds, *Metabolic Polymorphisms and Susceptibility to Cancer* (IARC Scientific Publications No. 148), Lyon, *IARC*Press, pp. 403–408

Vora, A.R., Yeoman, C.M. & Hayter, J.P. (2000) Alcohol, tobacco and paan use and understanding of oral cancer risk among Asian males in Leicester. *Br. dent. J.*, **188**, 444–451

Wahi, P.N. (1968) The epidemiology of oral and oropharyngeal cancer. A report of the study in Mainpuri district, Uttar Pradesh, India. *Bull. World Health Organ.*, **38**, 495–521

Wahi, P.N., Kehar, U. & Lahiri, B. (1965) Factors influencing oral and oropharyngeal cancers in India. *Br. J. Cancer*, **19**, 642–660

Wahi, P.N., Lahiri, B. & Kehar, U. (1966) Epidemiology of oral and oropharyngeal cancer. A study of regional factors in Uttar Pradesh. *J. Indian med. Assoc.*, **46**, 175–181

Walker, E.A., Pignatelli, B. & Friesen, M. (1982) The role of phenols in catalysis of nitrosamine formation. *J. Sci. Food Agric.*, **33**, 81–88

Wang, C.K. & Hwang, L.S. (1993) [Analysis of the phenolic compounds in betel quid.] *J. Chin. agric. chem. Soc.*, **31**, 623–632 (in Chinese)

Wang, C.-K. & Peng, C.-H. (1996) The mutagenicities of alkaloids and *N*-nitrosoguvacoline from betel quid. *Mutat. Res.*, **360**, 165–171

Wang, C.-K. & Wu, M.-J. (1996) [The separation of phenolics from *Piper betle* leaf and the effect on the mutagenicity of arecoline.] *J. Chin. agric. chem. Soc.*, **34**, 638–647 (in Chinese)

Wang, C.-K. & Hwang, L.-S. (1997) Effect of betel quid on catecholamine secretion from adrenal chromaffin cells. *Proc. natl Sci. Counc. Repub. China B*, **21**, 129–136

Wang, C.-K., Su, H.-Y. & Lii, C.-K. (1999) Chemical composition and toxicity of Taiwanese betel quid extract. *Food. chem. Toxicol.*, **37**, 135–144

Wang, C.-K., Chen, S.-L. & Wu, M.-G. (2001) Inhibitory effect of betel quid on the volatility of methyl mercaptan. *J. agric. Food Chem.*, **49**, 1979–1983

Wani, M.K., Yarber, R.H., Ahmed, A., Hengesteg, A. & Robbins, K.T. (2001) Cancer induction in the DMBA hamster cheek-pouch: A modified technique using a promoter. *Laryngoscope*, **111**, 204–206

Warnakulasuriya, K.A.A.S. (1990) Smoking and chewing habits in Sri Lanka: Implications for oral cancer and precancer. In: Gupta, P.C., Hammer J.E. & Murti P.R., *Control of Tobacco Related Cancer and Other Diseases*, Oxford University Press, Bombay, 1992, pp 113–118

Warnakulasuriya, K.A.A.S. (1992) Smoking and chewing habits in Sri Lanka: Implications for oral cancer and precancer. In: Gupta, P.C., Hamner, J.E., III & Murti, P.R., eds, *Control of Tobacco-related Cancers and Other Diseases*, Mumbai, Oxford University Press, pp. 113–118

Warnakulasuriya, K.A.A.S. (1996) Ethnicity, race and oral cancer. In: Bedi, R., Bhal, V. & Raja, R.R., eds, *Dentists, Patients and Ethnic Minorities*, London, Faculty of General Dental Practitioners (UK), Department of Health, pp. 57–65

Warnakulasuriya, S. (2002) Areca nut use following migration and its consequences. *Addict. Biol.*, **7**, 127–132

Warnakulasuriya, K.A.A.S. & Johnson, N.W. (1996) Epidemiology and risk factors for oral cancer: Rising trends in Europe and possible effects of migration. *Int. dent. J.*, **46**, 245–250

Warnakulasuriya, K.A.A.S., Ekanayake, A.N.I, Sivayoham, S., Stjernsward, J., Pindborg, J.J., Sobin, L.H. & Perera, K.S.G.P. (1984) Utilization of primary health care workers for early detection of oral cancer and precancer cases in Sri Lanka. *Bull. World Health Org.*, **62**, 243–250

Warnakulasuriya, K.A.A.S., Johnson, N.W., Linklater, K.M. & Bell, J. (1999) Cancer of mouth, pharynx and nasopharynx in Asian and Chinese immigrants resident in Thames regions. *Oral Oncol.*, **35**, 471–475

Warnakulasuriya, S., Trivedy, C. & Peters, T.J. (2002) Areca nut use: An independent risk factor for oral cancer. *Br. med. J.*, **324**, 799–800

Wary, K.K. & Sharan, R.N. (1988) Aqueous extract of betel-nut of North-East India induces DNA-strand breaks and enhances rate of cell proliferation in vitro. Effect of betel-nut extract in vitro. *Cancer Res. clin. Oncol.*, **114**, 579–582

Wary, K.K. & Sharan, R.N. (1991) Cytotoxic and cytostatic effects of arecoline and sodium nitrite on human cells *in vitro*. *Int. J. Cancer*, **47**, 396–400

Wasnik, K.S., Ughade, S.N., Zodpey, S.P. & Ingole, D.L. (1998) Tobacco consumption practices and risk of oropharyngeal cancer: A case–control study in central India. *Southeast Asian J. trop. Med. public Health*, **29**, 827–834

Weerapradist, W. & Boonpuknavig, V. (1983) Effect of betel nut on the buccal mucosa of the hamster cheek pouch: Comparative histological study of Thai and Indian betel nut and di-methyl benzanthracene (DMBA). *J. dent. Assoc. Thailand*, **33**, 53–66

Wei, Y.Y. & Chung, C. (1997) Elemental analysis of Taiwanese areca nut and limes with INAA. *J. Radioanal. nucl. Chem.*, **217**, 45–51

Wenke, G. & Hoffmann, D. (1983) A study of betel quid carcinogenesis. 1. On the *in vitro* N-nitrosation of arecoline. *Carcinogenesis*, **4**, 169–172

Wenke, G., Brunnemann, K.D., Hoffmann, D. & Bhide, S.V. (1984) A study of betel quid carcinogenesis. IV. Analysis of the saliva of betel chewers: A preliminary report. *J. Cancer Res. clin. Oncol.*, **108**, 110–113

Williams, R.L. & Carter, M.K. (1965) The saluretic effects of arecoline hydrochloride. *Arch. int. Pharmacodyn.*, **157**, 90–98

Williams, S.A., Summers, R.M., Ahmed, I.A. & Prendergast, M.J. (1996) Caries experience, tooth loss and oral health-related behaviours among Bangladeshi women resident in West Yorkshire, UK. *Community dent. Health*, **13**, 150–156

Williams, W.M., Hayakawa, T., Grange, E. & Rapoport, S.I. (1998) Arecoline stimulation of radio-labeled arachidonate incorporation from plasma into brain microvessels of awake rat. *Neurochem. Res.*, **23**, 551–555

Williams, S., Malik, A., Chowdhury, S. & Chauhan, S. (2002) Sociocultural aspects of areca nut use. *Addict. Biol.*, **7**, 147–154

Winstock, A.R., Trivedy, C.R., Warnakulasuriya, K.A.A.S. & Peters, T.J. (2000) A dependency syndrome related to areca nut use: Some medical and psychological aspects among areca nut users in the Gujarat community in the UK. *Addict. Biol.*, **5**, 173–179

Wong, T.Y., Jin, Y.T., Chen, H.O. & Lin, L.M. (1992) Studies on Taiwan betel quid carcinogenicity in hamster cheek-pouch. *Chinese dent. J.*, **11**, 155–162

Wong, Y.K., Liu, T.Y., Chang. K.W., Lin, S.C., Chao, T.W., Li, P.L. & Chang, C.S. (1998) *p53* Alterations in betel quid- and tobacco-associated oral squamous cell carcinomas from Taiwan. *J. oral Pathol. Med.*, **27**, 243–248

Wu, K.-D., Chuang, R.-B., Wu, F.-L.L., Hsu, W.-A., Jan, I.-S. & Tsai, K.-S. (1996) The milk-alkali syndrome caused by betelnuts in oyster shell paste. *Clin. Toxicol.*, **34**, 741–745

Wu, M.-T., Lee, Y.-C., Chen, C.-J., Yang, P.-W., Lee, C.-J., Wu, D.-C., Hsu, H.-K., Ho, C.K., Kao, E.L. & Lee, J.M. (2001) Risk of betel chewing for oesophageal cancer in Taiwan. *Br. J. Cancer*, **85**, 658–660

Wu, M.-T., Lee, J.-M., Wu, D.-C., Ho, C.-K., Wang, Y.-T., Lee, Y.-C., Hsu, H.-K. & Kao, E.-L. (2002) Genetic polymorphisms of cytochrome P4501A1 and oesophageal squamous-cell carcinoma in Taiwan. *Br. J. Cancer*, **87**, 529–532

Wu, M.-T., Wang, Y.-T., Ho, C.-K., Wu, D.-C., Lee, Y.-C., Hsu, H.-K., Kao, E.-L. & Lee, J.-M. (2003) *SULT1A1* polymorphism and esophageal cancer in males. *Int. J. Cancer*, **103**, 101–104

van Wyk, C.W., Stander, I., Padayachee, A. & Grobler-Rabie, A.F. (1993) The areca nut chewing habit and oral squamous cell carcinoma in South African Indians. A retrospective study. *S. Afr. med. J.*, **83**, 425–429

van Wyk, C.W., Olivier, A., de Miranda, C.M., van der Bijl, P. & Grobler-Rabie, A.F. (1994) Observations on the effect of areca nut extracts on oral fibroblast proliferation. *J. oral Pathol. Med.*, **23**, 145–148

van Wyk, C.W., Olivier, A., Hoal-van Helden, E.G. & Grobler-Rabie, A.F. (1995) Growth of oral and skin fibroblasts from patients with oral submucous fibrosis. *J. oral Pathol. Med.*, **24**, 349–353

van Wyk, C.W., de Miranda, C.M., Olivier, A. & van der Bijl, P. (1996) The effect of baked areca nut extract on the growth of buccal mucosa fibroblasts from healthy non-areca nut chewers. *J. dent. Assoc. S. Afr.*, **51**, 29–31

Xie, D.-P., Li, W., Qu, S.-Y., Zheng, T.-Z., Yang, Y.-L., Ding, Y.-H., Wei, Y.-L. & Chen, L.-B. (2002) Effects of areca on contraction of colonic muscle strips in rats. *World J. Gastroenterol.*, **8**, 350–352

Yan, J.J., Tzeng, C.C. & Jin, Y.T. (1996) Overexpression of p53 protein in squamous cell carcinomas of buccal mucosa and tongue in Taiwan: An immunohistochemical and clinicopathological study. *Oral Pathol. Med.*, **25**, 55–59

Yang, J.A., Huber, S.A. & Lucas, Z.J. (1979) Inhibition of DNA synthesis in cultured lymphocytes and tumor cells by extracts of betel nut, tobacco and miang leaf, plant substances associated with cancer of the ororespiratory epithelium. *Cancer Res.*, **39**, 4802–4809

Yang, M.S., Su, I.H., Wen, J.K. & Ko, Y.C. (1996) Prevalence and related risk factors of betel quid chewing by adolescent students in southern Taiwan. *J. oral Pathol. Med.*, **25**, 69–71

Yang, M.-S. Chang, F.-T. Chen S.-S. Lee, C.-H & Ko, Y.-C. (1999) Betel quid chewing and risk of adverse pregnancy outcomes among aborigines in southern Taiwan. *Public Health*, **113**, 189–192

Yang, M.-S., Chung, T.-C., Yang, M.-J., Hsu T.-Y. & Ko, Y.-C. (2001) Betel quid chewing and risk of adverse birth outcomes among aborigines in eastern Taiwan. *J. Toxicol. environ. Health*, **A64**, 465–472

Yang, Y.-H., Lee, H.-Y., Tung, S. & Shieh, T.-Y. (2001) Epidemiological survey of oral submucous fibrosis and leukoplakia in aborigines of Taiwan. *J. oral Pathol. Med.*, **30**, 213–219

Yang, C.Y., Meng, C.L., van der Bijl, P. & Lee, H.K. (2002) The effect of betel nut extract on cell growth and prostaglandin endoperoxide synthase in human epidermoid carcinoma cells. *Prostaglandins other Lipid Mediat.*, **67**, 181–195

Yeh, C.-J. (1997) Fatigue root fracture: A spontaneous root fracture in non-endodontically treated teeth. *Br. dent. J.*, **182**, 261–266

Yeole, B.B., Kurkure, A.P., Advani, S.H. & Lizzy, S. (2001) An assessment of cancer incidence patterns in Parsi and non-Parsi populations, Greater Mumbai. *Asian Pacific J. Cancer Prev.*, **2**, 293–298

Yi, M., Rosin, M.P. & Anderson, C.K. (1990) Response of fibroblast cultures from ataxia-telangiectasia patients to oxidative stress. *Cancer Lett.*, **54**, 43–50

Yoshinaga, K., Rice, C., Krenn, J. & Pilot, R.L. (1979) Effects of nicotine on early pregnancy in the rat. *Biol. Reprod.*, **20**, 294–303

Ysaol, J., Chilton, J.I. & Callaghan, P. (1996) A survey of betel nut chewing in Palau. *Isla J. Micrones. Stud.*, **4**, 244–255

Zafarulla, M.Y.M. (1985) Oral submucous fibrosis. *Dent. Update*, September, 527–529

Zaidi, S.H.M., Jafarey, N.A. & Aijaz Ali, S. (1974) Cancer trends in Karachi. *J. Pakistan. med. Assoc.*, **24**, 87–93

Zaidi, J.H., Arif, M., Fatima, I. & Qureshi, I.H. (2002) Radiochemical neutron activation analysis for trace elements of basic ingredients of pan. *J. radioanal. nucl. Chem.*, **253**, 459–464

Zain, R., Ikeda, N. & Yaacob M.B.H. (1995) *Oral Mucosal Lesions Survey of Adults in Malaysia*, Kuala Lampur, Ministry of Health

Zain, R.B., Ikeda, N., Razak, I.A., Axéll, T., Majid, Z.A., Gupta, P.C. & Yaacob, M. (1997) A national epidemiological survey of oral mucosal lesions in Malaysia. *Community dent. oral Epidemiol.*, **25**, 377–383

Zain, R.B., Ikeda, N., Gupta, P.C., Warnakulasuriya, K.A.A.S., van Wyk, C.W., Shrestha, P. & Axéll, T. (1999) Oral mucosal lesions associated with betel quid, areca nut and tobacco chewing habits: Consensus from a workshop held in Kuala Lampur, Malaysia, November 25–27, 1996. *J. oral Pathol. Med.*, **28**, 1–4

Znaor, A., Brennan, P., Gajalakshmi, V., Mathew, A., Shanta, V., Varghese, C. & Boffetta, P. (2003) Independent and combined effects of tobacco smoking, chewing and alcohol drinking on the risk of oral, pharyngeal and esophageal cancers in Indian men. *Int. J. Cancer*, **105**, 681–686

# SOME ARECA-NUT-DERIVED *N*-NITROSAMINES

# SOME ARECA-NUT-DERIVED *N*-NITROSAMINES

## 1. Exposure Data

### 1.1 Chemical and physical data

#### 1.1.1 *Synonyms and structural and molecular formulae*

| Chemical name [Chem. Abstr. Services Reg. No.] | Chem. Abstr. Name [Synonym] IUPAC Systematic Name | Structural and molecular formulae and molecular weight | | |
|---|---|---|---|---|
| 3-Methylnitrosamino-propionaldehyde [85502-23-4] | Propanal, 3-(methyl-nitrosoamino) [MNPA] 3-(Methylnitrosamino)-propionaldehyde | $C_4H_8N_2O_2$ | $H_3C-N(N=O)-CH_2CH_2CHO$ | Mol. wt: 116.1 |
| 3-Methylnitrosamino-propionitrile [60153-49-3] | Propanenitrile, 3-(methyl-nitroso-amino) [MNPN] 3-(Methylnitrosamino)-propionitrile | $C_4H_7N_3O$ | $CH_3-N(N=O)-CH_2CH_2C\equiv N$ | Mol. wt: 113.1 |
| *N*-Nitrosoguvacine [55557-01-2] | 3-Pyridinecarboxylic acid, 1,2,5,6-tetrahydro-1-nitroso- [NGC; nitrosoguvacine] 1,2,5,6-Tetrahydro-1-nitrosonicotinic acid | $C_6H_8N_2O_3$ | (tetrahydropyridine with C(=O)OH and N–N=O) | Mol. wt: 156.1 |
| *N*-Nitrosoguvacoline [55557-02-3] | 3-Pyridinecarboxylic acid, 1,2,5,6-tetra-hydro-1-nitroso-, methyl ester [NG; NGL; nitrosoguvacoline] Methyl 1,2,5,6-tetra-hydro-1-nitrosonicotinate | $C_7H_{10}N_2O_3$ | (tetrahydropyridine with C(=O)OCH$_3$ and N–N=O) | Mol. wt: 170.2 |

## 1.1.2 Chemical and physical properties

| Chemical/ Physical property | MNPA | MNPN | NGC | NGL |
|---|---|---|---|---|
| Description | No data | Light-yellow liquid (Chang et al. 1976) | Colourless, crystalline solid (Lijinsky & Taylor, 1976) | Yellow oil (Lijinsky & Taylor, 1976) |
| Melting-point | No data | No data | 175.5–177 °C (Lijinsky & Taylor, 1976) | No data |
| Boiling-point | No data | 102–103 °C (0.04 mm Hg) (Chang et al., 1976); 97 °C (0.075 mm Hg) (Wenke & Hoffmann, 1983) | No data | 137–178 °C (4 mm Hg) (Lijinsky & Taylor, 1976) |
| Spectroscopy data | NMR, UV and MS data have been reported (Wenke & Hoffmann, 1983; Nishikawa et al., 1992) | IR, NMR and MS data have been reported (Chang et al., 1976; Wenke & Hoffmann, 1983). MS data reported for MNPN isolated from saliva of betel-quid chewers (Prokopczyk et al., 1987) | MS data have been reported (Rainey et al., 1978) | MS data have been reported (Rainey et al., 1978) |
| Synthetic compound | Synthetic MNPA is a mixture of E- and Z-isomers in a ratio of 1.4 (Wenke & Hoffmann, 1983) | Synthetic MNPN is a mixture of E- and Z-isomers in a ratio of 1.7 (Wenke & Hoffmann, 1983) | | Synthetic NGL is a mixture of E- and Z-isomers in a ratio of 2.5 (Wenke & Hoffmann, 1983) |

MNPA, 3-methylnitrosaminopropionaldehyde; MNPN, 3-methylnitrosaminopropionitrile; NGC, *N*-nitrosoguvacine; NGL, *N*-nitrosoguvacoline; NMR, $^1$H-nuclear magnetic resonance; UV, ultraviolet; MS, mass spectrometry; IR, infrared

## 1.2 Production

3-Methylnitrosaminopropionaldehyde (MNPA) was prepared by Wenke and Hoffmann (1983) by the reaction of MNPA diethyl acetal with nitrite, followed by hydrolysis. 3-Methylnitrosaminopropionitrile (MNPN) was prepared by Chang et al. (1976) by the reaction of sodium nitrite with a solution of MNPN hydrochloride. *N*-Nitrosoguvacine (NGC) was prepared by Lijinsky and Taylor (1976) by nitrosation of guvacine that was synthesized from 3-carbethoxy-4-piperidone by hydrogenation to the piperidonol, followed by dehydration and de-esterification with hydrogen chloride gas at 200 °C, followed by esterification with diazomethane. *N*-Nitrosoguvacoline (NGL) was also prepared by Lijinsky and Taylor (1976) using the same process as that for NGC.

In in-vitro experiments, *N*-nitrosation of arecoline, the major alkaloid of the areca nut, resulted in the formation of NGL, MNPN and MNPA (Wenke & Hoffmann, 1983).

No evidence was found that any of these compounds has ever been produced in commercial quantities or has any use other than as a laboratory chemical.

## 1.3 Occurrence

NGL, MNPN and MNPA were not detected in three samples of betel quid without tobacco or in three samples of betel quid with tobacco. NGC was detected in one of each of the three samples with and without tobacco (Nair et al., 1985).

NGL, NGC and MNPN were found in the saliva of chewers of betel quid with tobacco at nanogram per millilitre levels (Table 1). NGL was also reported in the saliva of three of eight smokers (up to 7.6 ng/mL; Wenke et al., 1984a). [The Working Group noted the possibility of analytical problems or the additional use of areca nut by the smokers.] MNPN in saliva was confirmed by mass spectroscopic analysis (Prokopczyk et al., 1987); MNPA was not detected in saliva or any other human biological fluid.

Table 1. Levels (range in ng/mL) of areca-nut-derived nitrosamines detected in the saliva[a] of chewers of betel quid with tobacco (BQ + T) and without tobacco (BQ)

| Nitrosamine | BQ + T (no.)[b] | BQ (no.)[b] | Reference |
|---|---|---|---|
| NGL | 4.3–45 (5)[c] | 2.2–9.5 (5)[c] | Wenke et al. (1984a) |
| | 0–7.1 (12) | 0–5.9 (12) | Nair et al. (1985) |
| | NR | 0–142 (9) | Stich et al. (1986) |
| | 3.1–23.5 (10) | 0.6–8.8 (10) | Nair et al. (1987) |
| NGC | 0–30.4 (6) | 0–26.6 (6) | Nair et al. (1985) |
| MNPN | NR | 0.5–11.4 (10) | Prokopczyk et al. (1987) |

NGL, $N$-nitrosoguvacoline; NGC, $N$-nitrosoguvacine; MNPN, 3-methyl-nitrosaminopropionitrile; NR, not reported
[a] Number in parentheses refers to number of samples
[b] The whole saliva or the supernatant was analysed.
[c] In ppb

In-vitro experiments support the hypothesis that, during the chewing of betel quid, nitrosation of arecoline, the major alkaloid of areca nut, produces NGL and MNPN. It was concluded that the conditions prevailing in the oral cavity of betel-quid chewers are likely to favour the formation of these compounds (see Monograph on Betel-quid and Areca-nut Chewing, Section 4.1.1). In-vitro nitrosation of betel quid with and without tobacco under neutral and acidic pH with nitrite in the presence of thiocyanate yielded both NGL and NGC; the formation of NGC was greater than that of NGL when betel quid without tobacco was nitrosated (Nair et al., 1985). Small amounts of crude phenolic extracts from fresh green areca fruit (< 60 mg/300 mL) significantly inhibited the formation of NGL from arecoline upon the addition of nitrite, whereas larger amounts (> 250 mg/300 mL) enhanced its formation (Wang & Peng, 1996).

## 1.4 Analysis

Wenke and Hoffmann (1983) reported a method for analysis of MNPN, MNPA and NGC by gas chromatography with a nitrosamine-selective thermal-energy analyser. Analysis of NGC and NGL has also been reported using similar techniques (Nair *et al.*, 1985).

## 2. Studies of Cancer in Humans

No data were available to the Working Group.

## 3. Studies of Cancer in Experimental Animals

### 3.1  3-Methylnitrosaminopropionaldehyde (MNPA)

*Subcutaneous administration*

*Rat*: Groups of 15 male and 15 female Fischer 344 rats, 7 weeks of age, received 45 subcutaneous injections of 6.57 mg [0.057 mmol] per animal MNPA (purity, > 99% on the basis of gas chromatography and high-performance liquid chromatography) in 0.3 mL tri-octanoin. A group of 12 male and 12 female rats received vehicle only and served as controls. The experiment was terminated 100 weeks after the first injection. Animals were killed at termination or earlier when moribund, and were autopsied and examined histologically. Four of 15 males and 1/14 females developed lung adenoma and one female rat developed lung adenocarcinoma. The total lung tumour incidence was significantly higher in treated groups (6/29) than in controls ($n = 24$), which developed no lung tumours during this period. Other tumours in the treated groups (males and females combined) were nasal papillomas (4/29), liver adenomas (4/29), forestomach papillomas (3/29), nephroblastoma (1/29) and leukaemia (3/29), none of which was found in control animals. A large variety of different tumours occurred in the control group (Nishikawa *et al.*, 1992).

### 3.2  3-Methylnitrosaminopropionitrile (MNPN)

#### 3.2.1  *Oral application*

*Rat*: MNPN (0.3 mL of a 15 mmol/L solution) was applied by oral swabbing to the oral cavity of 30 male Fischer 344 rats, 10 weeks of age, three times a week for 1 week, once a day for the next 3 weeks and then twice daily until the end of the bioassay (54 weeks). Animals were autopsied and examined histologically. A control group of 30 animals received water alone applied by oral swabbing. In the treated group, 2/30 animals developed lung adenoma and 2/30 developed lung adenocarcinoma, 10/30 and 14/30 developed nasal cavity adenoma and carcinoma, respectively, 1/30 and 2/30 developed liver adenoma and carcinoma, respectively, 2/30 developed oesophageal papilloma and 1/30 developed oral cavity papilloma. None of 30 control animals developed these lesions (Prokopczyk et al., 1991).

### 3.2.2 Subcutaneous administration

*Rat*: A group of 15 male and 15 female Fischer 344 rats, 7 weeks of age, received thrice-weekly subcutaneous injections of 2.13 mg [0.019 mmol] per animal MNPN (purity, > 99% as determined by high-performance liquid chromatography) in 0.3 mL saline for 20 weeks (total dose, 129 mg per rat or 646 mg/kg bw). A group of 12 males and 12 females served as vehicle controls. The experiment was terminated after 24 weeks because of significant weight loss in the treated animals. Animals were killed at termination or earlier when moribund, and autopsy and histological examination of gross lesions in major organs were carried out. Statistically significant increases in tumour incidence were observed for the following neoplasms: (i) papillomas of the oesophagus in 12/15 treated males ($p < 0.01$) and 14/15 treated females ($p < 0.01$); 3/15 males and 2/15 females treated with MNPN also developed carcinomas of the oesophagus (significant at $p < 0.05$ for both sexes combined); (ii) papillomas of the nasal cavity in 11/15 treated males ($p < 0.01$) and 9/15 treated females ($p < 0.01$); and (iii) papillomas and carcinomas of the tongue in 5/15 treated males ($p < 0.05$) and 6/15 treated females ($p < 0.05$). No tumour was seen in controls (Wenke et al., 1984b).

Groups of 21 male and 21 female Fischer 344 rats, 7 weeks of age, received thrice-weekly subcutaneous injections of 0.53 or 2.13 mg/kg bw MNPN in saline for 20 weeks (cumulative dose, 6.4 and 25.7 mg per rat, respectively). A group of 12 male and 12 female rats received saline only and served as controls. Animals were autopsied and gross lesions and major organs were analysed histologically. At the termination of the experiment at 106 weeks, 18/21 male ($p < 0.01$) and 15/21 ($p < 0.01$) female rats had developed nasal carcinomas at the higher dose, whereas only one nasal papilloma had developed with the lower dose. A nasal papilloma was also observed in the control group. The lower dose induced liver tumours [histology not mentioned] in 9/21 male rats, whereas only 1/12 control males developed this tumour. No liver tumours were observed in female rats treated with MNPN, but 3/12 female control rats developed liver tumours. A large variety of other tumours occurred in control and experimental groups (Prokopczyk et al., 1987)

### 3.2.3 Administration with known carcinogens or modifiers of cancer risk

*Mouse*: In a tumour initiation–promotion experiment, a group of 19 female SEN mice, 50–55 days of age, received topical applications of 0.1 mg MNPN in 100 μL acetone every other day for 20 days, amounting to a total dose of 1 mg MNPN. After a 10-day interval, animals were treated with 2 μg 12-*O*-tetradecanoylphorbol-13-acetate in

100 μL acetone twice weekly for 20 weeks. A group of 20 vehicle-treated mice served as controls. Of the MNPN-treated mice, 89% (17/19) developed skin tumours, as did 20% (4/20) of the vehicle-treated controls. Lung adenomas were also found in 89% (17/19) of the MNPN-treated mice but not in the controls. The incidences of both skin tumours and lung adenomas were statistically significant ($p < 0.001$) when compared with the controls (Prokopczyk et al., 1991). [The Working Group noted the absence of a group treated with MNPN only and of an adequate histological description of the skin lesions.]

## 3.3 N-Nitrosoguvacoline (NGL)

### 3.3.1 Oral administration

*Rat:* A group of 15 male and 15 female Sprague-Dawley rats, 8–10 weeks of age, was given drinking-water containing 150 mg/L NGL (no impurity detected by silica-gel thin-layer chromatography) on 5 days per week for 50 weeks (total dose, 750 mg per rat). All animals survived until the end of treatment and were subsequently observed until death or killed at 133 weeks. At 100 weeks, 12 males and nine females were still alive; the four survivors (one male and three females) were killed at 133 weeks. Thirty female and 26 male rats served as untreated [matched or historical, not specified] controls. No statistically significant increase in tumour incidence was found (27 tumours in 30 NGL-treated rats versus 97 tumours in 56 control animals) (Lijinsky & Taylor, 1976). [The Working Group noted that mortality data for the control group were not provided.]

A group of 30 male Fischer 344 rats, 8 weeks of age, received 20 ppm [mg/L] NGL (purity > 99% on the basis of gas chromatography and high-performance liquid chromatography) in the drinking-water for 128 weeks (cumulative dose of NGL, 4.1 mmol/kg). All animals survived until the end of the experiment. Of the treated animals, 4/30 ($p < 0.05$) developed acinar adenoma of pancreas (exocrine pancreas) compared with 1/80 untreated controls (Rivenson et al., 1988).

### 3.3.2 Administration with known carcinogens or modifiers of cancer risk

*Rat*: A group of 30 male Fischer 344 rats, 8 weeks of age, was given 20 ppm [mg/L] NGL concomitantly with 1 ppm 4-(methylnitrosamino)-1-(3-pyridyl)-1-butanone (NNK) in the drinking-water (approximate total doses, 4.1 mmol/kg NGL and 0.17 mmol/kg NNK). Tumour yields observed in these rats were not significantly different from those in rats given NNK only (Rivenson et al., 1988).

# 4. Other Data Relevant to an Evaluation of Carcinogenicity and its Mechanisms

## 4.1 Absorption, distribution, metabolism and excretion

### 4.1.1 *Humans*

NGL, NGC and MNPN have been detected in saliva (see Section 1.3).

### 4.1.2 *Experimental systems*

*N*-Nitrosonipecotic acid (NNIP) was identified as a major urinary metabolite of NGL in rats. When male BDIV rats were given NGL (50 or 500 µg by stomach tube), urinary NNIP accounted for 66% of the dose in each case. NGC (2.9–4.7% of the dose) was also identified in urine. Only 0.8–1.1% of the dose was excreted in the 24-h faeces (Ohshima *et al.*, 1989). In hamsters treated with areca nut and nitrite, NNIP was detected in urine (1.9 ± 0.9 ng/mL; range, 0.57–2.85 ng/mL), indicating endogenous formation of NGL and/or NGC. NNIP was not detected in the urine of hamsters treated with nitrite or areca nut alone (Ernst *et al.*, 1987).

NNIP was identified as a major urinary metabolite of NGC in rats. When male BDIV rats were given NGC (50 or 500 µg by stomach tube), urinary NNIP accounted for 82–84% of the dose in the 24-h urine, and 1.6–3.1% of the dose in the 24-h faeces. Unchanged urinary NGC accounted for 2.1–7.6% of the dose. Unchanged NGC (0.5% of the dose) was also observed in the 24-h faeces after administration of the higher dose (Ohshima *et al.*, 1989).

## 4.2 Toxic effects

### 4.2.1 *Humans*

No data were available to the Working Group.

### 4.2.2 *Experimental systems*

No toxic effects were reported in rats administered NGL in the drinking-water (0.88 mM [150 mg/L] for 50 weeks; Lijinsky & Taylor, 1976; or 20 ppm [315 mg/rat] for 106 weeks; Rivenson *et al.*, 1988). NGL (1.7 mM [289 mg/L]) caused a 50% decrease in the colony-forming efficiency of human buccal epithelial cells (Sundqvist *et al.*, 1989).

NGC (up to 5 mM [780 mg/L]) had no significant effect on survival of human buccal epithelial cells (Sundqvist *et al.*, 1989).

No toxic effects were reported in male and female Fischer 344 rats treated with 60 subcutaneous injections of MNPN (2.13 mg, 0.019 mmol) thrice weekly over 20 weeks. This dose was highly carcinogenic, however (see Section 3.2) (Wenke *et al.*, 1984). No toxic effects were reported in male Fischer 344 rats in which the oral cavity was swabbed with MNPN twice daily up to 5 days per week (0.3 mL of a 15 mmol solution) for 54 weeks. The total dose of MNPN was approximately 259 mg [2.31 mmol] per rat. This dose was carcinogenic (see Section 3.2) (Prokopczyk *et al.*, 1991). MNPN (up to 5 mM) had no significant effect on survival of human buccal epithelial cells (Sundqvist *et al.*, 1989).

Male and female Fischer 344 rats, 7 weeks of age, received 45 subcutaneous injections of MNPA (6.57 mg, 0.057 mmol, in 0.3 mL trioctanoin) thrice weekly for 15 weeks. The total dose of MNPA per rat was approximately 296 mg (2.6 mmol). Weight gain in treated females was significantly lower than that in controls. Marked liver hydropic degeneration was noted in a female rat that died during week 10. The authors concluded that MNPA was hepatotoxic in females (Nishikawa *et al.*, 1992). MNPA (0.15 mM) decreased the colony-forming efficiency of cultured human buccal epithelial cells by 50%; it also (80 µM) decreased low-molecular-weight thiols in these cells by 25% (Sundqvist *et al.*, 1989).

## 4.3 Reproductive and developmental effects

No data were available to the Working Group.

## 4.4 Genetic and related effects

### 4.4.1 *Humans*

No data were available to the Working Group.

### 4.4.2 *Experimental systems*

Results of genotoxicity tests of NGL, NGC, MNPN and MNPA are summarized in Table 2.

In the presence of an exogenous metabolic activation system, NGL was mutagenic to *Salmonella typhimurium* strain TA1535 but only weakly mutagenic to strains TA100 and TA98. Mixed results were obtained in the absence of metabolic activation. It did not cause sex-linked recessive lethal mutations in mature sperm or spermatids of *Drosophila melanogaster*, nor did it induce DNA single-strand breaks in human buccal epithelial cells.

NGC was inactive in *S. typhimurium* TA1535, and did not induce DNA single-strand breaks in human buccal epithelial cells.

MNPN did not induce DNA single-strand breaks in human buccal epithelial cells.

## Table 2. Genetic and related effects of areca-nut-derived nitrosamines

| Test system | Result[a] Without exogenous metabolic system | Result[a] With exogenous metabolic system | Dose[b] (LED or HID) | Reference |
|---|---|---|---|---|
| **NGL** | | | | |
| *Salmonella typhimurium* TA100, reverse mutation | + | (+) | 24 μmol [4 mg/plate] | Wang & Peng (1996) |
| *Salmonella typhimurium* TA1535, reverse mutation | – | + | 200 μg/plate | Rao et al. (1977) |
| *Salmonella typhimurium* TA98, reverse mutation | (+)[c] | (+) | 24 μmol [4 mg/plate] | Wang & Peng (1996) |
| *Drosophila melanogaster*, sex-linked recessive lethal mutation | – | | 20 mM [3400 mg/mL] | Nix et al. (1979) |
| DNA single-strand breaks, human buccal epithelial cells *in vitro* | – | NT | 5 mM [850 μg/mL] | Sundqvist et al. (1989) |
| **NGC** | | | | |
| *Salmonella typhimurium* TA1535, reverse mutation | – | – | 600 μg/plate | Rao et al. (1977) |
| DNA single-strand breaks, human buccal epithelial cells *in vitro* | – | NT | 5 mM [780 μg/mL] | Sundqvist et al. (1989) |
| **MNPN** | | | | |
| DNA single-strand breaks, human buccal epithelial cells *in vitro* | + | NT | 5 mM [565 μg/mL] | Sundqvist et al. (1989) |
| **MNPA** | | | | |
| *Salmonella typhimurium* TA100, TA1535, TA104, reverse mutation | NT | – | 0.4 μmol [46.4 μg]/plate | Chung et al. (1994) |
| DNA single-strand breaks, human buccal epithelial cells *in vitro* | + | NT | 0.3 mM [34.8 μg/mL] | Sundqvist et al. (1989); Sundqvist & Grafstrom (1992) |
| DNA–protein cross-links, human buccal epithelial cells *in vitro* | + | NT | 0.1 mM [11.6 μg/mL] | Sundqvist & Grafstrom (1992) |

NGL, *N*-nitrosoguvacoline; NGC, *N*-nitrosoguvacine; MNPN, 3-methylnitrosaminopropionitrile; MNPA, 3-methylnitrosaminopropionaldehyde

[a] +, positive; (+), weakly positive; –, negative; NT, not tested
[b] LED, lowest effective dose; HID, highest ineffective dose unless otherwise stated; in-vitro tests, μg/mL
[c] The lowest effective dose tested without an exogenous metabolic system (15 μmol/plate [2.5 mg/plate]) was weakly positive; the dose of 24 μmol was not tested without exogenous system.

**Figure 1. Intermediates involved in the α-hydroxylation of 3-methylnitrosamino-propionitrile (MNPN) and their reaction products with deoxyguanosine (dg)**

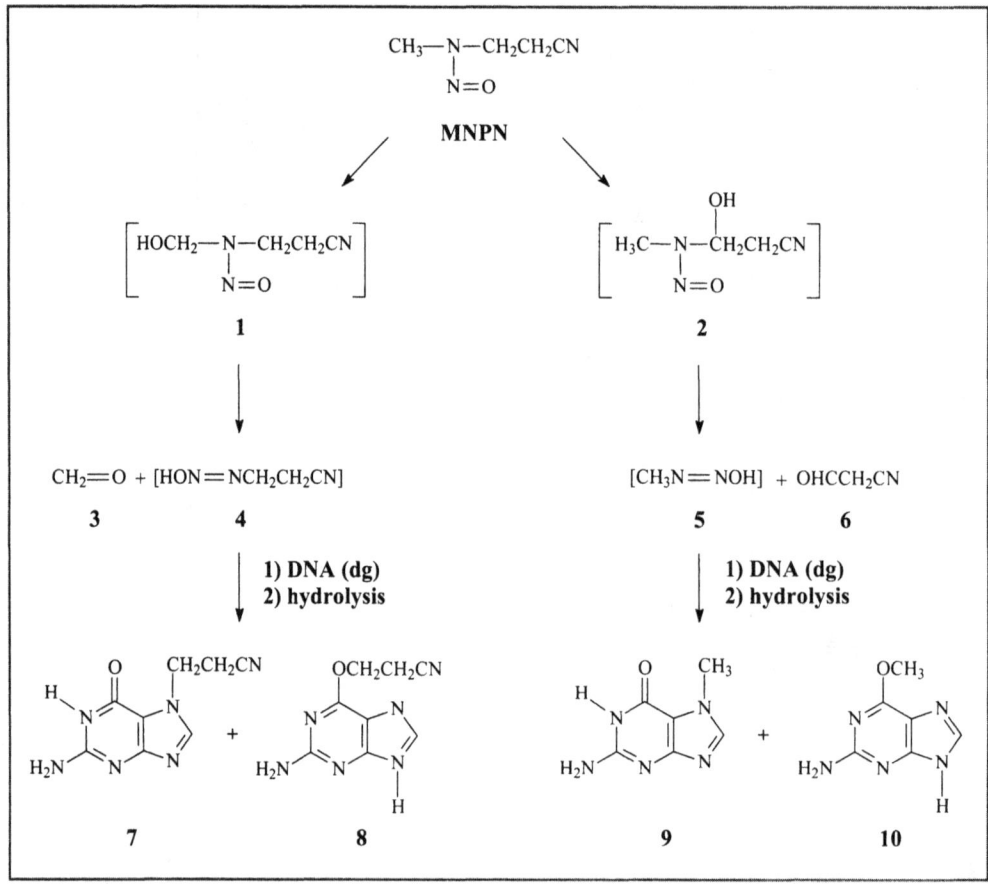

Adapted from Prokopczyk et al. (1988)

MNPA was not mutagenic in the presence of rat liver 9000 × g supernatant in *S. typhimurium*. It also induced DNA–protein cross-links at concentrations of 0.1 mM and higher and a significant increase in the levels of DNA single-strand breaks in human buccal epithelial cells in a dose-dependent manner (0.1–1.0 mM). 3-(Carbethoxynitrosamino)-propionaldehyde, a model compound precursor for α-methyl hydroxylation of MNPA, reacted with deoxyguanosine or DNA to form cyclic 1,$N^2$-propanodeoxyguanosine adducts identical to those derived by the reaction of acrolein with deoxyguanosine and was mutagenic in *S. typhimurium* strains TA100, TA104 and TA1535 without metabolic activation (Chung et al., 1994).

Male Fischer 344 rats were given a single intravenous or subcutaneous injection of MNPN (45 mg/kg, 0.4 mmol/kg) in saline or were administered MNPN by swabbing of the oral cavity (250 mg/kg, 2.21 mmol/kg) and were killed 0.5–36 h later. 7-Methylguanine (**9**) and $O^6$-methylguanine (**10**) (Figure 1) were detected in DNA of the liver, oesophagus and nasal mucosa. Levels were higher in the liver and nasal mucosa than in the oesophagus. Adducts **9** and **10** were also detected in DNA of the oral cavity after swabbing. These adducts resulted from α-methylene hydroxylation of MNPN via intermediate **2** (Figure 1) (Prokopczyk et al., 1987).

Male Fischer 344 rats were given a single subcutaneous injection of MNPN (45 mg/kg, 0.4 mmol/kg) and killed 2–36 h later. 7-(2-Cyanoethyl)guanine (**7**), $O^6$-(2-cyanoethyl)guanine (**8**), 7-methylguanine (**9**) and $O^6$-methylguanine (**10**) were detected in the DNA of the liver, nasal mucosa and oesophagus. Adduct ratios (**9**:**7**) ranged from 3.4 to 7.1 in the liver, 1.5 to 2.2 in nasal mucosa and 0.8 to 1.7 in the oesophagus. Levels of adducts **7** and **9** were higher in the DNA of the liver and nasal mucosa than in that of the oesophagus. Adduct ratios (**10**:**8**) ranged from 0.49 to 1.23 in liver and from 0.91 to 3.0 in nasal mucosa. Levels of adducts **8** and **10** were higher in the DNA of the liver and nasal mucosa than in that of the oesophagus; in these latter tissues, the level of adduct **10** was very low, while adduct **8** was not detected. Adducts **7** and **8** result from α-methyl hydroxylation of MNPN (Figure 1; Prokopczyk et al., 1988).

## 5. Summary of Data Reported and Evaluation

### 5.1 Exposure data

*N*-Nitrosoguvacoline, *N*-nitrosoguvacine and 3-methylnitrosopropionitrile have been found in the saliva of betel-quid chewers. Thus, there is some evidence that chewers are exposed to these compounds.

### 5.2 Human carcinogenicity data

No data were available to the Working Group.

### 5.3 Animal carcinogenicity data

Following subcutaneous administration of 3-methylnitrosaminopropionaldehyde to rats, the incidence of lung adenoma and adenocarcinoma was significantly increased in both males and females. A variety of other benign and malignant tumours was also observed.

Application of 3-methylnitrosopropionitrile to the oral cavity of male rats produced adenomas and adenocarcinomas in lung and nasal cavity, adenomas and carcinomas in the liver and papillomas in the oesophagus and oral cavity.

Subcutaneous administration of 3-methylnitrosaminopropionitrile to rats induced papillomas and carcinomas of the oesophagus and the tongue and papillomas of the nasal cavity in males and females in a short-term experiment, and an increased incidence of nasal carcinomas in male and female rats and of liver tumours in male rats in a long-term experiment.

In an initiation–promotion study on mouse skin, initiation with 3-methylnitrosopropionitrile led to the development of skin tumours and lung adenomas.

Addition of *N*-nitrosoguvacoline to the drinking-water of rats induced pancreatic adenomas in males in one study, but no increase in tumours in males or females in another.

## 5.4 Other relevant data

*N*-Nitrosoguvacoline and *N*-nitrosoguvacine are metabolized in rats to *N*-nitrosonipecotic acid, which is excreted in the urine. *N*-Nitrosonipecotic acid has been detected in the urine of hamsters treated with areca nut plus nitrite, indicating the endogenous formation of *N*-nitrosoguvacoline and *N*-nitrosoguvacine.

3-Methylnitrosopropionitrile induced liver toxicity in female rats.

*N*-Nitrosoguvacoline but not *N*-nitrosoguvacine was mutagenic to bacteria. 3-Methylnitrosaminopropionitrile caused single-strand breaks and DNA–protein cross-links in human buccal epithelial cells. DNA methylation and cyanoethylation were observed in rats treated with 3-methylnitrosaminopropionitrile. These studies demonstrate that *N*-nitrosoguvacoline, *N*-nitrosoguvacine and 3-methylnitrosaminopropionitrile are genotoxic.

## 5.5 Evaluation

There is *inadequate evidence* in humans for the carcinogenicity of *N*-nitrosoguvacoline, *N*-nitrosoguvacine and 3-methylnitrosaminopropionitrile.

There is *sufficient evidence* in experimental animals for the carcinogenicity of 3-methylnitrosaminopropionitrile.

There is *limited evidence* in experimental animals for the carcinogenicity of 3-methylnitrosaminopropionaldehyde.

There is *inadequate evidence* in experimental animals for the carcinogenicity of *N*-nitrosoguvacoline and *N*-nitrosoguvacine.

### Overall evaluation

*N*-Nitrosoguvacoline is *not classifiable as to its carcinogenicity to humans (Group 3)*.
*N*-Nitrosoguvacine is *not classifiable as to its carcinogenicity to humans (Group 3)*.
3-Methylnitrosaminopropionitrile is *possibly carcinogenic to humans (Group 2B)*.
3-Methylnitrosaminopropionaldehyde is *not classifiable as to its carcinogenicity to humans (Group 3)*.

## 6. References

Chang, S.K., Harrington, G.W., Veale, H.S. & Swern, D. (1976) The unusually mild and facile basic hydrolysis of N-nitroso-2-(methylamino)acetonitrile. *J. org. Chem.*, **41**, 3752–3755

Chung, F.L., Krzeminski, J., Wang, M., Chen, H.J. & Prokopczyk, B. (1994) Formation of the acrolein-derived 1,$N^2$-propanodeoxyguanosine adducts in DNA upon reaction with 3-(N-carbethoxy-N-nitrosamino)propionaldehyde. *Chem. Res. Toxicol.*, **7**, 62–67

Ernst, H., Ohshima, H., Bartsch, H., Mohr, U. & Reichart, P. (1987) Tumorigenicity study in Syrian hamsters fed areca nut together with nitrite. *Carcinogenesis*, **8**, 1843–1845

Lijinsky, W. & Taylor, H.W. (1976) Carcinogenicity test of two unsaturated derivatives of N-nitrosopiperidine in Sprague-Dawley rats. *J. natl Cancer Inst.*, **57**, 1315–1317

Nair, J., Ohshima, H., Friesen, M., Croisy, A., Bhide, S.V. & Bartsch, H. (1985) Tobacco-specific and betel nut-specific N-nitroso compounds: Occurrence in saliva and urine of betel quid chewers and formation *in vitro* by nitrosation of betel quid. *Carcinogenesis*, **6**, 295–303

Nair, J., Nair, U.J., Ohshima, H., Bhide, S.V. & Bartsch, H. (1987) Endogenous nitrosation in the oral cavity of chewers while chewing betel quid with or without tobacco. In: Bartsch, H., O'Neill, I.K. & Schulte-Hermann, R., eds, *Relevance of N-Nitroso Compounds to Human Cancer: Exposures and Mechanisms* (IARC Scientific Publications No. 84), Lyon, IARCPress, pp. 465–469

Nishikawa, A., Prokopczyk, B., Rivenson, A., Zang, E. & Hoffmann, D. (1992) A study of betel quid carcinogenesis. VIII. Carcinogenicity of 3-(methylnitrosamino)propionaldehyde in F344 rats. *Carcinogenesis*, **13**, 369–372

Nix, C.E., Brewen, B., Wilkerson, R., Lijinsky, W. & Epler, J.L. (1979) Effects of N-nitrosopiperidine substitutions on mutagenicity in *Drosophila melanogaster*. *Mutat. Res.*, **67**, 27–38

Ohshima, H., Friesen, M. & Bartsch, H. (1989) Identification in rats of N-nitrosonipecotic acid as a major urinary metabolite of the areca-nut alkaloid-derived nitrosamines, N-nitrosoguvacoline and N-nitrosoguvacine. *Cancer Lett.*, **44**, 211–216

Prokopczyk, B., Rivenson, A., Bertinato, P., Brunnemann, K.D. & Hoffmann, D. (1987) 3-(Methylnitrosamino)proprionitrile: Occurrence in saliva of betel quid chewers, carcinogenicity, and DNA methylation in F344 rats. *Cancer Res.*, **47**, 467–471

Prokopczyk, B., Bertinato, P. & Hoffmann, D. (1988) Cyanoethylation of DNA *in vivo* by 3-(methylnitrosamino)propionitrile, an *Areca*-derived carcinogen. *Cancer Res.*, **48**, 6780–6784

Prokopczyk, B., Rivenson, A. & Hoffmann, D. (1991) A study of betel quid carcinogenesis. IX. Comparative carcinogenicity of 3-(methylnitrosamino)propionitrile and 4-(methylnitrosamino)-1-(3-pyridyl)-1-butanone upon local application to mouse skin and rat oral mucosa. *Cancer Lett.*, **60**, 153–157

Rainey, W.T., Christie, W.H. & Lijinsky, W. (1978) Mass spectrometry of N-nitrosamines. *Biochem. mass Spectrom.*, **5**, 395–408

Rao, T.K., Hardigree, A.A., Young, J.A., Lijinsky, W. & Epler, J.L. (1977) Mutagenicity of N-nitrosopiperidines with *Salmonella typhimurium*/microsomal activation system. *Mutat. Res.*, **56**, 131–145

Rivenson, A., Hoffmann, D., Prokopczyk, B., Amin, S. & Hecht, S.S. (1988) Induction of lung and exocrine pancreas tumors in F344 rats by tobacco-specific and *Areca*-derived *N*-nitrosamines. *Cancer Res.*, **48**, 6912–6917

Stich, H.F., Rosin, M.P. & Brunnemann, K.D. (1986) Oral lesions, genotoxicity and nitrosamines in betel quid chewers with no obvious increase in oral cancer risk. *Cancer Lett.*, **31**, 15–25

Sundqvist, K. & Grafstrom, R.C. (1992) Effects of areca nut on growth, differentiation and formation of DNA damage in cultured human buccal epithelial cells. *Int. J. Cancer*, **52**, 305–310

Sundqvist, K., Liu, Y., Nair, J., Bartsch, H., Arvidson, K. & Grafstrom, R.C. (1989) Cytotoxic and genotoxic effects of areca nut-related compounds in cultured human buccal epithelial cells. *Cancer Res.*, **49**, 5294–5298

Wang, C.-K. & Peng, C.-H. (1996) The mutagenicities of alkaloids and *N*-nitrosoguvacoline from betel quid. *Mutat. Res*, **360**, 165–171

Wenke, G. & Hoffmann, D. (1983) A study of betel quid carcinogenesis. 1. On the in vitro *N*-nitrosation of arecoline. *Carcinogenesis*, **4**, 169–172

Wenke, G., Brunnemann, K.D., Hoffmann, D. & Bhide, S.V. (1984a) A study of betel quid carcinogenesis. IV. Analysis of the saliva of betel chewers. A preliminary report. *J. Cancer Res. clin. Oncol.*, **108**, 110–113

Wenke, G., Rivenson, A. & Hoffmann, D. (1984b) A study of betel quid carcinogenesis. III. 3-(Methylnitrosamino)propionitrile, a powerful carcinogen in F344 rats. *Carcinogenesis*, **5**, 1137–1140

# GLOSSARY A — TERMS USED IN THE MONOGRAPHS

*Areca catechu* L.: see **areca nut** (Figure 1)
**Areca fruit**: fruit of the palm *Areca catechu* L. — see **areca nut**
**Areca nut**: nut from the fruit of the *Areca catechu* L. (Palmaceae) tree, a palm native to South Asia. The fruit is green when unripe and orange-yellow in colour when ripe and is the size of a small egg. The nut (seed) is separated from the fibrous pericarp and used fresh or dried, or processed by roasting, sun drying, boiling, soaking in water or fermenting. The unripe green areca fruit may also be used. Synonyms include **supari** (in Hindi and other languages in India), *puwak* (Sri Lanka), *gua* (in Sylheti), *mak* (Thailand), *pinang* (Sarawak and Malaysia), *daka* (Papua New Guinea), *pugua* (Guam) and *Kun-ywet* (Myanmar). The term 'areca' is derived by the Portuguese from *Malayalam atrekka* and from the Tamil *aakkay*. (Figure 2)
**Betel inflorescence**: flower of the vine *Piper betle* L.
**Betel leaf**: leaf of the vine *Piper betle* L. (note the difference in spelling between the Latin term '*betle*' and English 'betel'). It is cultivated in hot, humid climates in Asia. Serves as the wrapping for **betel quid**. (Figure 3)
**Betel nut**: the term 'betel nut', although commonly used in the scientific literature, has caused considerable confusion and should be avoided. The correct term is **areca nut** because betel vine and areca palm are different plants.
**Betel quid**: usually prepared by smearing a **betel leaf** with **slaked lime**, to which pieces of **areca nut** are added. **Catechu** may be added. Crushed leaves of cured tobacco and flavouring agents may also be added. The ingredients are folded in the betel leaf and chewed. Known as *paan* in Hindi and other languages in India and *buyo* in the Philippines. Betel quid may be prepared differently in different parts of the world. See *lao-hwa* and **stem quid**. (Figure 4)
*Bidi*: hand-rolled Indian cigarette consisting of flaked tobacco rolled in temburni leaf
*Buyo*: mixture consisting of **betel leaves**, **areca nut**, slaked lime and tobacco or any combination of these constituents. See **betel quid**
**Catechu**: astringent, reddish-brown substance which is often smeared on the betel leaf used to wrap the betel quid ingredients. In general, two types of catechu are used, depending on the plant from which the catechu has been extracted. Also known as pale or black catechu, *kattha*, *dok can*, *gambir* and **cutch**. In northern Thailand, **catechu** may be extracted from another plant and is referred to as *nang ko*.
*Chuna*: see **slaked lime**. Also spelt *chunam*
**Cutch**: see **catechu**

*Gambir*: ***gambir*** is a woody, climbing shrub native to China and other parts of southeast Asia. The plant consists of a thin, wooden stem that is reddish-brown in color, with broad green leaves. Most of the stem branches also have hook-like appendages, which the plant uses to attach itself to a surface. The medicinal part of gambir is a watery extract, which is taken from the plant's leaves and young shoots. The main ingredients in the extract are tannins and catechins. Gambir acts mainly as a sedative; it dilates peripheral blood vessels and lowers blood pressure. It is also used to treat hypertension, dizziness and anxiety. In traditional Chinese medicine, gambir is used to calm wind to relieve convulsions; calm the liver; and remove (or clear away) heat.

*Gudaku*: paste consisting of powdered tobacco, molasses and other ingredients. Also spelt ***Gudakhu***

*Gutka*: commercial preparation of **areca nut** and powdered tobacco, **slaked lime**, **catechu** and other ingredients. Also spelt ***gutkha*** (Figure 5)

*Kattha*: see **catechu**

**Khaini**: mixture of tobacco and **slaked lime** mixed in the palm of the hand

**Lao-hwa quid**: specific Taiwanese term for unripe areca nut split in half, with inflorescence of *Piper betle* L. inserted in the middle and **slaked lime** added

**Lime**: see **slaked lime**

*Mainpuri* **tobacco**: mixture of **areca nut**, **slaked lime** and tobacco. Other ingredients may be added. The name *Mainpuri* is derived from an area in the northern part of India.

*Mawa*: mixture of predominantly **areca nut** pieces with some tobacco and **slaked lime**

*Mishri*: roasted or half-burnt tobacco prepared by baking on a hot metal plate and powdered. Also known as ***masheri*** or ***misheri***

*Nang ko*: see **catechu**

*Naswar*: mixture of powdered tobacco, **slaked lime** and indigo. Popular in Afghanistan and Pakistan. Also spelt ***nasswar, niswar***

*Paan*: see **betel quid**. Also spelt *pan*

*Pan masala*: commercial preparation containing **areca nut**, **slaked lime**, **catechu** and other ingredients, but without tobacco. (Figure 5)

*Piper betle* L.: see **betel leaf**

**Slaked lime**: prepared from coral, sea shells (shell lime) or quarried limestone and mixed with water. Red and white varieties are available in Taiwan, China, Thailand and Myanmar. Also known in India as ***chuna*** or ***chunam***

**Stem quid**: specific Taiwanese name for betel quid consisting of unripe **areca nut** split in half, with stem of inflorescence inserted in the middle and **slaked lime** added

*Supari*: see **areca nut**

*Tambula*: Sanskrit term referring to **betel leaf**, **betel quid** or **areca nut**. Also called betel *thambool*

*Tamol*: fermented form of **areca nut**

*Zarda*: tobacco leaf broken into small pieces and boiled in water with **slaked lime** and spices until evaporation, then dried and coloured with vegetable dyes; usually chewed mixed with **areca nut** and spices

# GLOSSARY B — PRECANCEROUS LESIONS AND CONDITIONS AND SOME OTHER BETEL QUID-ASSOCIATED LESIONS

**Lichenoid lesions**: clinically resemble idiopathic oral lichen planus but represent type IV contact hypersensitivity reactions. In areca-nut chewers, they are found at the site of quid placement and are unilateral in nature.

**Betel chewer's mucosa (BCM)**: brownish-red discoloration of the oral mucosa, often accompanied by encrustation with quid particles, which are not easily removed, and show a tendency for desquamation and peeling. The underlying area of the mucosa assumes a wrinkled appearance. The lesion is usually localized and associated with the site of quid placement in the buccal cavity (Figure 6).

**Erythroplakia**: a bright red lesion of the oral mucosa that cannot be characterized clinically or pathologically as any other definable lesion (Axéll et al., 1984; WHO, 1996).

**Oral leukoplakia**: predominantly white patch or plaque on the oral mucosa that cannot be characterized clinically or pathologically as any other disease and is not associated with any physical or chemical causative agent except tobacco (Axéll et al., 1984). Based on clinical appearance, leukoplakia can be divided into two main subtypes: homogeneous leukoplakia (white) and non-homogeneous — including speckled or nodular — leukoplakia (red/white) (Figure 7).

**Oral lichen planus**: a chronic inflammatory disease of the skin and the oral mucosa of unknown etiology, although alterations in cell-mediated immunity may be important. Clinically, six types of oral lichen planus are described: papular, reticular, plaque-like, atrophic, erosive (ulcerative) and bullous. Malignant transformation has been observed in up to 2–3% of patients.

**Oral submucous fibrosis (OSF)**: chronic disorder characterized by fibrosis of the lining mucosa of the upper digestive tract involving the oral cavity, oro- and hypopharynx and the upper third of the oesophagus (Johnson et al., 1997). The fibrosis involves the lamina propria and the submucosa and may often extend into the underlying musculature, resulting in the deposition of dense fibrous bands. These bands give rise to the limited mouth opening, which is a hallmark of this disorder (Figure 8).

**Precancerous conditions**: a generalized state associated with a significantly increased risk for cancer (WHO, 1996).

**Precancerous lesions**: a morphologically altered tissue in which cancer is more likely to occur than in its apparently normal counterpart (WHO, 1996).

**Figure 1.** *Arecacatechu L.* palm

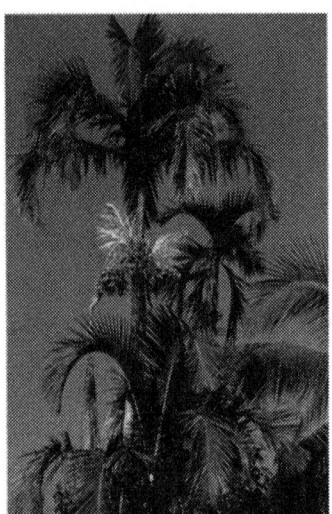

**Figure 3. Betel leaves (*Piper betle L.*)**

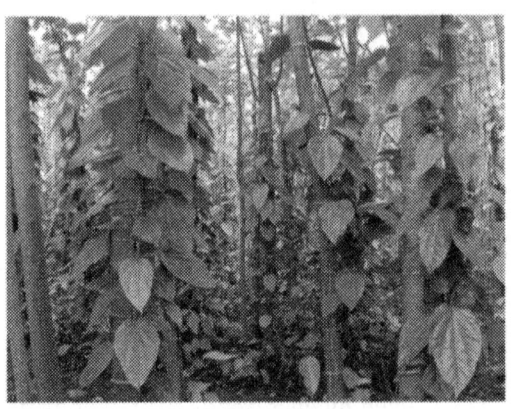

**Figure 2. Areca nuts (a) unripe, (b) raw, lime-coated and dried and (c) cut open to reveal the nut and husk**

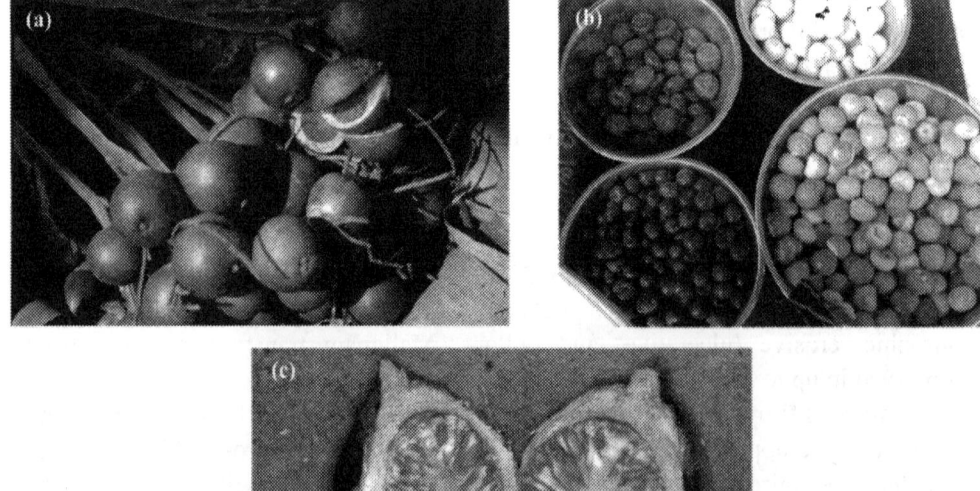

Figures 1, 2(a) and 2(c) provided by Peter Reichart; figures 2(b) and 3 provided by the Nargis Dutt Memorial Cancer Hospital, Barshi, Solapur District, Maharashtra, India

# Figure 4. Preparation of betel quid

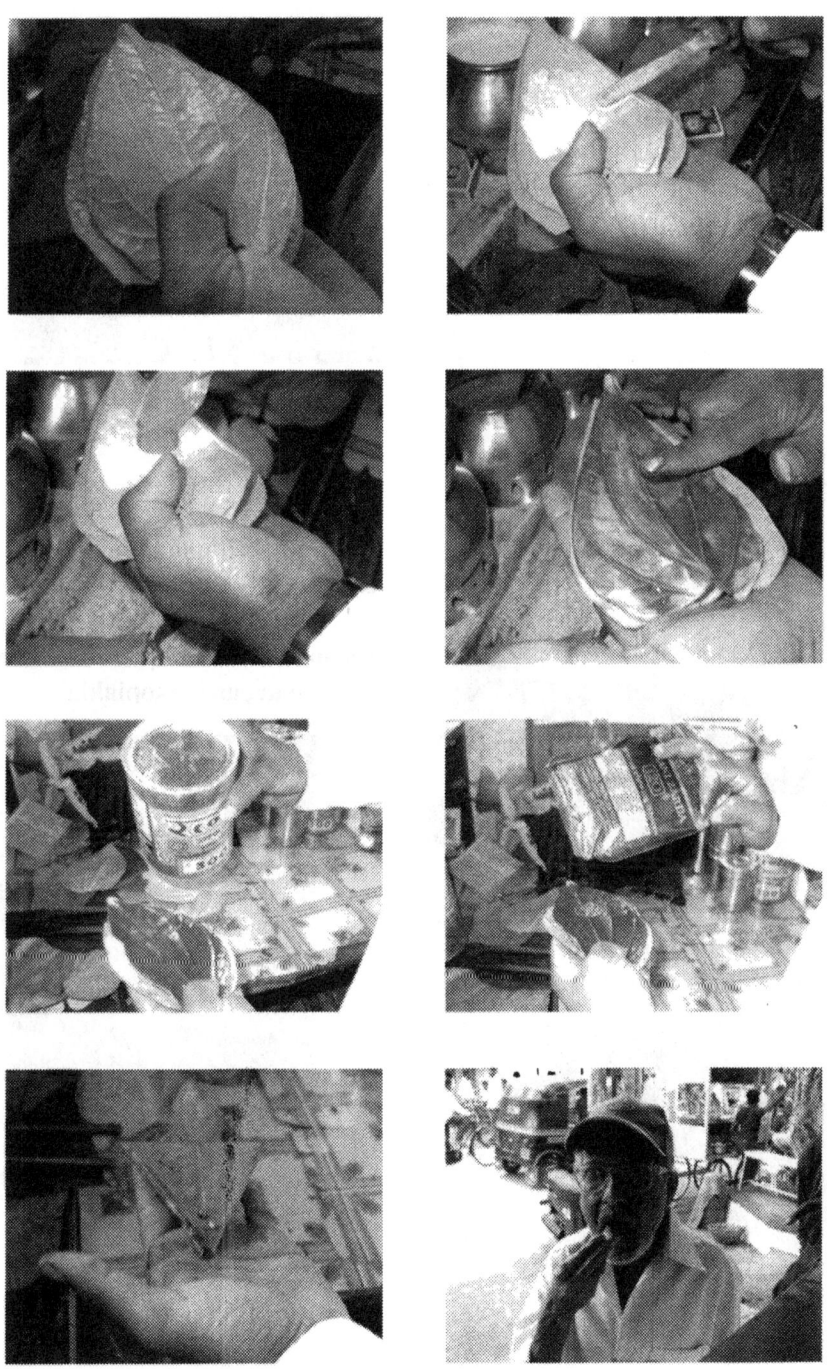

Provided by the Nargis Dutt Memorial Cancer Hospital, Barshi, Solapur District, Maharashtra, India

Figure 5. Shop in India selling a variety of commercial preparations of areca nut products (*gutka*, *pan masala* and *supari*)

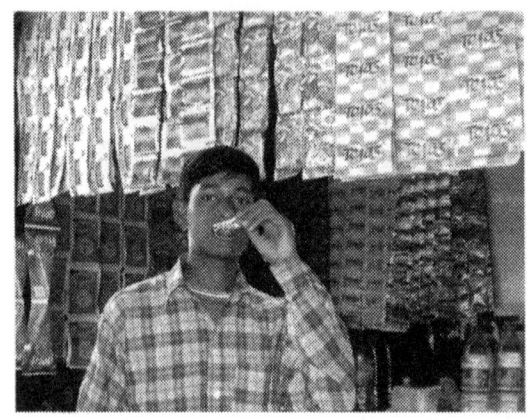

Figure 6. Betel chewer's mucosa with brownish flakes and homogeneous leukoplakia of the right cheek

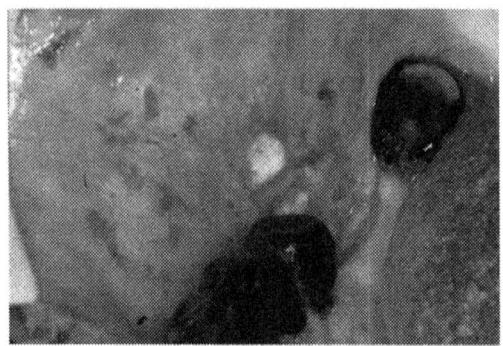

Figure 7. Whitish lesion of the right cheek with some brownish adherent flakes of the betel quid. The white lesions correspond to an extended homogeneous leukoplakia.

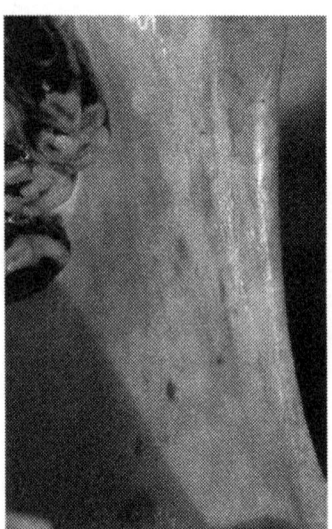

Figure 8. Betel chewer's mucosa with initial oral submucous fibrosis (white bands and plaques in the buccal mucosa)

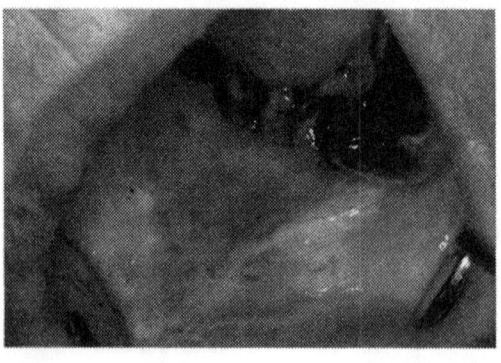

Figure 5 provided by the Nargis Dutt Memorial Cancer Hospital, Barshi, Solapur District, Maharashtra, India; figures 6, 7 and 8 provided by Peter Reichart

# CUMULATIVE CROSS INDEX TO *IARC MONOGRAPHS ON THE EVALUATION OF CARCINOGENIC RISKS TO HUMANS*

The volume, page and year of publication are given. References to corrigenda are given in parentheses.

## A

| | |
|---|---|
| A-α-C | *40*, 245 (1986); *Suppl. 7*, 56 (1987) |
| Acetaldehyde | *36*, 101 (1985) (*corr. 42*, 263); *Suppl. 7*, 77 (1987); *71*, 319 (1999) |
| Acetaldehyde formylmethylhydrazone (*see* Gyromitrin) | |
| Acetamide | *7*, 197 (1974); *Suppl. 7*, 56, 389 (1987); *71*, 1211 (1999) |
| Acetaminophen (*see* Paracetamol) | |
| Aciclovir | *76*, 47 (2000) |
| Acid mists (*see* Sulfuric acid and other strong inorganic acids, occupational exposures to mists and vapours from) | |
| Acridine orange | *16*, 145 (1978); *Suppl. 7*, 56 (1987) |
| Acriflavinium chloride | *13*, 31 (1977); *Suppl. 7*, 56 (1987) |
| Acrolein | *19*, 479 (1979); *36*, 133 (1985); *Suppl. 7*, 78 (1987); *63*, 337 (1995) (*corr. 65*, 549) |
| Acrylamide | *39*, 41 (1986); *Suppl. 7*, 56 (1987); *60*, 389 (1994) |
| Acrylic acid | *19*, 47 (1979); *Suppl. 7*, 56 (1987); *71*, 1223 (1999) |
| Acrylic fibres | *19*, 86 (1979); *Suppl. 7*, 56 (1987) |
| Acrylonitrile | *19*, 73 (1979); *Suppl. 7*, 79 (1987); *71*, 43 (1999) |
| Acrylonitrile-butadiene-styrene copolymers | *19*, 91 (1979); *Suppl. 7*, 56 (1987) |
| Actinolite (*see* Asbestos) | |
| Actinomycin D (*see also* Actinomycins) | *Suppl. 7*, 80 (1987) |
| Actinomycins | *10*, 29 (1976) (*corr. 42*, 255) |
| Adriamycin | *10*, 43 (1976); *Suppl. 7*, 82 (1987) |
| AF-2 | *31*, 47 (1983); *Suppl. 7*, 56 (1987) |
| Aflatoxins | *1*, 145 (1972) (*corr. 42*, 251); *10*, 51 (1976); *Suppl. 7*, 83 (1987); *56*, 245 (1993); *82*, 171 (2002) |
| Aflatoxin B$_1$ (*see* Aflatoxins) | |
| Aflatoxin B$_2$ (*see* Aflatoxins) | |
| Aflatoxin G$_1$ (*see* Aflatoxins) | |
| Aflatoxin G$_2$ (*see* Aflatoxins) | |
| Aflatoxin M$_1$ (*see* Aflatoxins) | |
| Agaritine | *31*, 63 (1983); *Suppl. 7*, 56 (1987) |
| Alcohol drinking | *44* (1988) |
| Aldicarb | *53*, 93 (1991) |

| | |
|---|---|
| Aldrin | 5, 25 (1974); *Suppl. 7*, 88 (1987) |
| Allyl chloride | 36, 39 (1985); *Suppl. 7*, 56 (1987); 71, 1231 (1999) |
| Allyl isothiocyanate | 36, 55 (1985); *Suppl. 7*, 56 (1987); 73, 37 (1999) |
| Allyl isovalerate | 36, 69 (1985); *Suppl. 7*, 56 (1987); 71, 1241 (1999) |
| Aluminium production | 34, 37 (1984); *Suppl. 7*, 89 (1987) |
| Amaranth | 8, 41 (1975); *Suppl. 7*, 56 (1987) |
| 5-Aminoacenaphthene | 16, 243 (1978); *Suppl. 7*, 56 (1987) |
| 2-Aminoanthraquinone | 27, 191 (1982); *Suppl. 7*, 56 (1987) |
| *para*-Aminoazobenzene | 8, 53 (1975); *Suppl. 7*, 56, 390 (1987) |
| *ortho*-Aminoazotoluene | 8, 61 (1975) (*corr.* 42, 254); *Suppl. 7*, 56 (1987) |
| *para*-Aminobenzoic acid | 16, 249 (1978); *Suppl. 7*, 56 (1987) |
| 4-Aminobiphenyl | 1, 74 (1972) (*corr.* 42, 251); *Suppl. 7*, 91 (1987) |
| 2-Amino-3,4-dimethylimidazo[4,5-*f*]quinoline (*see* MeIQ) | |
| 2-Amino-3,8-dimethylimidazo[4,5-*f*]quinoxaline (*see* MeIQx) | |
| 3-Amino-1,4-dimethyl-5*H*-pyrido[4,3-*b*]indole (*see* Trp-P-1) | |
| 2-Aminodipyrido[1,2-*a*:3′,2′-*d*]imidazole (*see* Glu-P-2) | |
| 1-Amino-2-methylanthraquinone | 27, 199 (1982); *Suppl. 7*, 57 (1987) |
| 2-Amino-3-methylimidazo[4,5-*f*]quinoline (*see* IQ) | |
| 2-Amino-6-methyldipyrido[1,2-*a*:3′,2′-*d*]imidazole (*see* Glu-P-1) | |
| 2-Amino-1-methyl-6-phenylimidazo[4,5-*b*]pyridine (*see* PhIP) | |
| 2-Amino-3-methyl-9*H*-pyrido[2,3-*b*]indole (*see* MeA-α-C) | |
| 3-Amino-1-methyl-5*H*-pyrido[4,3-*b*]indole (*see* Trp-P-2) | |
| 2-Amino-5-(5-nitro-2-furyl)-1,3,4-thiadiazole | 7, 143 (1974); *Suppl. 7*, 57 (1987) |
| 2-Amino-4-nitrophenol | 57, 167 (1993) |
| 2-Amino-5-nitrophenol | 57, 177 (1993) |
| 4-Amino-2-nitrophenol | 16, 43 (1978); *Suppl. 7*, 57 (1987) |
| 2-Amino-5-nitrothiazole | 31, 71 (1983); *Suppl. 7*, 57 (1987) |
| 2-Amino-9*H*-pyrido[2,3-*b*]indole (*see* A-α-C) | |
| 11-Aminoundecanoic acid | 39, 239 (1986); *Suppl. 7*, 57 (1987) |
| Amitrole | 7, 31 (1974); 41, 293 (1986) (*corr.* 52, 513; *Suppl. 7*, 92 (1987); 79, 381 (2001) |
| Ammonium potassium selenide (*see* Selenium and selenium compounds) | |
| Amorphous silica (*see also* Silica) | 42, 39 (1987); *Suppl. 7*, 341 (1987); 68, 41 (1997) (*corr.* 81, 383) |
| Amosite (*see* Asbestos) | |
| Ampicillin | 50, 153 (1990) |
| Amsacrine | 76, 317 (2000) |
| Anabolic steroids (*see* Androgenic (anabolic) steroids) | |
| Anaesthetics, volatile | 11, 285 (1976); *Suppl. 7*, 93 (1987) |
| Analgesic mixtures containing phenacetin (*see also* Phenacetin) | *Suppl. 7*, 310 (1987) |
| Androgenic (anabolic) steroids | *Suppl. 7*, 96 (1987) |
| Angelicin and some synthetic derivatives (*see also* Angelicins) | 40, 291 (1986) |
| Angelicin plus ultraviolet radiation (*see also* Angelicin and some synthetic derivatives) | *Suppl. 7*, 57 (1987) |
| Angelicins | *Suppl. 7*, 57 (1987) |
| Aniline | 4, 27 (1974) (*corr.* 42, 252); 27, 39 (1982); *Suppl. 7*, 99 (1987) |

| | |
|---|---|
| *ortho*-Anisidine | *27*, 63 (1982); *Suppl. 7*, 57 (1987); *73*, 49 (1999) |
| *para*-Anisidine | *27*, 65 (1982); *Suppl. 7*, 57 (1987) |
| Anthanthrene | *32*, 95 (1983); *Suppl. 7*, 57 (1987) |
| Anthophyllite (*see* Asbestos) | |
| Anthracene | *32*, 105 (1983); *Suppl. 7*, 57 (1987) |
| Anthranilic acid | *16*, 265 (1978); *Suppl. 7*, 57 (1987) |
| Anthraquinones | *82*, 129 (2002) |
| Antimony trioxide | *47*, 291 (1989) |
| Antimony trisulfide | *47*, 291 (1989) |
| ANTU (*see* 1-Naphthylthiourea) | |
| Apholate | *9*, 31 (1975); *Suppl. 7*, 57 (1987) |
| *para*-Aramid fibrils | *68*, 409 (1997) |
| Aramite® | *5*, 39 (1974); *Suppl. 7*, 57 (1987) |
| Areca nut (*see also* Betel quid) | *85*, 39 (2004) |
| *Aristolochia* species (*see also* Traditional herbal medicines) | *82*, 69 (2002) |
| Aristolochic acids | *82*, 69 (2002) |
| Arsanilic acid (*see* Arsenic and arsenic compounds) | |
| Arsenic and arsenic compounds | *1*, 41 (1972); *2*, 48 (1973); *23*, 39 (1980); *Suppl. 7*, 100 (1987) |
| Arsenic in drinking-water | *84* (2004) |
| Arsenic pentoxide (*see* Arsenic and arsenic compounds) | |
| Arsenic trioxide (*see* Arsenic in drinking-water) | |
| Arsenic trisulfide (*see* Arsenic in drinking-water) | |
| Arsine (*see* Arsenic and arsenic compounds) | |
| Asbestos | *2*, 17 (1973) (*corr. 42*, 252); *14* (1977) (*corr. 42*, 256); *Suppl. 7*, 106 (1987) (*corr. 45*, 283) |
| Atrazine | *53*, 441 (1991); *73*, 59 (1999) |
| Attapulgite (*see* Palygorskite) | |
| Auramine (technical-grade) | *1*, 69 (1972) (*corr. 42*, 251); *Suppl. 7*, 118 (1987) |
| Auramine, manufacture of (*see also* Auramine, technical-grade) | *Suppl. 7*, 118 (1987) |
| Aurothioglucose | *13*, 39 (1977); *Suppl. 7*, 57 (1987) |
| Azacitidine | *26*, 37 (1981); *Suppl. 7*, 57 (1987); *50*, 47 (1990) |
| 5-Azacytidine (*see* Azacitidine) | |
| Azaserine | *10*, 73 (1976) (*corr. 42*, 255); *Suppl. 7*, 57 (1987) |
| Azathioprine | *26*, 47 (1981); *Suppl. 7*, 119 (1987) |
| Aziridine | *9*, 37 (1975); *Suppl. 7*, 58 (1987); *71*, 337 (1999) |
| 2-(1-Aziridinyl)ethanol | *9*, 47 (1975); *Suppl. 7*, 58 (1987) |
| Aziridyl benzoquinone | *9*, 51 (1975); *Suppl. 7*, 58 (1987) |
| Azobenzene | *8*, 75 (1975); *Suppl. 7*, 58 (1987) |
| AZT (*see* Zidovudine) | |

## B

| | |
|---|---|
| Barium chromate (*see* Chromium and chromium compounds) | |
| Basic chromic sulfate (*see* Chromium and chromium compounds) | |
| BCNU (*see* Bischloroethyl nitrosourea) | |
| Benz[*a*]acridine | *32*, 123 (1983); *Suppl. 7*, 58 (1987) |

| | |
|---|---|
| Benz[c]acridine | 3, 241 (1973); 32, 129 (1983); Suppl. 7, 58 (1987) |
| Benzal chloride (see also α-Chlorinated toluenes and benzoyl chloride) | 29, 65 (1982); Suppl. 7, 148 (1987); 71, 453 (1999) |
| Benz[a]anthracene | 3, 45 (1973); 32, 135 (1983); Suppl. 7, 58 (1987) |
| Benzene | 7, 203 (1974) (corr. 42, 254); 29, 93, 391 (1982); Suppl. 7, 120 (1987) |
| Benzidine | 1, 80 (1972); 29, 149, 391 (1982); Suppl. 7, 123 (1987) |
| Benzidine-based dyes | Suppl. 7, 125 (1987) |
| Benzo[b]fluoranthene | 3, 69 (1973); 32, 147 (1983); Suppl. 7, 58 (1987) |
| Benzo[j]fluoranthene | 3, 82 (1973); 32, 155 (1983); Suppl. 7, 58 (1987) |
| Benzo[k]fluoranthene | 32, 163 (1983); Suppl. 7, 58 (1987) |
| Benzo[ghi]fluoranthene | 32, 171 (1983); Suppl. 7, 58 (1987) |
| Benzo[a]fluorene | 32, 177 (1983); Suppl. 7, 58 (1987) |
| Benzo[b]fluorene | 32, 183 (1983); Suppl. 7, 58 (1987) |
| Benzo[c]fluorene | 32, 189 (1983); Suppl. 7, 58 (1987) |
| Benzofuran | 63, 431 (1995) |
| Benzo[ghi]perylene | 32, 195 (1983); Suppl. 7, 58 (1987) |
| Benzo[c]phenanthrene | 32, 205 (1983); Suppl. 7, 58 (1987) |
| Benzo[a]pyrene | 3, 91 (1973); 32, 211 (1983) (corr. 68, 477); Suppl. 7, 58 (1987) |
| Benzo[e]pyrene | 3, 137 (1973); 32, 225 (1983); Suppl. 7, 58 (1987) |
| 1,4-Benzoquinone (see para-Quinone) | |
| 1,4-Benzoquinone dioxime | 29, 185 (1982); Suppl. 7, 58 (1987); 71, 1251 (1999) |
| Benzotrichloride (see also α-Chlorinated toluenes and benzoyl chloride) | 29, 73 (1982); Suppl. 7, 148 (1987); 71, 453 (1999) |
| Benzoyl chloride (see also α-Chlorinated toluenes and benzoyl chloride) | 29, 83 (1982) (corr. 42, 261); Suppl. 7, 126 (1987); 71, 453 (1999) |
| Benzoyl peroxide | 36, 267 (1985); Suppl. 7, 58 (1987); 71, 345 (1999) |
| Benzyl acetate | 40, 109 (1986); Suppl. 7, 58 (1987); 71, 1255 (1999) |
| Benzyl chloride (see also α-Chlorinated toluenes and benzoyl chloride) | 11, 217 (1976) (corr. 42, 256); 29, 49 (1982); Suppl. 7, 148 (1987); 71, 453 (1999) |
| Benzyl violet 4B | 16, 153 (1978); Suppl. 7, 58 (1987) |
| Bertrandite (see Beryllium and beryllium compounds) | |
| Beryllium and beryllium compounds | 1, 17 (1972); 23, 143 (1980) (corr. 42, 260); Suppl. 7, 127 (1987); 58, 41 (1993) |
| Beryllium acetate (see Beryllium and beryllium compounds) | |
| Beryllium acetate, basic (see Beryllium and beryllium compounds) | |
| Beryllium-aluminium alloy (see Beryllium and beryllium compounds) | |
| Beryllium carbonate (see Beryllium and beryllium compounds) | |
| Beryllium chloride (see Beryllium and beryllium compounds) | |
| Beryllium-copper alloy (see Beryllium and beryllium compounds) | |
| Beryllium-copper-cobalt alloy (see Beryllium and beryllium compounds) | |

Beryllium fluoride (see Beryllium and beryllium compounds)
Beryllium hydroxide (see Beryllium and beryllium compounds)
Beryllium-nickel alloy (see Beryllium and beryllium compounds)
Beryllium oxide (see Beryllium and beryllium compounds)
Beryllium phosphate (see Beryllium and beryllium compounds)
Beryllium silicate (see Beryllium and beryllium compounds)
Beryllium sulfate (see Beryllium and beryllium compounds)
Beryl ore (see Beryllium and beryllium compounds)

| | |
|---|---|
| Betel quid with tobacco | 37, 141 (1985); Suppl. 7, 128 (1987); 85, 39 (2004) |
| Betel quid without tobacco | 37, 141 (1985); Suppl. 7, 128 (1987); 85, 39 (2004) |
| BHA (see Butylated hydroxyanisole) | |
| BHT (see Butylated hydroxytoluene) | |
| Bis(1-aziridinyl)morpholinophosphine sulfide | 9, 55 (1975); Suppl. 7, 58 (1987) |
| 2,2-Bis(bromomethyl)propane-1,3-diol | 77, 455 (2000) |
| Bis(2-chloroethyl)ether | 9, 117 (1975); Suppl. 7, 58 (1987); 71, 1265 (1999) |
| N,N-Bis(2-chloroethyl)-2-naphthylamine | 4, 119 (1974) (corr. 42, 253); Suppl. 7, 130 (1987) |
| Bischloroethyl nitrosourea (see also Chloroethyl nitrosoureas) | 26, 79 (1981); Suppl. 7, 150 (1987) |
| 1,2-Bis(chloromethoxy)ethane | 15, 31 (1977); Suppl. 7, 58 (1987); 71, 1271 (1999) |
| 1,4-Bis(chloromethoxymethyl)benzene | 15, 37 (1977); Suppl. 7, 58 (1987); 71, 1273 (1999) |
| Bis(chloromethyl)ether | 4, 231 (1974) (corr. 42, 253); Suppl. 7, 131 (1987) |
| Bis(2-chloro-1-methylethyl)ether | 41, 149 (1986); Suppl. 7, 59 (1987); 71, 1275 (1999) |
| Bis(2,3-epoxycyclopentyl)ether | 47, 231 (1989); 71, 1281 (1999) |
| Bisphenol A diglycidyl ether (see also Glycidyl ethers) | 71, 1285 (1999) |
| Bisulfites (see Sulfur dioxide and some sulfites, bisulfites and metabisulfites) | |
| Bitumens | 35, 39 (1985); Suppl. 7, 133 (1987) |
| Bleomycins (see also Etoposide) | 26, 97 (1981); Suppl. 7, 134 (1987) |
| Blue VRS | 16, 163 (1978); Suppl. 7, 59 (1987) |
| Boot and shoe manufacture and repair | 25, 249 (1981); Suppl. 7, 232 (1987) |
| Bracken fern | 40, 47 (1986); Suppl. 7, 135 (1987) |
| Brilliant Blue FCF, disodium salt | 16, 171 (1978) (corr. 42, 257); Suppl. 7, 59 (1987) |
| Bromochloroacetonitrile (see also Halogenated acetonitriles) | 71, 1291 (1999) |
| Bromodichloromethane | 52, 179 (1991); 71, 1295 (1999) |
| Bromoethane | 52, 299 (1991); 71, 1305 (1999) |
| Bromoform | 52, 213 (1991); 71, 1309 (1999) |
| 1,3-Butadiene | 39, 155 (1986) (corr. 42, 264 Suppl. 7, 136 (1987); 54, 237 (1992); 71, 109 (1999) |
| 1,4-Butanediol dimethanesulfonate | 4, 247 (1974); Suppl. 7, 137 (1987) |
| n-Butyl acrylate | 39, 67 (1986); Suppl. 7, 59 (1987); 71, 359 (1999) |
| Butylated hydroxyanisole | 40, 123 (1986); Suppl. 7, 59 (1987) |
| Butylated hydroxytoluene | 40, 161 (1986); Suppl. 7, 59 (1987) |

Butyl benzyl phthalate                                      *29*, 193 (1982) (*corr. 42*, 261);
                                                            *Suppl. 7*, 59 (1987); *73*, 115 (1999)
β-Butyrolactone                                             *11*, 225 (1976); *Suppl. 7*, 59
                                                            (1987); *71*, 1317 (1999)
γ-Butyrolactone                                             *11*, 231 (1976); *Suppl. 7*, 59
                                                            (1987); *71*, 367 (1999)


## C

Cabinet-making (*see* Furniture and cabinet-making)
Cadmium acetate (*see* Cadmium and cadmium compounds)
Cadmium and cadmium compounds                               *2*, 74 (1973); *11*, 39 (1976)
                                                            (*corr. 42*, 255); *Suppl. 7*, 139
                                                            (1987); *58*, 119 (1993)

Cadmium chloride (*see* Cadmium and cadmium compounds)
Cadmium oxide (*see* Cadmium and cadmium compounds)
Cadmium sulfate (*see* Cadmium and cadmium compounds)
Cadmium sulfide (*see* Cadmium and cadmium compounds)
Caffeic acid                                                *56*, 115 (1993)
Caffeine                                                    *51*, 291 (1991)
Calcium arsenate (*see* Arsenic in drinking-water)
Calcium chromate (*see* Chromium and chromium compounds)
Calcium cyclamate (*see* Cyclamates)
Calcium saccharin (*see* Saccharin)
Cantharidin                                                 *10*, 79 (1976); *Suppl. 7*, 59 (1987)
Caprolactam                                                 *19*, 115 (1979) (*corr. 42*, 258);
                                                            *39*, 247 (1986) (*corr. 42*, 264);
                                                            *Suppl. 7*, 59, 390 (1987); *71*, 383
                                                            (1999)
Captafol                                                    *53*, 353 (1991)
Captan                                                      *30*, 295 (1983); *Suppl. 7*, 59 (1987)
Carbaryl                                                    *12*, 37 (1976); *Suppl. 7*, 59 (1987)
Carbazole                                                   *32*, 239 (1983); *Suppl. 7*, 59
                                                            (1987); *71*, 1319 (1999)
3-Carbethoxypsoralen                                        *40*, 317 (1986); *Suppl. 7*, 59 (1987)
Carbon black                                                *3*, 22 (1973); *33*, 35 (1984);
                                                            *Suppl. 7*, 142 (1987); *65*, 149
                                                            (1996)
Carbon tetrachloride                                        *1*, 53 (1972); *20*, 371 (1979);
                                                            *Suppl. 7*, 143 (1987); *71*, 401
                                                            (1999)
Carmoisine                                                  *8*, 83 (1975); *Suppl. 7*, 59 (1987)
Carpentry and joinery                                       *25*, 139 (1981); *Suppl. 7*, 378
                                                            (1987)
Carrageenan                                                 *10*, 181 (1976) (*corr. 42*, 255); *31*,
                                                            79 (1983); *Suppl. 7*, 59 (1987)

*Cassia occidentalis* (*see* Traditional herbal medicines)
Catechol                                                    *15*, 155 (1977); *Suppl. 7*, 59
                                                            (1987); *71*, 433 (1999)

CCNU (*see* 1-(2-Chloroethyl)-3-cyclohexyl-1-nitrosourea)
Ceramic fibres (*see* Man-made vitreous fibres)
Chemotherapy, combined, including alkylating agents (*see* MOPP and
    other combined chemotherapy including alkylating agents)

| | |
|---|---|
| Chloral (*see also* Chloral hydrate) | *63*, 245 (1995) |
| Chloral hydrate | *63*, 245 (1995); *84* (2004) |
| Chlorambucil | *9*, 125 (1975); *26*, 115 (1981); *Suppl. 7*, 144 (1987) |
| Chloramine | *84* (2004) |
| Chloramphenicol | *10*, 85 (1976); *Suppl. 7*, 145 (1987); *50*, 169 (1990) |
| Chlordane (*see also* Chlordane/Heptachlor) | *20*, 45 (1979) (*corr. 42*, 258) |
| Chlordane and Heptachlor | *Suppl. 7*, 146 (1987); *53*, 115 (1991); *79*, 411 (2001) |
| Chlordecone | *20*, 67 (1979); *Suppl. 7*, 59 (1987) |
| Chlordimeform | *30*, 61 (1983); *Suppl. 7*, 59 (1987) |
| Chlorendic acid | *48*, 45 (1990) |
| Chlorinated dibenzodioxins (other than TCDD) (*see also* Polychlorinated dibenzo-*para*-dioxins) | *15*, 41 (1977); *Suppl. 7*, 59 (1987) |
| Chlorinated drinking-water | *52*, 45 (1991) |
| Chlorinated paraffins | *48*, 55 (1990) |
| α-Chlorinated toluenes and benzoyl chloride | *Suppl. 7*, 148 (1987); *71*, 453 (1999) |
| Chlormadinone acetate | *6*, 149 (1974); *21*, 365 (1979); *Suppl. 7*, 291, 301 (1987); *72*, 49 (1999) |
| Chlornaphazine (*see N,N*-Bis(2-chloroethyl)-2-naphthylamine) | |
| Chloroacetonitrile (*see also* Halogenated acetonitriles) | *71*, 1325 (1999) |
| *para*-Chloroaniline | *57*, 305 (1993) |
| Chlorobenzilate | *5*, 75 (1974); *30*, 73 (1983); *Suppl. 7*, 60 (1987) |
| Chlorodibromomethane | *52*, 243 (1991); *71*, 1331 (1999) |
| Chlorodifluoromethane | *41*, 237 (1986) (*corr. 51*, 483); *Suppl. 7*, 149 (1987); *71*, 1339 (1999) |
| Chloroethane | *52*, 315 (1991); *71*, 1345 (1999) |
| 1-(2-Chloroethyl)-3-cyclohexyl-1-nitrosourea (*see also* Chloroethyl nitrosoureas) | *26*, 137 (1981) (*corr. 42*, 260); *Suppl. 7*, 150 (1987) |
| 1-(2-Chloroethyl)-3-(4-methylcyclohexyl)-1-nitrosourea (*see also* Chloroethyl nitrosoureas) | *Suppl. 7*, 150 (1987) |
| Chloroethyl nitrosoureas | *Suppl. 7*, 150 (1987) |
| Chlorofluoromethane | *41*, 229 (1986); *Suppl. 7*, 60 (1987); *71*, 1351 (1999) |
| Chloroform | *1*, 61 (1972); *20*, 401 (1979); *Suppl. 7*, 152 (1987); *73*, 131 (1999) |
| 3-Chloro-4-(dichloromethyl)-5-hydroxy-2(5*H*)-furanone | *84* (2004) |
| Chloromethyl methyl ether (technical-grade) (*see also* Bis(chloromethyl)ether) | *4*, 239 (1974); *Suppl. 7*, 131 (1987) |
| (4-Chloro-2-methylphenoxy)acetic acid (*see* MCPA) | |
| 1-Chloro-2-methylpropene | *63*, 315 (1995) |
| 3-Chloro-2-methylpropene | *63*, 325 (1995) |
| 2-Chloronitrobenzene | *65*, 263 (1996) |
| 3-Chloronitrobenzene | *65*, 263 (1996) |
| 4-Chloronitrobenzene | *65*, 263 (1996) |
| Chlorophenols (*see also* Polychlorophenols and their sodium salts) | *Suppl. 7*, 154 (1987) |
| Chlorophenols (occupational exposures to) | *41*, 319 (1986) |
| Chlorophenoxy herbicides | *Suppl. 7*, 156 (1987) |

Chlorophenoxy herbicides (occupational exposures to)     *41*, 357 (1986)
4-Chloro-*ortho*-phenylenediamine     *27*, 81 (1982); *Suppl. 7*, 60 (1987)
4-Chloro-*meta*-phenylenediamine     *27*, 82 (1982); *Suppl. 7*, 60 (1987)
Chloroprene     *19*, 131 (1979); *Suppl. 7*, 160 (1987); *71*, 227 (1999)
Chloropropham     *12*, 55 (1976); *Suppl. 7*, 60 (1987)
Chloroquine     *13*, 47 (1977); *Suppl. 7*, 60 (1987)
Chlorothalonil     *30*, 319 (1983); *Suppl. 7*, 60 (1987); *73*, 183 (1999)
*para*-Chloro-*ortho*-toluidine and its strong acid salts (*see also* Chlordimeform)     *16*, 277 (1978); *30*, 65 (1983); *Suppl. 7*, 60 (1987); *48*, 123 (1990); *77*, 323 (2000)
4-Chloro-*ortho*-toluidine (see *para*-chloro-*ortho*-toluidine)
5-Chloro-*ortho*-toluidine     *77*, 341 (2000)
Chlorotrianisene (*see also* Nonsteroidal oestrogens)     *21*, 139 (1979); *Suppl. 7*, 280 (1987)
2-Chloro-1,1,1-trifluoroethane     *41*, 253 (1986); *Suppl. 7*, 60 (1987); *71*, 1355 (1999)
Chlorozotocin     *50*, 65 (1990)
Cholesterol     *10*, 99 (1976); *31*, 95 (1983); *Suppl. 7*, 161 (1987)
Chromic acetate (*see* Chromium and chromium compounds)
Chromic chloride (*see* Chromium and chromium compounds)
Chromic oxide (*see* Chromium and chromium compounds)
Chromic phosphate (*see* Chromium and chromium compounds)
Chromite ore (*see* Chromium and chromium compounds)
Chromium and chromium compounds (*see also* Implants, surgical)     *2*, 100 (1973); *23*, 205 (1980); *Suppl. 7*, 165 (1987); *49*, 49 (1990) (*corr. 51*, 483)
Chromium carbonyl (*see* Chromium and chromium compounds)
Chromium potassium sulfate (*see* Chromium and chromium compounds)
Chromium sulfate (*see* Chromium and chromium compounds)
Chromium trioxide (*see* Chromium and chromium compounds)
Chrysazin (*see* Dantron)
Chrysene     *3*, 159 (1973); *32*, 247 (1983); *Suppl. 7*, 60 (1987)
Chrysoidine     *8*, 91 (1975); *Suppl. 7*, 169 (1987)
Chrysotile (*see* Asbestos)
CI Acid Orange 3     *57*, 121 (1993)
CI Acid Red 114     *57*, 247 (1993)
CI Basic Red 9 (*see also* Magenta)     *57*, 215 (1993)
Ciclosporin     *50*, 77 (1990)
CI Direct Blue 15     *57*, 235 (1993)
CI Disperse Yellow 3 (see Disperse Yellow 3)
Cimetidine     *50*, 235 (1990)
Cinnamyl anthranilate     *16*, 287 (1978); *31*, 133 (1983); *Suppl. 7*, 60 (1987); *77*, 177 (2000)
CI Pigment Red 3     *57*, 259 (1993)
CI Pigment Red 53:1 (*see* D&C Red No. 9)
Cisplatin (*see also* Etoposide)     *26*, 151 (1981); *Suppl. 7*, 170 (1987)
Citrinin     *40*, 67 (1986); *Suppl. 7*, 60 (1987)
Citrus Red No. 2     *8*, 101 (1975) (*corr. 42*, 254); *Suppl. 7*, 60 (1987)

| | |
|---|---|
| Clinoptilolite (*see* Zeolites) | |
| Clofibrate | 24, 39 (1980); *Suppl. 7*, 171 (1987); 66, 391 (1996) |
| Clomiphene citrate | 21, 551 (1979); *Suppl. 7*, 172 (1987) |
| *Clonorchis sinensis* (infection with) | 61, 121 (1994) |
| Coal dust | 68, 337 (1997) |
| Coal gasification | 34, 65 (1984); *Suppl. 7*, 173 (1987) |
| Coal-tar pitches (*see also* Coal-tars) | 35, 83 (1985); *Suppl. 7*, 174 (1987) |
| Coal-tars | 35, 83 (1985); *Suppl. 7*, 175 (1987) |
| Cobalt[III] acetate (*see* Cobalt and cobalt compounds) | |
| Cobalt-aluminium-chromium spinel (*see* Cobalt and cobalt compounds) | |
| Cobalt and cobalt compounds (*see also* Implants, surgical) | 52, 363 (1991) |
| Cobalt[II] chloride (*see* Cobalt and cobalt compounds) | |
| Cobalt-chromium alloy (*see* Chromium and chromium compounds) | |
| Cobalt-chromium-molybdenum alloys (*see* Cobalt and cobalt compounds) | |
| Cobalt metal powder (*see* Cobalt and cobalt compounds) | |
| Cobalt naphthenate (*see* Cobalt and cobalt compounds) | |
| Cobalt[II] oxide (*see* Cobalt and cobalt compounds) | |
| Cobalt[II,III] oxide (*see* Cobalt and cobalt compounds) | |
| Cobalt[II] sulfide (*see* Cobalt and cobalt compounds) | |
| Coffee | 51, 41 (1991) (*corr.* 52, 513) |
| Coke production | 34, 101 (1984); *Suppl. 7*, 176 (1987) |
| Combined oral contraceptives (*see* Oral contraceptives, combined) | |
| Conjugated equine oestrogens | 72, 399 (1999) |
| Conjugated oestrogens (*see also* Steroidal oestrogens) | 21, 147 (1979); *Suppl. 7*, 283 (1987) |
| Continuous glass filament (*see* Man-made vitreous fibres) | |
| Contraceptives, oral (*see* Oral contraceptives, combined; Sequential oral contraceptives) | |
| Copper 8-hydroxyquinoline | 15, 103 (1977); *Suppl. 7*, 61 (1987) |
| Coronene | 32, 263 (1983); *Suppl. 7*, 61 (1987) |
| Coumarin | 10, 113 (1976); *Suppl. 7*, 61 (1987); 77, 193 (2000) |
| Creosotes (*see also* Coal-tars) | 35, 83 (1985); *Suppl. 7*, 177 (1987) |
| *meta*-Cresidine | 27, 91 (1982); *Suppl. 7*, 61 (1987) |
| *para*-Cresidine | 27, 92 (1982); *Suppl. 7*, 61 (1987) |
| Cristobalite (*see* Crystalline silica) | |
| Crocidolite (*see* Asbestos) | |
| Crotonaldehyde | 63, 373 (1995) (*corr.* 65, 549) |
| Crude oil | 45, 119 (1989) |
| Crystalline silica (*see also* Silica) | 42, 39 (1987); *Suppl. 7*, 341 (1987); 68, 41 (1997) (*corr.* 81, 383) |
| Cycasin (*see also* Methylazoxymethanol) | 1, 157 (1972) (*corr.* 42, 251); 10, 121 (1976); *Suppl. 7*, 61 (1987) |
| Cyclamates | 22, 55 (1980); *Suppl. 7*, 178 (1987); 73, 195 (1999) |
| Cyclamic acid (*see* Cyclamates) | |
| Cyclochlorotine | 10, 139 (1976); *Suppl. 7*, 61 (1987) |
| Cyclohexanone | 47, 157 (1989); 71, 1359 (1999) |
| Cyclohexylamine (*see* Cyclamates) | |
| Cyclopenta[*cd*]pyrene | 32, 269 (1983); *Suppl. 7*, 61 (1987) |

Cyclopropane (see Anaesthetics, volatile)
Cyclophosphamide                                        9, 135 (1975); 26, 165 (1981);
                                                        Suppl. 7, 182 (1987)
Cyproterone acetate                                     72, 49 (1999)

# D

2,4-D (see also Chlorophenoxy herbicides; Chlorophenoxy    15, 111 (1977)
   herbicides, occupational exposures to)
Dacarbazine                                             26, 203 (1981); Suppl. 7, 184
                                                        (1987)
Dantron                                                 50, 265 (1990) (corr. 59, 257)
D&C Red No. 9                                           8, 107 (1975); Suppl. 7, 61 (1987);
                                                        57, 203 (1993)
Dapsone                                                 24, 59 (1980); Suppl. 7, 185 (1987)
Daunomycin                                              10, 145 (1976); Suppl. 7, 61 (1987)
DDD (see DDT)
DDE (see DDT)
DDT                                                     5, 83 (1974) (corr. 42, 253);
                                                        Suppl. 7, 186 (1987); 53, 179
                                                        (1991)
Decabromodiphenyl oxide                                 48, 73 (1990); 71, 1365 (1999)
Deltamethrin                                            53, 251 (1991)
Deoxynivalenol (see Toxins derived from *Fusarium graminearum*,
   *F. culmorum* and *F. crookwellense*)
Diacetylaminoazotoluene                                 8, 113 (1975); Suppl. 7, 61 (1987)
N,N'-Diacetylbenzidine                                  16, 293 (1978); Suppl. 7, 61 (1987)
Diallate                                                12, 69 (1976); 30, 235 (1983);
                                                        Suppl. 7, 61 (1987)
2,4-Diaminoanisole and its salts                        16, 51 (1978); 27, 103 (1982);
                                                        Suppl. 7, 61 (1987); 79, 619 (2001)
4,4'-Diaminodiphenyl ether                              16, 301 (1978); 29, 203 (1982);
                                                        Suppl. 7, 61 (1987)
1,2-Diamino-4-nitrobenzene                              16, 63 (1978); Suppl. 7, 61 (1987)
1,4-Diamino-2-nitrobenzene                              16, 73 (1978); Suppl. 7, 61 (1987);
                                                        57, 185 (1993)
2,6-Diamino-3-(phenylazo)pyridine (see Phenazopyridine hydrochloride)
2,4-Diaminotoluene (see also Toluene diisocyanates)     16, 83 (1978); Suppl. 7, 61 (1987)
2,5-Diaminotoluene (see also Toluene diisocyanates)     16, 97 (1978); Suppl. 7, 61 (1987)
ortho-Dianisidine (see 3,3'-Dimethoxybenzidine)
Diatomaceous earth, uncalcined (see Amorphous silica)
Diazepam                                                13, 57 (1977); Suppl. 7, 189
                                                        (1987); 66, 37 (1996)
Diazomethane                                            7, 223 (1974); Suppl. 7, 61 (1987)
Dibenz[a,h]acridine                                     3, 247 (1973); 32, 277 (1983);
                                                        Suppl. 7, 61 (1987)
Dibenz[a,j]acridine                                     3, 254 (1973); 32, 283 (1983);
                                                        Suppl. 7, 61 (1987)
Dibenz[a,c]anthracene                                   32, 289 (1983) (corr. 42, 262);
                                                        Suppl. 7, 61 (1987)
Dibenz[a,h]anthracene                                   3, 178 (1973) (corr. 43, 261);
                                                        32, 299 (1983); Suppl. 7, 61 (1987)
Dibenz[a,j]anthracene                                   32, 309 (1983); Suppl. 7, 61 (1987)

| | |
|---|---|
| 7H-Dibenzo[c,g]carbazole | 3, 260 (1973); 32, 315 (1983); Suppl. 7, 61 (1987) |
| Dibenzodioxins, chlorinated (other than TCDD) (see Chlorinated dibenzodioxins (other than TCDD)) | |
| Dibenzo[a,e]fluoranthene | 32, 321 (1983); Suppl. 7, 61 (1987) |
| Dibenzo[h,rst]pentaphene | 3, 197 (1973); Suppl. 7, 62 (1987) |
| Dibenzo[a,e]pyrene | 3, 201 (1973); 32, 327 (1983); Suppl. 7, 62 (1987) |
| Dibenzo[a,h]pyrene | 3, 207 (1973); 32, 331 (1983); Suppl. 7, 62 (1987) |
| Dibenzo[a,i]pyrene | 3, 215 (1973); 32, 337 (1983); Suppl. 7, 62 (1987) |
| Dibenzo[a,l]pyrene | 3, 224 (1973); 32, 343 (1983); Suppl. 7, 62 (1987) |
| Dibenzo-para-dioxin | 69, 33 (1997) |
| Dibromoacetonitrile (see also Halogenated acetonitriles) | 71, 1369 (1999) |
| 1,2-Dibromo-3-chloropropane | 15, 139 (1977); 20, 83 (1979); Suppl. 7, 191 (1987); 71, 479 (1999) |
| 1,2-Dibromoethane (see Ethylene dibromide) | |
| 2,3-Dibromopropan-1-ol | 77, 439 (2000) |
| Dichloroacetic acid | 63, 271 (1995); 84 (2004) |
| Dichloroacetonitrile (see also Halogenated acetonitriles) | 71, 1375 (1999) |
| Dichloroacetylene | 39, 369 (1986); Suppl. 7, 62 (1987); 71, 1381 (1999) |
| ortho-Dichlorobenzene | 7, 231 (1974); 29, 213 (1982); Suppl. 7, 192 (1987); 73, 223 (1999) |
| meta-Dichlorobenzene | 73, 223 (1999) |
| para-Dichlorobenzene | 7, 231 (1974); 29, 215 (1982); Suppl. 7, 192 (1987); 73, 223 (1999) |
| 3,3′-Dichlorobenzidine | 4, 49 (1974); 29, 239 (1982); Suppl. 7, 193 (1987) |
| trans-1,4-Dichlorobutene | 15, 149 (1977); Suppl. 7, 62 (1987); 71, 1389 (1999) |
| 3,3′-Dichloro-4,4′-diaminodiphenyl ether | 16, 309 (1978); Suppl. 7, 62 (1987) |
| 1,2-Dichloroethane | 20, 429 (1979); Suppl. 7, 62 (1987); 71, 501 (1999) |
| Dichloromethane | 20, 449 (1979); 41, 43 (1986); Suppl. 7, 194 (1987); 71, 251 (1999) |
| 2,4-Dichlorophenol (see Chlorophenols; Chlorophenols, occupational exposures to; Polychlorophenols and their sodium salts) | |
| (2,4-Dichlorophenoxy)acetic acid (see 2,4-D) | |
| 2,6-Dichloro-para-phenylenediamine | 39, 325 (1986); Suppl. 7, 62 (1987) |
| 1,2-Dichloropropane | 41, 131 (1986); Suppl. 7, 62 (1987); 71, 1393 (1999) |
| 1,3-Dichloropropene (technical-grade) | 41, 113 (1986); Suppl. 7, 195 (1987); 71, 933 (1999) |
| Dichlorvos | 20, 97 (1979); Suppl. 7, 62 (1987); 53, 267 (1991) |
| Dicofol | 30, 87 (1983); Suppl. 7, 62 (1987) |
| Dicyclohexylamine (see Cyclamates) | |
| Didanosine | 76, 153 (2000) |
| Dieldrin | 5, 125 (1974); Suppl. 7, 196 (1987) |

| | |
|---|---|
| Dienoestrol (see also Nonsteroidal oestrogens) | 21, 161 (1979); Suppl. 7, 278 (1987) |
| Diepoxybutane (see also 1,3-Butadiene) | 11, 115 (1976) (corr. 42, 255); Suppl. 7, 62 (1987); 71, 109 (1999) |
| Diesel and gasoline engine exhausts | 46, 41 (1989) |
| Diesel fuels | 45, 219 (1989) (corr. 47, 505) |
| Diethanolamine | 77, 349 (2000) |
| Diethyl ether (see Anaesthetics, volatile) | |
| Di(2-ethylhexyl) adipate | 29, 257 (1982); Suppl. 7, 62 (1987); 77, 149 (2000) |
| Di(2-ethylhexyl) phthalate | 29, 269 (1982) (corr. 42, 261); Suppl. 7, 62 (1987); 77, 41 (2000) |
| 1,2-Diethylhydrazine | 4, 153 (1974); Suppl. 7, 62 (1987); 71, 1401 (1999) |
| Diethylstilboestrol | 6, 55 (1974); 21, 173 (1979) (corr. 42, 259); Suppl. 7, 273 (1987) |
| Diethylstilboestrol dipropionate (see Diethylstilboestrol) | |
| Diethyl sulfate | 4, 277 (1974); Suppl. 7, 198 (1987); 54, 213 (1992); 71, 1405 (1999) |
| N,N′-Diethylthiourea | 79, 649 (2001) |
| Diglycidyl resorcinol ether | 11, 125 (1976); 36, 181 (1985); Suppl. 7, 62 (1987); 71, 1417 (1999) |
| Dihydrosafrole | 1, 170 (1972); 10, 233 (1976) Suppl. 7, 62 (1987) |
| 1,8-Dihydroxyanthraquinone (see Dantron) | |
| Dihydroxybenzenes (see Catechol; Hydroquinone; Resorcinol) | |
| 1,3-Dihydroxy-2-hydroxymethylanthraquinone | 82, 129 (2002) |
| Dihydroxymethylfuratrizine | 24, 77 (1980); Suppl. 7, 62 (1987) |
| Diisopropyl sulfate | 54, 229 (1992); 71, 1421 (1999) |
| Dimethisterone (see also Progestins; Sequential oral contraceptives) | 6, 167 (1974); 21, 377 (1979)) |
| Dimethoxane | 15, 177 (1977); Suppl. 7, 62 (1987) |
| 3,3′-Dimethoxybenzidine | 4, 41 (1974); Suppl. 7, 198 (1987) |
| 3,3′-Dimethoxybenzidine-4,4′-diisocyanate | 39, 279 (1986); Suppl. 7, 62 (1987) |
| para-Dimethylaminoazobenzene | 8, 125 (1975); Suppl. 7, 62 (1987) |
| para-Dimethylaminoazobenzenediazo sodium sulfonate | 8, 147 (1975); Suppl. 7, 62 (1987) |
| trans-2-[(Dimethylamino)methylimino]-5-[2-(5-nitro-2-furyl)-vinyl]-1,3,4-oxadiazole | 7, 147 (1974) (corr. 42, 253); Suppl. 7, 62 (1987) |
| 4,4′-Dimethylangelicin plus ultraviolet radiation (see also Angelicin and some synthetic derivatives) | Suppl. 7, 57 (1987) |
| 4,5′-Dimethylangelicin plus ultraviolet radiation (see also Angelicin and some synthetic derivatives) | Suppl. 7, 57 (1987) |
| 2,6-Dimethylaniline | 57, 323 (1993) |
| N,N-Dimethylaniline | 57, 337 (1993) |
| Dimethylarsinic acid (see Arsenic and arsenic compounds) | |
| 3,3′-Dimethylbenzidine | 1, 87 (1972); Suppl. 7, 62 (1987) |
| Dimethylcarbamoyl chloride | 12, 77 (1976); Suppl. 7, 199 (1987); 71, 531 (1999) |
| Dimethylformamide | 47, 171 (1989); 71, 545 (1999) |
| 1,1-Dimethylhydrazine | 4, 137 (1974); Suppl. 7, 62 (1987); 71, 1425 (1999) |

| | |
|---|---|
| 1,2-Dimethylhydrazine | 4, 145 (1974) (corr. 42, 253); Suppl. 7, 62 (1987); 71, 947 (1999) |
| Dimethyl hydrogen phosphite | 48, 85 (1990); 71, 1437 (1999) |
| 1,4-Dimethylphenanthrene | 32, 349 (1983); Suppl. 7, 62 (1987) |
| Dimethyl sulfate | 4, 271 (1974); Suppl. 7, 200 (1987); 71, 575 (1999) |
| 3,7-Dinitrofluoranthene | 46, 189 (1989); 65, 297 (1996) |
| 3,9-Dinitrofluoranthene | 46, 195 (1989); 65, 297 (1996) |
| 1,3-Dinitropyrene | 46, 201 (1989) |
| 1,6-Dinitropyrene | 46, 215 (1989) |
| 1,8-Dinitropyrene | 33, 171 (1984); Suppl. 7, 63 (1987); 46, 231 (1989) |
| Dinitrosopentamethylenetetramine | 11, 241 (1976); Suppl. 7, 63 (1987) |
| 2,4-Dinitrotoluene | 65, 309 (1996) (corr. 66, 485) |
| 2,6-Dinitrotoluene | 65, 309 (1996) (corr. 66, 485) |
| 3,5-Dinitrotoluene | 65, 309 (1996) |
| 1,4-Dioxane | 11, 247 (1976); Suppl. 7, 201 (1987); 71, 589 (1999) |
| 2,4′-Diphenyldiamine | 16, 313 (1978); Suppl. 7, 63 (1987) |
| Direct Black 38 (*see also* Benzidine-based dyes) | 29, 295 (1982) (corr. 42, 261) |
| Direct Blue 6 (*see also* Benzidine-based dyes) | 29, 311 (1982) |
| Direct Brown 95 (*see also* Benzidine-based dyes) | 29, 321 (1982) |
| Disperse Blue 1 | 48, 139 (1990) |
| Disperse Yellow 3 | 8, 97 (1975); Suppl. 7, 60 (1987); 48, 149 (1990) |
| Disulfiram | 12, 85 (1976); Suppl. 7, 63 (1987) |
| Dithranol | 13, 75 (1977); Suppl. 7, 63 (1987) |
| Divinyl ether (*see* Anaesthetics, volatile) | |
| Doxefazepam | 66, 97 (1996) |
| Doxylamine succinate | 79, 145 (2001) |
| Droloxifene | 66, 241 (1996) |
| Dry cleaning | 63, 33 (1995) |
| Dulcin | 12, 97 (1976); Suppl. 7, 63 (1987) |

## E

| | |
|---|---|
| Endrin | 5, 157 (1974); Suppl. 7, 63 (1987) |
| Enflurane (*see* Anaesthetics, volatile) | |
| Eosin | 15, 183 (1977); Suppl. 7, 63 (1987) |
| Epichlorohydrin | 11, 131 (1976) (corr. 42, 256); Suppl. 7, 202 (1987); 71, 603 (1999) |
| 1,2-Epoxybutane | 47, 217 (1989); 71, 629 (1999) |
| 1-Epoxyethyl-3,4-epoxycyclohexane (*see* 4-Vinylcyclohexene diepoxide) | |
| 3,4-Epoxy-6-methylcyclohexylmethyl 3,4-epoxy-6-methyl-cyclohexane carboxylate | 11, 147 (1976); Suppl. 7, 63 (1987); 71, 1441 (1999) |
| *cis*-9,10-Epoxystearic acid | 11, 153 (1976); Suppl. 7, 63 (1987); 71, 1443 (1999) |
| Epstein-Barr virus | 70, 47 (1997) |
| *d*-Equilenin | 72, 399 (1999) |
| Equilin | 72, 399 (1999) |
| Erionite | 42, 225 (1987); Suppl. 7, 203 (1987) |

| | |
|---|---|
| Estazolam | 66, 105 (1996) |
| Ethinyloestradiol | 6, 77 (1974); 21, 233 (1979); Suppl. 7, 286 (1987); 72, 49 (1999) |
| Ethionamide | 13, 83 (1977); Suppl. 7, 63 (1987) |
| Ethyl acrylate | 19, 57 (1979); 39, 81 (1986); Suppl. 7, 63 (1987); 71, 1447 (1999) |
| Ethylbenzene | 77, 227 (2000) |
| Ethylene | 19, 157 (1979); Suppl. 7, 63 (1987); 60, 45 (1994); 71, 1447 (1999) |
| Ethylene dibromide | 15, 195 (1977); Suppl. 7, 204 (1987); 71, 641 (1999) |
| Ethylene oxide | 11, 157 (1976); 36, 189 (1985) (corr. 42, 263); Suppl. 7, 205 (1987); 60, 73 (1994) |
| Ethylene sulfide | 11, 257 (1976); Suppl. 7, 63 (1987) |
| Ethylenethiourea | 7, 45 (1974); Suppl. 7, 207 (1987); 79, 659 (2001) |
| 2-Ethylhexyl acrylate | 60, 475 (1994) |
| Ethyl methanesulfonate | 7, 245 (1974); Suppl. 7, 63 (1987) |
| N-Ethyl-N-nitrosourea | 1, 135 (1972); 17, 191 (1978); Suppl. 7, 63 (1987) |
| Ethyl selenac (see also Selenium and selenium compounds) | 12, 107 (1976); Suppl. 7, 63 (1987) |
| Ethyl tellurac | 12, 115 (1976); Suppl. 7, 63 (1987) |
| Ethynodiol diacetate | 6, 173 (1974); 21, 387 (1979); Suppl. 7, 292 (1987); 72, 49 (1999) |
| Etoposide | 76, 177 (2000) |
| Eugenol | 36, 75 (1985); Suppl. 7, 63 (1987) |
| Evans blue | 8, 151 (1975); Suppl. 7, 63 (1987) |
| Extremely low-frequency electric fields | 80 (2002) |
| Extremely low-frequency magnetic fields | 80 (2002) |

# F

| | |
|---|---|
| Fast Green FCF | 16, 187 (1978); Suppl. 7, 63 (1987) |
| Fenvalerate | 53, 309 (1991) |
| Ferbam | 12, 121 (1976) (corr. 42, 256); Suppl. 7, 63 (1987) |
| Ferric oxide | 1, 29 (1972); Suppl. 7, 216 (1987) |
| Ferrochromium (see Chromium and chromium compounds) | |
| Fluometuron | 30, 245 (1983); Suppl. 7, 63 (1987) |
| Fluoranthene | 32, 355 (1983); Suppl. 7, 63 (1987) |
| Fluorene | 32, 365 (1983); Suppl. 7, 63 (1987) |
| Fluorescent lighting (exposure to) (see Ultraviolet radiation) | |
| Fluorides (inorganic, used in drinking-water) | 27, 237 (1982); Suppl. 7, 208 (1987) |
| 5-Fluorouracil | 26, 217 (1981); Suppl. 7, 210 (1987) |
| Fluorspar (see Fluorides) | |
| Fluosilicic acid (see Fluorides) | |
| Fluroxene (see Anaesthetics, volatile) | |

| | |
|---|---|
| Foreign bodies | *74* (1999) |
| Formaldehyde | *29*, 345 (1982); *Suppl. 7*, 211 (1987); *62*, 217 (1995) (*corr. 65*, 549; *corr. 66*, 485) |
| 2-(2-Formylhydrazino)-4-(5-nitro-2-furyl)thiazole | *7*, 151 (1974) (*corr. 42*, 253); *Suppl. 7*, 63 (1987) |
| Frusemide (*see* Furosemide) | |
| Fuel oils (heating oils) | *45*, 239 (1989) (*corr. 47*, 505) |
| Fumonisin B$_1$ (*see* also Toxins derived from *Fusarium moniliforme*) | *82*, 301 (2002) |
| Fumonisin B$_2$ (*see* Toxins derived from *Fusarium moniliforme*) | |
| Furan | *63*, 393 (1995) |
| Furazolidone | *31*, 141 (1983); *Suppl. 7*, 63 (1987) |
| Furfural | *63*, 409 (1995) |
| Furniture and cabinet-making | *25*, 99 (1981); *Suppl. 7*, 380 (1987) |
| Furosemide | *50*, 277 (1990) |
| 2-(2-Furyl)-3-(5-nitro-2-furyl)acrylamide (*see* AF-2) | |
| Fusarenon-X (*see* Toxins derived from *Fusarium graminearum, F. culmorum* and *F. crookwellense*) | |
| Fusarenone-X (*see* Toxins derived from *Fusarium graminearum, F. culmorum* and *F. crookwellense*) | |
| Fusarin C (*see* Toxins derived from *Fusarium moniliforme*) | |

## G

| | |
|---|---|
| Gamma (γ)-radiation | *75*, 121 (2000) |
| Gasoline | *45*, 159 (1989) (*corr. 47*, 505) |
| Gasoline engine exhaust (*see* Diesel and gasoline engine exhausts) | |
| Gemfibrozil | *66*, 427 (1996) |
| Glass fibres (*see* Man-made mineral fibres) | |
| Glass manufacturing industry, occupational exposures in | *58*, 347 (1993) |
| Glass wool (*see* Man-made vitreous fibres) | |
| Glass filaments (*see* Man-made mineral fibres) | |
| Glu-P-1 | *40*, 223 (1986); *Suppl. 7*, 64 (1987) |
| Glu-P-2 | *40*, 235 (1986); *Suppl. 7*, 64 (1987) |
| L-Glutamic acid, 5-[2-(4-hydroxymethyl)phenylhydrazide] (*see* Agaritine) | |
| Glycidaldehyde | *11*, 175 (1976); *Suppl. 7*, 64 (1987); *71*, 1459 (1999) |
| Glycidol | *77*, 469 (2000) |
| Glycidyl ethers | *47*, 237 (1989); *71*, 1285, 1417, 1525, 1539 (1999) |
| Glycidyl oleate | *11*, 183 (1976); *Suppl. 7*, 64 (1987) |
| Glycidyl stearate | *11*, 187 (1976); *Suppl. 7*, 64 (1987) |
| Griseofulvin | *10*, 153 (1976); *Suppl. 7*, 64, 391 (1987); *79*, 289 (2001) |
| Guinea Green B | *16*, 199 (1978); *Suppl. 7*, 64 (1987) |
| Gyromitrin | *31*, 163 (1983); *Suppl. 7*, 64, 391 (1987) |

## H

| | |
|---|---|
| Haematite | *1*, 29 (1972); *Suppl. 7*, 216 (1987) |
| Haematite and ferric oxide | *Suppl. 7*, 216 (1987) |
| Haematite mining, underground, with exposure to radon | *1*, 29 (1972); *Suppl. 7*, 216 (1987) |
| Hairdressers and barbers (occupational exposure as) | *57*, 43 (1993) |
| Hair dyes, epidemiology of | *16*, 29 (1978); *27*, 307 (1982); |
| Halogenated acetonitriles | *52*, 269 (1991); *71*, 1325, 1369, 1375, 1533 (1999) |
| Halothane (*see* Anaesthetics, volatile) | |
| HC Blue No. 1 | *57*, 129 (1993) |
| HC Blue No. 2 | *57*, 143 (1993) |
| α-HCH (*see* Hexachlorocyclohexanes) | |
| β-HCH (*see* Hexachlorocyclohexanes) | |
| γ-HCH (*see* Hexachlorocyclohexanes) | |
| HC Red No. 3 | *57*, 153 (1993) |
| HC Yellow No. 4 | *57*, 159 (1993) |
| Heating oils (*see* Fuel oils) | |
| *Helicobacter pylori* (infection with) | *61*, 177 (1994) |
| Hepatitis B virus | *59*, 45 (1994) |
| Hepatitis C virus | *59*, 165 (1994) |
| Hepatitis D virus | *59*, 223 (1994) |
| Heptachlor (*see also* Chlordane/Heptachlor) | *5*, 173 (1974); *20*, 129 (1979) |
| Hexachlorobenzene | *20*, 155 (1979); *Suppl. 7*, 219 (1987); *79*, 493 (2001) |
| Hexachlorobutadiene | *20*, 179 (1979); *Suppl. 7*, 64 (1987); *73*, 277 (1999) |
| Hexachlorocyclohexanes | *5*, 47 (1974); *20*, 195 (1979) (*corr. 42*, 258); *Suppl. 7*, 220 (1987) |
| Hexachlorocyclohexane, technical-grade (*see* Hexachlorocyclohexanes) | |
| Hexachloroethane | *20*, 467 (1979); *Suppl. 7*, 64 (1987); *73*, 295 (1999) |
| Hexachlorophene | *20*, 241 (1979); *Suppl. 7*, 64 (1987) |
| Hexamethylphosphoramide | *15*, 211 (1977); *Suppl. 7*, 64 (1987); *71*, 1465 (1999) |
| Hexoestrol (*see also* Nonsteroidal oestrogens) | *Suppl. 7*, 279 (1987) |
| Hormonal contraceptives, progestogens only | *72*, 339 (1999) |
| Human herpesvirus 8 | *70*, 375 (1997) |
| Human immunodeficiency viruses | *67*, 31 (1996) |
| Human papillomaviruses | *64* (1995) (*corr. 66*, 485) |
| Human T-cell lymphotropic viruses | *67*, 261 (1996) |
| Hycanthone mesylate | *13*, 91 (1977); *Suppl. 7*, 64 (1987) |
| Hydralazine | *24*, 85 (1980); *Suppl. 7*, 222 (1987) |
| Hydrazine | *4*, 127 (1974); *Suppl. 7*, 223 (1987); *71*, 991 (1999) |
| Hydrochloric acid | *54*, 189 (1992) |
| Hydrochlorothiazide | *50*, 293 (1990) |
| Hydrogen peroxide | *36*, 285 (1985); *Suppl. 7*, 64 (1987); *71*, 671 (1999) |
| Hydroquinone | *15*, 155 (1977); *Suppl. 7*, 64 (1987); *71*, 691 (1999) |
| 1-Hydroxyanthraquinone | *82*, 129 (2002) |
| 4-Hydroxyazobenzene | *8*, 157 (1975); *Suppl. 7*, 64 (1987) |

| | |
|---|---|
| 17α-Hydroxyprogesterone caproate (*see also* Progestins) | *21*, 399 (1979) (*corr. 42*, 259) |
| 8-Hydroxyquinoline | *13*, 101 (1977); *Suppl. 7*, 64 (1987) |
| 8-Hydroxysenkirkine | *10*, 265 (1976); *Suppl. 7*, 64 (1987) |
| Hydroxyurea | *76*, 347 (2000) |
| Hypochlorite salts | *52*, 159 (1991) |

# I

| | |
|---|---|
| Implants, surgical | *74*, 1999 |
| Indeno[1,2,3-*cd*]pyrene | *3*, 229 (1973); *32*, 373 (1983); *Suppl. 7*, 64 (1987) |
| Inorganic acids (*see* Sulfuric acid and other strong inorganic acids, occupational exposures to mists and vapours from) | |
| Insecticides, occupational exposures in spraying and application of | *53*, 45 (1991) |
| Insulation glass wool (*see* Man-made vitreous fibres) | |
| Involuntary smoking | *83*, 1189 (2004) |
| Ionizing radiation (*see* Neutrons, γ- and X-radiation) | |
| IQ | *40*, 261 (1986); *Suppl. 7*, 64 (1987); *56*, 165 (1993) |
| Iron and steel founding | *34*, 133 (1984); *Suppl. 7*, 224 (1987) |
| Iron-dextran complex | *2*, 161 (1973); *Suppl. 7*, 226 (1987) |
| Iron-dextrin complex | *2*, 161 (1973) (*corr. 42*, 252); *Suppl. 7*, 64 (1987) |
| Iron oxide (*see* Ferric oxide) | |
| Iron oxide, saccharated (*see* Saccharated iron oxide) | |
| Iron sorbitol-citric acid complex | *2*, 161 (1973); *Suppl. 7*, 64 (1987) |
| Isatidine | *10*, 269 (1976); *Suppl. 7*, 65 (1987) |
| Isoflurane (*see* Anaesthetics, volatile) | |
| Isoniazid (*see* Isonicotinic acid hydrazide) | |
| Isonicotinic acid hydrazide | *4*, 159 (1974); *Suppl. 7*, 227 (1987) |
| Isophosphamide | *26*, 237 (1981); *Suppl. 7*, 65 (1987) |
| Isoprene | *60*, 215 (1994); *71*, 1015 (1999) |
| Isopropanol | *15*, 223 (1977); *Suppl. 7*, 229 (1987); *71*, 1027 (1999) |
| Isopropanol manufacture (strong-acid process) (*see also* Isopropanol; Sulfuric acid and other strong inorganic acids, occupational exposures to mists and vapours from) | *Suppl. 7*, 229 (1987) |
| Isopropyl oils | *15*, 223 (1977); *Suppl. 7*, 229 (1987); *71*, 1483 (1999) |
| Isosafrole | *1*, 169 (1972); *10*, 232 (1976); *Suppl. 7*, 65 (1987) |

# J

| | |
|---|---|
| Jacobine | *10*, 275 (1976); *Suppl. 7*, 65 (1987) |
| Jet fuel | *45*, 203 (1989) |
| Joinery (*see* Carpentry and joinery) | |

## K

| | |
|---|---|
| Kaempferol | *31*, 171 (1983); *Suppl. 7*, 65 (1987) |
| Kaposi's sarcoma herpesvirus | *70*, 375 (1997) |
| Kepone (*see* Chlordecone) | |
| Kojic acid | *79*, 605 (2001) |

## L

| | |
|---|---|
| Lasiocarpine | *10*, 281 (1976); *Suppl. 7*, 65 (1987) |
| Lauroyl peroxide | *36*, 315 (1985); *Suppl. 7*, 65 (1987); *71*, 1485 (1999) |
| Lead acetate (*see* Lead and lead compounds) | |
| Lead and lead compounds (*see also* Foreign bodies) | *1*, 40 (1972) (*corr. 42*, 251); *2*, 52, 150 (1973); *12*, 131 (1976); *23*, 40, 208, 209, 325 (1980); *Suppl. 7*, 230 (1987) |
| Lead arsenate (*see* Arsenic and arsenic compounds) | |
| Lead carbonate (*see* Lead and lead compounds) | |
| Lead chloride (*see* Lead and lead compounds) | |
| Lead chromate (*see* Chromium and chromium compounds) | |
| Lead chromate oxide (*see* Chromium and chromium compounds) | |
| Lead naphthenate (*see* Lead and lead compounds) | |
| Lead nitrate (*see* Lead and lead compounds) | |
| Lead oxide (*see* Lead and lead compounds) | |
| Lead phosphate (*see* Lead and lead compounds) | |
| Lead subacetate (*see* Lead and lead compounds) | |
| Lead tetroxide (*see* Lead and lead compounds) | |
| Leather goods manufacture | *25*, 279 (1981); *Suppl. 7*, 235 (1987) |
| Leather industries | *25*, 199 (1981); *Suppl. 7*, 232 (1987) |
| Leather tanning and processing | *25*, 201 (1981); *Suppl. 7*, 236 (1987) |
| Ledate (*see also* Lead and lead compounds) | *12*, 131 (1976) |
| Levonorgestrel | *72*, 49 (1999) |
| Light Green SF | *16*, 209 (1978); *Suppl. 7*, 65 (1987) |
| *d*-Limonene | *56*, 135 (1993); *73*, 307 (1999) |
| Lindane (*see* Hexachlorocyclohexanes) | |
| Liver flukes (*see* Clonorchis sinensis, Opisthorchis felineus and Opisthorchis viverrini) | |
| Lucidin (*see* 1,3-Dihydro-2-hydroxymethylanthraquinone) | |
| Lumber and sawmill industries (including logging) | *25*, 49 (1981); *Suppl. 7*, 383 (1987) |
| Luteoskyrin | *10*, 163 (1976); *Suppl. 7*, 65 (1987) |
| Lynoestrenol | *21*, 407 (1979); *Suppl. 7*, 293 (1987); *72*, 49 (1999) |

## M

| | |
|---|---|
| Madder root (*see also* Rubia tinctorum) | *82*, 129 (2002) |

| | |
|---|---|
| Magenta | 4, 57 (1974) (corr. 42, 252); Suppl. 7, 238 (1987); 57, 215 (1993) |
| Magenta, manufacture of (see also Magenta) | Suppl. 7, 238 (1987); 57, 215 (1993) |
| Malathion | 30, 103 (1983); Suppl. 7, 65 (1987) |
| Maleic hydrazide | 4, 173 (1974) (corr. 42, 253); Suppl. 7, 65 (1987) |
| Malonaldehyde | 36, 163 (1985); Suppl. 7, 65 (1987); 71, 1037 (1999) |
| Malondialdehyde (see Malonaldehyde) | |
| Maneb | 12, 137 (1976); Suppl. 7, 65 (1987) |
| Man-made mineral fibres (see Man-made vitreous fibres) | |
| Man-made vitreous fibres | 43, 39 (1988); 81 (2002) |
| Mannomustine | 9, 157 (1975); Suppl. 7, 65 (1987) |
| Mate | 51, 273 (1991) |
| MCPA (see also Chlorophenoxy herbicides; Chlorophenoxy herbicides, occupational exposures to) | 30, 255 (1983) |
| MeA-α-C | 40, 253 (1986); Suppl. 7, 65 (1987) |
| Medphalan | 9, 168 (1975); Suppl. 7, 65 (1987) |
| Medroxyprogesterone acetate | 6, 157 (1974); 21, 417 (1979) (corr. 42, 259); Suppl. 7, 289 (1987); 72, 339 (1999) |
| Megestrol acetate | Suppl. 7, 293 (1987); 72, 49 (1999) |
| MeIQ | 40, 275 (1986); Suppl. 7, 65 (1987); 56, 197 (1993) |
| MeIQx | 40, 283 (1986); Suppl. 7, 65 (1987) 56, 211 (1993) |
| Melamine | 39, 333 (1986); Suppl. 7, 65 (1987); 73, 329 (1999) |
| Melphalan | 9, 167 (1975); Suppl. 7, 239 (1987) |
| 6-Mercaptopurine | 26, 249 (1981); Suppl. 7, 240 (1987) |
| Mercuric chloride (see Mercury and mercury compounds) | |
| Mercury and mercury compounds | 58, 239 (1993) |
| Merphalan | 9, 169 (1975); Suppl. 7, 65 (1987) |
| Mestranol | 6, 87 (1974); 21, 257 (1979) (corr. 42, 259); Suppl. 7, 288 (1987); 72, 49 (1999) |
| Metabisulfites (see Sulfur dioxide and some sulfites, bisulfites and metabisulfites) | |
| Metallic mercury (see Mercury and mercury compounds) | |
| Methanearsonic acid, disodium salt (see Arsenic and arsenic compounds) | |
| Methanearsonic acid, monosodium salt (see Arsenic and arsenic compounds) | |
| Methimazole | 79, 53 (2001) |
| Methotrexate | 26, 267 (1981); Suppl. 7, 241 (1987) |
| Methoxsalen (see 8-Methoxypsoralen) | |
| Methoxychlor | 5, 193 (1974); 20, 259 (1979); Suppl. 7, 66 (1987) |
| Methoxyflurane (see Anaesthetics, volatile) | |
| 5-Methoxypsoralen | 40, 327 (1986); Suppl. 7, 242 (1987) |

8-Methoxypsoralen (see also 8-Methoxypsoralen plus ultraviolet radiation) — *24*, 101 (1980)

8-Methoxypsoralen plus ultraviolet radiation — *Suppl. 7*, 243 (1987)

Methyl acrylate — *19*, 52 (1979); *39*, 99 (1986); *Suppl. 7*, 66 (1987); *71*, 1489 (1999)

5-Methylangelicin plus ultraviolet radiation (see also Angelicin and some synthetic derivatives) — *Suppl. 7*, 57 (1987)

2-Methylaziridine — *9*, 61 (1975); *Suppl. 7*, 66 (1987); *71*, 1497 (1999)

Methylazoxymethanol acetate (see also Cycasin) — *1*, 164 (1972); *10*, 131 (1976); *Suppl. 7*, 66 (1987)

Methyl bromide — *41*, 187 (1986) (corr. *45*, 283); *Suppl. 7*, 245 (1987); *71*, 721 (1999)

Methyl *tert*-butyl ether — *73*, 339 (1999)

Methyl carbamate — *12*, 151 (1976); *Suppl. 7*, 66 (1987)

Methyl-CCNU (see 1-(2-Chloroethyl)-3-(4-methylcyclohexyl)-1-nitrosourea)

Methyl chloride — *41*, 161 (1986); *Suppl. 7*, 246 (1987); *71*, 737 (1999)

1-, 2-, 3-, 4-, 5- and 6-Methylchrysenes — *32*, 379 (1983); *Suppl. 7*, 66 (1987)

*N*-Methyl-*N*,4-dinitrosoaniline — *1*, 141 (1972); *Suppl. 7*, 66 (1987)

4,4′-Methylene bis(2-chloroaniline) — *4*, 65 (1974) (corr. *42*, 252); *Suppl. 7*, 246 (1987); *57*, 271 (1993)

4,4′-Methylene bis(*N,N*-dimethyl)benzenamine — *27*, 119 (1982); *Suppl. 7*, 66 (1987)

4,4′-Methylene bis(2-methylaniline) — *4*, 73 (1974); *Suppl. 7*, 248 (1987)

4,4′-Methylenedianiline — *4*, 79 (1974) (corr. *42*, 252); *39*, 347 (1986); *Suppl. 7*, 66 (1987)

4,4′-Methylenediphenyl diisocyanate — *19*, 314 (1979); *Suppl. 7*, 66 (1987); *71*, 1049 (1999)

2-Methylfluoranthene — *32*, 399 (1983); *Suppl. 7*, 66 (1987)

3-Methylfluoranthene — *32*, 399 (1983); *Suppl. 7*, 66 (1987)

Methylglyoxal — *51*, 443 (1991)

Methyl iodide — *15*, 245 (1977); *41*, 213 (1986); *Suppl. 7*, 66 (1987); *71*, 1503 (1999)

Methylmercury chloride (see Mercury and mercury compounds)

Methylmercury compounds (see Mercury and mercury compounds)

Methyl methacrylate — *19*, 187 (1979); *Suppl. 7*, 66 (1987); *60*, 445 (1994)

Methyl methanesulfonate — *7*, 253 (1974); *Suppl. 7*, 66 (1987); *71*, 1059 (1999)

2-Methyl-1-nitroanthraquinone — *27*, 205 (1982); *Suppl. 7*, 66 (1987)

*N*-Methyl-*N*′-nitro-*N*-nitrosoguanidine — *4*, 183 (1974); *Suppl. 7*, 248 (1987)

3-Methylnitrosaminopropionaldehyde [see 3-(*N*-Nitrosomethylamino)-propionaldehyde]

3-Methylnitrosaminopropionitrile [see 3-(*N*-Nitrosomethylamino)-propionitrile]

4-(Methylnitrosamino)-4-(3-pyridyl)-1-butanal [see 4-(*N*-Nitrosomethylamino)-4-(3-pyridyl)-1-butanal]

4-(Methylnitrosamino)-1-(3-pyridyl)-1-butanone [see 4-(-Nitrosomethylamino)-1-(3-pyridyl)-1-butanone]

# CUMULATIVE INDEX

| | |
|---|---|
| N-Methyl-N-nitrosourea | 1, 125 (1972); 17, 227 (1978); Suppl. 7, 66 (1987) |
| N-Methyl-N-nitrosourethane | 4, 211 (1974); Suppl. 7, 66 (1987) |
| N-Methylolacrylamide | 60, 435 (1994) |
| Methyl parathion | 30, 131 (1983); Suppl. 7, 66, 392 (1987) |
| 1-Methylphenanthrene | 32, 405 (1983); Suppl. 7, 66 (1987) |
| 7-Methylpyrido[3,4-c]psoralen | 40, 349 (1986); Suppl. 7, 71 (1987) |
| Methyl red | 8, 161 (1975); Suppl. 7, 66 (1987) |
| Methyl selenac (see also Selenium and selenium compounds) | 12, 161 (1976); Suppl. 7, 66 (1987) |
| Methylthiouracil | 7, 53 (1974); Suppl. 7, 66 (1987); 79, 75 (2001) |
| Metronidazole | 13, 113 (1977); Suppl. 7, 250 (1987) |
| Mineral oils | 3, 30 (1973); 33, 87 (1984) (corr. 42, 262); Suppl. 7, 252 (1987) |
| Mirex | 5, 203 (1974); 20, 283 (1979) (corr. 42, 258); Suppl. 7, 66 (1987) |
| Mists and vapours from sulfuric acid and other strong inorganic acids | 54, 41 (1992) |
| Mitomycin C | 10, 171 (1976); Suppl. 7, 67 (1987) |
| Mitoxantrone | 76, 289 (2000) |
| MNNG (see N-Methyl-N'-nitro-N-nitrosoguanidine) | |
| MOCA (see 4,4'-Methylene bis(2-chloroaniline)) | |
| Modacrylic fibres | 19, 86 (1979); Suppl. 7, 67 (1987) |
| Monochloramine (see Chloramine) | |
| Monocrotaline | 10, 291 (1976); Suppl. 7, 67 (1987) |
| Monuron | 12, 167 (1976); Suppl. 7, 67 (1987); 53, 467 (1991) |
| MOPP and other combined chemotherapy including alkylating agents | Suppl. 7, 254 (1987) |
| Mordanite (see Zeolites) | |
| Morinda officinalis (see also Traditional herbal medicines) | 82, 129 (2002) |
| Morpholine | 47, 199 (1989); 71, 1511 (1999) |
| 5-(Morpholinomethyl)-3-[(5-nitrofurfurylidene)amino]-2-oxazolidinone | 7, 161 (1974); Suppl. 7, 67 (1987) |
| Musk ambrette | 65, 477 (1996) |
| Musk xylene | 65, 477 (1996) |
| Mustard gas | 9, 181 (1975) (corr. 42, 254); Suppl. 7, 259 (1987) |
| Myleran (see 1,4-Butanediol dimethanesulfonate) | |

# N

| | |
|---|---|
| Nafenopin | 24, 125 (1980); Suppl. 7, 67 (1987) |
| Naphthalene | 82, 367 (2002) |
| 1,5-Naphthalenediamine | 27, 127 (1982); Suppl. 7, 67 (1987) |
| 1,5-Naphthalene diisocyanate | 19, 311 (1979); Suppl. 7, 67 (1987); 71, 1515 (1999) |
| 1-Naphthylamine | 4, 87 (1974) (corr. 42, 253); Suppl. 7, 260 (1987) |
| 2-Naphthylamine | 4, 97 (1974); Suppl. 7, 261 (1987) |

| | |
|---|---|
| 1-Naphthylthiourea | *30*, 347 (1983); *Suppl. 7*, 263 (1987) |
| Neutrons | *75*, 361 (2000) |
| Nickel acetate (*see* Nickel and nickel compounds) | |
| Nickel ammonium sulfate (*see* Nickel and nickel compounds) | |
| Nickel and nickel compounds (*see also* Implants, surgical) | *2*, 126 (1973) (*corr. 42*, 252); *11*, 75 (1976); *Suppl. 7*, 264 (1987) (*corr. 45*, 283); *49*, 257 (1990) (*corr. 67*, 395) |
| Nickel carbonate (*see* Nickel and nickel compounds) | |
| Nickel carbonyl (*see* Nickel and nickel compounds) | |
| Nickel chloride (*see* Nickel and nickel compounds) | |
| Nickel-gallium alloy (*see* Nickel and nickel compounds) | |
| Nickel hydroxide (*see* Nickel and nickel compounds) | |
| Nickelocene (*see* Nickel and nickel compounds) | |
| Nickel oxide (*see* Nickel and nickel compounds) | |
| Nickel subsulfide (*see* Nickel and nickel compounds) | |
| Nickel sulfate (*see* Nickel and nickel compounds) | |
| Niridazole | *13*, 123 (1977); *Suppl. 7*, 67 (1987) |
| Nithiazide | *31*, 179 (1983); *Suppl. 7*, 67 (1987) |
| Nitrilotriacetic acid and its salts | *48*, 181 (1990); *73*, 385 (1999) |
| 5-Nitroacenaphthene | *16*, 319 (1978); *Suppl. 7*, 67 (1987) |
| 5-Nitro-*ortho*-anisidine | *27*, 133 (1982); *Suppl. 7*, 67 (1987) |
| 2-Nitroanisole | *65*, 369 (1996) |
| 9-Nitroanthracene | *33*, 179 (1984); *Suppl. 7*, 67 (1987) |
| 7-Nitrobenz[*a*]anthracene | *46*, 247 (1989) |
| Nitrobenzene | *65*, 381 (1996) |
| 6-Nitrobenzo[*a*]pyrene | *33*, 187 (1984); *Suppl. 7*, 67 (1987); *46*, 255 (1989) |
| 4-Nitrobiphenyl | *4*, 113 (1974); *Suppl. 7*, 67 (1987) |
| 6-Nitrochrysene | *33*, 195 (1984); *Suppl. 7*, 67 (1987); *46*, 267 (1989) |
| Nitrofen (technical-grade) | *30*, 271 (1983); *Suppl. 7*, 67 (1987) |
| 3-Nitrofluoranthene | *33*, 201 (1984); *Suppl. 7*, 67 (1987) |
| 2-Nitrofluorene | *46*, 277 (1989) |
| Nitrofural | *7*, 171 (1974); *Suppl. 7*, 67 (1987); *50*, 195 (1990) |
| 5-Nitro-2-furaldehyde semicarbazone (*see* Nitrofural) | |
| Nitrofurantoin | *50*, 211 (1990) |
| Nitrofurazone (*see* Nitrofural) | |
| 1-[(5-Nitrofurfurylidene)amino]-2-imidazolidinone | *7*, 181 (1974); *Suppl. 7*, 67 (1987) |
| *N*-[4-(5-Nitro-2-furyl)-2-thiazolyl]acetamide | *1*, 181 (1972); *7*, 185 (1974); *Suppl. 7*, 67 (1987) |
| Nitrogen mustard | *9*, 193 (1975); *Suppl. 7*, 269 (1987) |
| Nitrogen mustard *N*-oxide | *9*, 209 (1975); *Suppl. 7*, 67 (1987) |
| Nitromethane | *77*, 487 (2000) |
| 1-Nitronaphthalene | *46*, 291 (1989) |
| 2-Nitronaphthalene | *46*, 303 (1989) |
| 3-Nitroperylene | *46*, 313 (1989) |
| 2-Nitro-*para*-phenylenediamine (*see* 1,4-Diamino-2-nitrobenzene) | |
| 2-Nitropropane | *29*, 331 (1982); *Suppl. 7*, 67 (1987); *71*, 1079 (1999) |
| 1-Nitropyrene | *33*, 209 (1984); *Suppl. 7*, 67 (1987); *46*, 321 (1989) |

| | |
|---|---|
| 2-Nitropyrene | *46*, 359 (1989) |
| 4-Nitropyrene | *46*, 367 (1989) |
| N-Nitrosatable drugs | 24, 297 (1980) (*corr.* 42, 260) |
| N-Nitrosatable pesticides | 30, 359 (1983) |
| N'-Nitrosoanabasine | 37, 225 (1985); *Suppl. 7*, 67 (1987) |
| N'-Nitrosoanatabine | 37, 233 (1985); *Suppl. 7*, 67 (1987) |
| N-Nitrosodi-n-butylamine | 4, 197 (1974); *17*, 51 (1978); *Suppl. 7*, 67 (1987) |
| N-Nitrosodiethanolamine | 17, 77 (1978); *Suppl. 7*, 67 (1987); 77, 403 (2000) |
| N-Nitrosodiethylamine | 1, 107 (1972) (*corr.* 42, 251); 17, 83 (1978) (*corr.* 42, 257); *Suppl. 7*, 67 (1987) |
| N-Nitrosodimethylamine | 1, 95 (1972); *17*, 125 (1978) (*corr.* 42, 257); *Suppl. 7*, 67 (1987) |
| N-Nitrosodiphenylamine | 27, 213 (1982); *Suppl. 7*, 67 (1987) |
| para-Nitrosodiphenylamine | 27, 227 (1982) (*corr.* 42, 261); *Suppl. 7*, 68 (1987) |
| N-Nitrosodi-n-propylamine | 17, 177 (1978); *Suppl. 7*, 68 (1987) |
| N-Nitroso-N-ethylurea (*see* N-Ethyl-N-nitrosourea) | |
| N-Nitrosofolic acid | 17, 217 (1978); *Suppl. 7*, 68 (1987) |
| N-Nitrosoguvacine | 37, 263 (1985); *Suppl. 7*, 68 (1987); *85*, 281 (2004) |
| N-Nitrosoguvacoline | 37, 263 (1985); *Suppl. 7*, 68 (1987); *85*, 281 (2004) |
| N-Nitrosohydroxyproline | 17, 304 (1978); *Suppl. 7*, 68 (1987) |
| 3-(N-Nitrosomethylamino)propionaldehyde | 37, 263 (1985); *Suppl. 7*, 68 (1987); *85*, 281 (2004) |
| 3-(N-Nitrosomethylamino)propionitrile | 37, 263 (1985); *Suppl. 7*, 68 (1987); *85*, 281 (2004) |
| 4-(N-Nitrosomethylamino)-4-(3-pyridyl)-1-butanal | 37, 205 (1985); *Suppl. 7*, 68 (1987) |
| 4-(N-Nitrosomethylamino)-1-(3-pyridyl)-1-butanone | 37, 209 (1985); *Suppl. 7*, 68 (1987) |
| N-Nitrosomethylethylamine | 17, 221 (1978); *Suppl. 7*, 68 (1987) |
| N-Nitroso-N-methylurea (*see* N-Methyl-N-nitrosourea) | |
| N-Nitroso-N-methylurethane (*see* N-Methyl-N-nitrosourethane) | 17, 257 (1978); *Suppl. 7*, 68 (1987) |
| N-Nitrosomethylvinylamine | 17, 263 (1978); *Suppl. 7*, 68 (1987) |
| N-Nitrosomorpholine | 17, 281 (1978); *37*, 241 (1985); *Suppl. 7*, 68 (1987) |
| N'-Nitrosonornicotine | |
| N-Nitrosopiperidine | 17, 287 (1978); *Suppl. 7*, 68 (1987) |
| N-Nitrosoproline | 17, 303 (1978); *Suppl. 7*, 68 (1987) |
| N-Nitrosopyrrolidine | 17, 313 (1978); *Suppl. 7*, 68 (1987) |
| N-Nitrososarcosine | 17, 327 (1978); *Suppl. 7*, 68 (1987) |
| Nitrosoureas, chloroethyl (*see* Chloroethyl nitrosoureas) | |
| 5-Nitro-ortho-toluidine | *48*, 169 (1990) |
| 2-Nitrotoluene | *65*, 409 (1996) |
| 3-Nitrotoluene | *65*, 409 (1996) |
| 4-Nitrotoluene | *65*, 409 (1996) |
| Nitrous oxide (*see* Anaesthetics, volatile) | |
| Nitrovin | 31, 185 (1983); *Suppl. 7*, 68 (1987) |
| Nivalenol (*see* Toxins derived from *Fusarium graminearum*, *F. culmorum* and *F. crookwellense*) | |
| NNA (*see* 4-(N-Nitrosomethylamino)-4-(3-pyridyl)-1-butanal) | |
| NNK (*see* 4-(N-Nitrosomethylamino)-1-(3-pyridyl)-1-butanone) | |

| | |
|---|---|
| Nonsteroidal oestrogens | *Suppl. 7*, 273 (1987) |
| Norethisterone | *6*, 179 (1974); *21*, 461 (1979); *Suppl. 7*, 294 (1987); *72*, 49 (1999) |
| Norethisterone acetate | *72*, 49 (1999) |
| Norethynodrel | *6*, 191 (1974); *21*, 461 (1979) (*corr. 42*, 259); *Suppl. 7*, 295 (1987); *72*, 49 (1999) |
| Norgestrel | *6*, 201 (1974); *21*, 479 (1979); *Suppl. 7*, 295 (1987); *72*, 49 (1999) |
| Nylon 6 | *19*, 120 (1979); *Suppl. 7*, 68 (1987) |

## O

| | |
|---|---|
| Ochratoxin A | *10*, 191 (1976); *31*, 191 (1983) (*corr. 42*, 262); *Suppl. 7*, 271 (1987); *56*, 489 (1993) |
| Oestradiol | *6*, 99 (1974); *21*, 279 (1979); *Suppl. 7*, 284 (1987); *72*, 399 (1999) |
| Oestradiol-17β (*see* Oestradiol) | |
| Oestradiol 3-benzoate (*see* Oestradiol) | |
| Oestradiol dipropionate (*see* Oestradiol) | |
| Oestradiol mustard | *9*, 217 (1975); *Suppl. 7*, 68 (1987) |
| Oestradiol valerate (*see* Oestradiol) | |
| Oestriol | *6*, 117 (1974); *21*, 327 (1979); *Suppl. 7*, 285 (1987); *72*, 399 (1999) |
| Oestrogen-progestin combinations (*see* Oestrogens, progestins (progestogens) and combinations) | |
| Oestrogen-progestin replacement therapy (*see* Post-menopausal oestrogen-progestogen therapy) | |
| Oestrogen replacement therapy (*see* Post-menopausal oestrogen therapy) | |
| Oestrogens (*see* Oestrogens, progestins and combinations) | |
| Oestrogens, conjugated (*see* Conjugated oestrogens) | |
| Oestrogens, nonsteroidal (*see* Nonsteroidal oestrogens) | |
| Oestrogens, progestins (progestogens) and combinations | *6* (1974); *21* (1979); *Suppl. 7*, 272 (1987); *72*, 49, 339, 399, 531 (1999) |
| Oestrogens, steroidal (*see* Steroidal oestrogens) | |
| Oestrone | *6*, 123 (1974); *21*, 343 (1979) (*corr. 42*, 259); *Suppl. 7*, 286 (1987); *72*, 399 (1999) |
| Oestrone benzoate (*see* Oestrone) | |
| Oil Orange SS | *8*, 165 (1975); *Suppl. 7*, 69 (1987) |
| *Opisthorchis felineus* (infection with) | *61*, 121 (1994) |
| *Opisthorchis viverrini* (infection with) | *61*, 121 (1994) |
| Oral contraceptives, combined | *Suppl. 7*, 297 (1987); *72*, 49 (1999) |
| Oral contraceptives, sequential (*see* Sequential oral contraceptives) | |
| Orange I | *8*, 173 (1975); *Suppl. 7*, 69 (1987) |
| Orange G | *8*, 181 (1975); *Suppl. 7*, 69 (1987) |
| Organolead compounds (*see also* Lead and lead compounds) | *Suppl. 7*, 230 (1987) |

| | |
|---|---|
| Oxazepam | *13*, 58 (1977); *Suppl. 7*, 69 (1987); *66*, 115 (1996) |
| Oxymetholone (*see also* Androgenic (anabolic) steroids) | *13*, 131 (1977) |
| Oxyphenbutazone | *13*, 185 (1977); *Suppl. 7*, 69 (1987) |

## P

| | |
|---|---|
| Paint manufacture and painting (occupational exposures in) | *47*, 329 (1989) |
| Palygorskite | *42*, 159 (1987); *Suppl. 7*, 117 (1987); *68*, 245 (1997) |
| Panfuran S (*see also* Dihydroxymethylfuratrizine) | *24*, 77 (1980); *Suppl. 7*, 69 (1987) |
| Paper manufacture (*see* Pulp and paper manufacture) | |
| Paracetamol | *50*, 307 (1990); *73*, 401 (1999) |
| Parasorbic acid | *10*, 199 (1976) (*corr. 42*, 255); *Suppl. 7*, 69 (1987) |
| Parathion | *30*, 153 (1983); *Suppl. 7*, 69 (1987) |
| Patulin | *10*, 205 (1976); *40*, 83 (1986); *Suppl. 7*, 69 (1987) |
| Penicillic acid | *10*, 211 (1976); *Suppl. 7*, 69 (1987) |
| Pentachloroethane | *41*, 99 (1986); *Suppl. 7*, 69 (1987); *71*, 1519 (1999) |
| Pentachloronitrobenzene (see Quintozene) | |
| Pentachlorophenol (*see also* Chlorophenols; Chlorophenols, occupational exposures to; Polychlorophenols and their sodium salts) | *20*, 303 (1979); *53*, 371 (1991) |
| Permethrin | *53*, 329 (1991) |
| Perylene | *32*, 411 (1983); *Suppl. 7*, 69 (1987) |
| Petasitenine | *31*, 207 (1983); *Suppl. 7*, 69 (1987) |
| Petasites japonicus (*see also* Pyrrolizidine alkaloids) | *10*, 333 (1976) |
| Petroleum refining (occupational exposures in) | *45*, 39 (1989) |
| Petroleum solvents | *47*, 43 (1989) |
| Phenacetin | *13*, 141 (1977); *24*, 135 (1980); *Suppl. 7*, 310 (1987) |
| Phenanthrene | *32*, 419 (1983); *Suppl. 7*, 69 (1987) |
| Phenazopyridine hydrochloride | *8*, 117 (1975); *24*, 163 (1980) (*corr. 42*, 260); *Suppl. 7*, 312 (1987) |
| Phenelzine sulfate | *24*, 175 (1980); *Suppl. 7*, 312 (1987) |
| Phenicarbazide | *12*, 177 (1976); *Suppl. 7*, 70 (1987) |
| Phenobarbital and its sodium salt | *13*, 157 (1977); *Suppl. 7*, 313 (1987); *79*, 161 (2001) |
| Phenol | *47*, 263 (1989) (*corr. 50*, 385); *71*, 749 (1999) |
| Phenolphthalein | *76*, 387 (2000) |
| Phenoxyacetic acid herbicides (*see* Chlorophenoxy herbicides) | |
| Phenoxybenzamine hydrochloride | *9*, 223 (1975); *24*, 185 (1980); *Suppl. 7*, 70 (1987) |
| Phenylbutazone | *13*, 183 (1977); *Suppl. 7*, 316 (1987) |
| *meta*-Phenylenediamine | *16*, 111 (1978); *Suppl. 7*, 70 (1987) |
| *para*-Phenylenediamine | *16*, 125 (1978); *Suppl. 7*, 70 (1987) |
| Phenyl glycidyl ether (*see also* Glycidyl ethers) | *71*, 1525 (1999) |

N-Phenyl-2-naphthylamine　　　　　　　　　　　　　　　16, 325 (1978) (corr. 42, 257);
　　　　　　　　　　　　　　　　　　　　　　　　　　　Suppl. 7, 318 (1987)
ortho-Phenylphenol　　　　　　　　　　　　　　　　　　30, 329 (1983); Suppl. 7, 70
　　　　　　　　　　　　　　　　　　　　　　　　　　　(1987); 73, 451 (1999)
Phenytoin　　　　　　　　　　　　　　　　　　　　　　13, 201 (1977); Suppl. 7, 319
　　　　　　　　　　　　　　　　　　　　　　　　　　　(1987); 66, 175 (1996)
Phillipsite (see Zeolites)
PhIP　　　　　　　　　　　　　　　　　　　　　　　　56, 229 (1993)
Pickled vegetables　　　　　　　　　　　　　　　　　　56, 83 (1993)
Picloram　　　　　　　　　　　　　　　　　　　　　　53, 481 (1991)
Piperazine oestrone sulfate (see Conjugated oestrogens)
Piperonyl butoxide　　　　　　　　　　　　　　　　　　30, 183 (1983); Suppl. 7, 70 (1987)
Pitches, coal-tar (see Coal-tar pitches)
Polyacrylic acid　　　　　　　　　　　　　　　　　　　19, 62 (1979); Suppl. 7, 70 (1987)
Polybrominated biphenyls　　　　　　　　　　　　　　　18, 107 (1978); 41, 261 (1986);
　　　　　　　　　　　　　　　　　　　　　　　　　　　Suppl. 7, 321 (1987)
Polychlorinated biphenyls　　　　　　　　　　　　　　　7, 261 (1974); 18, 43 (1978)
　　　　　　　　　　　　　　　　　　　　　　　　　　　(corr. 42, 258); Suppl. 7, 322
　　　　　　　　　　　　　　　　　　　　　　　　　　　(1987)
Polychlorinated camphenes (see Toxaphene)
Polychlorinated dibenzo-para-dioxins (other than　　　　69, 33 (1997)
　　2,3,7,8-tetrachlorodibenzodioxin)
Polychlorinated dibenzofurans　　　　　　　　　　　　　69, 345 (1997)
Polychlorophenols and their sodium salts　　　　　　　　71, 769 (1999)
Polychloroprene　　　　　　　　　　　　　　　　　　　19, 141 (1979); Suppl. 7, 70 (1987)
Polyethylene (see also Implants, surgical)　　　　　　　　19, 164 (1979); Suppl. 7, 70 (1987)
Poly(glycolic acid) (see Implants, surgical)
Polymethylene polyphenyl isocyanate (see also 4,4'-Methylenediphenyl　19, 314 (1979); Suppl. 7, 70 (1987)
　　diisocyanate)
Polymethyl methacrylate (see also Implants, surgical)　　19, 195 (1979); Suppl. 7, 70 (1987)
Polyoestradiol phosphate (see Oestradiol-17β)
Polypropylene (see also Implants, surgical)　　　　　　　19, 218 (1979); Suppl. 7, 70 (1987)
Polystyrene (see also Implants, surgical)　　　　　　　　19, 245 (1979); Suppl. 7, 70 (1987)
Polytetrafluoroethylene (see also Implants, surgical)　　19, 288 (1979); Suppl. 7, 70 (1987)
Polyurethane foams (see also Implants, surgical)　　　　19, 320 (1979); Suppl. 7, 70 (1987)
Polyvinyl acetate (see also Implants, surgical)　　　　　19, 346 (1979); Suppl. 7, 70 (1987)
Polyvinyl alcohol (see also Implants, surgical)　　　　　19, 351 (1979); Suppl. 7, 70 (1987)
Polyvinyl chloride (see also Implants, surgical)　　　　　7, 306 (1974); 19, 402 (1979);
　　　　　　　　　　　　　　　　　　　　　　　　　　　Suppl. 7, 70 (1987)
Polyvinyl pyrrolidone　　　　　　　　　　　　　　　　　19, 463 (1979); Suppl. 7, 70
　　　　　　　　　　　　　　　　　　　　　　　　　　　(1987); 71, 1181 (1999)
Ponceau MX　　　　　　　　　　　　　　　　　　　　　8, 189 (1975); Suppl. 7, 70 (1987)
Ponceau 3R　　　　　　　　　　　　　　　　　　　　　8, 199 (1975); Suppl. 7, 70 (1987)
Ponceau SX　　　　　　　　　　　　　　　　　　　　　8, 207 (1975); Suppl. 7, 70 (1987)
Post-menopausal oestrogen therapy　　　　　　　　　　　Suppl. 7, 280 (1987); 72, 399
　　　　　　　　　　　　　　　　　　　　　　　　　　　(1999)
Post-menopausal oestrogen-progestogen therapy　　　　　Suppl. 7, 308 (1987); 72, 531
　　　　　　　　　　　　　　　　　　　　　　　　　　　(1999)
Potassium arsenate (see Arsenic and arsenic compounds)
Potassium arsenite (see Arsenic and arsenic compounds)
Potassium bis(2-hydroxyethyl)dithiocarbamate　　　　　　12, 183 (1976); Suppl. 7, 70 (1987)
Potassium bromate　　　　　　　　　　　　　　　　　　40, 207 (1986); Suppl. 7, 70 (1987);
　　　　　　　　　　　　　　　　　　　　　　　　　　　73, 481 (1999)
Potassium chromate (see Chromium and chromium compounds)

Potassium dichromate (*see* Chromium and chromium compounds)
Prazepam — 66, 143 (1996)
Prednimustine — 50, 115 (1990)
Prednisone — 26, 293 (1981); *Suppl. 7*, 326 (1987)

Printing processes and printing inks — 65, 33 (1996)
Procarbazine hydrochloride — 26, 311 (1981); *Suppl. 7*, 327 (1987)

Proflavine salts — 24, 195 (1980); *Suppl. 7*, 70 (1987)
Progesterone (*see also* Progestins; Combined oral contraceptives) — 6, 135 (1974); 21, 491 (1979) (*corr.* 42, 259)

Progestins (*see* Progestogens)
Progestogens — *Suppl. 7*, 289 (1987); 72, 49, 339, 531 (1999)

Pronetalol hydrochloride — 13, 227 (1977) (*corr.* 42, 256); *Suppl. 7*, 70 (1987)
1,3-Propane sultone — 4, 253 (1974) (*corr.* 42, 253); *Suppl. 7*, 70 (1987); 71, 1095 (1999)

Propham — 12, 189 (1976); *Suppl. 7*, 70 (1987)
β-Propiolactone — 4, 259 (1974) (*corr.* 42, 253); *Suppl. 7*, 70 (1987); 71, 1103 (1999)

$n$-Propyl carbamate — 12, 201 (1976); *Suppl. 7*, 70 (1987)
Propylene — 19, 213 (1979); *Suppl. 7*, 71 (1987); 60, 161 (1994)

Propyleneimine (*see* 2-Methylaziridine)
Propylene oxide — 11, 191 (1976); 36, 227 (1985) (*corr.* 42, 263); *Suppl. 7*, 328 (1987); 60, 181 (1994)

Propylthiouracil — 7, 67 (1974); *Suppl. 7*, 329 (1987); 79, 91 (2001)

Ptaquiloside (*see also* Bracken fern) — 40, 55 (1986); *Suppl. 7*, 71 (1987)
Pulp and paper manufacture — 25, 157 (1981); *Suppl. 7*, 385 (1987)

Pyrene — 32, 431 (1983); *Suppl. 7*, 71 (1987)
Pyridine — 77, 503 (2000)
Pyrido[3,4-*c*]psoralen — 40, 349 (1986); *Suppl. 7*, 71 (1987)
Pyrimethamine — 13, 233 (1977); *Suppl. 7*, 71 (1987)
Pyrrolizidine alkaloids (*see* Hydroxysenkirkine; Isatidine; Jacobine; Lasiocarpine; Monocrotaline; Retrorsine; Riddelliine; Seneciphylline; Senkirkine)

# Q

Quartz (*see* Crystalline silica)
Quercetin (*see also* Bracken fern) — 31, 213 (1983); *Suppl. 7*, 71 (1987); 73, 497 (1999)

*para*-Quinone — 15, 255 (1977); *Suppl. 7*, 71 (1987); 71, 1245 (1999)

Quintozene — 5, 211 (1974); *Suppl. 7*, 71 (1987)

**R**

| | |
|---|---|
| Radiation (see gamma-radiation, neutrons, ultraviolet radiation, X-radiation) | |
| Radionuclides, internally deposited | 78 (2001) |
| Radon | 43, 173 (1988) (corr. 45, 283) |
| Refractory ceramic fibres (see Man-made vitreous fibres) | |
| Reserpine | 10, 217 (1976); 24, 211 (1980) (corr. 42, 260); Suppl. 7, 330 (1987) |
| Resorcinol | 15, 155 (1977); Suppl. 7, 71 (1987); 71, 1119 (1990) |
| Retrorsine | 10, 303 (1976); Suppl. 7, 71 (1987) |
| Rhodamine B | 16, 221 (1978); Suppl. 7, 71 (1987) |
| Rhodamine 6G | 16, 233 (1978); Suppl. 7, 71 (1987) |
| Riddelliine | 10, 313 (1976); Suppl. 7, 71 (1987); 82, 153 (2002) |
| Rifampicin | 24, 243 (1980); Suppl. 7, 71 (1987) |
| Ripazepam | 66, 157 (1996) |
| Rock (stone) wool (see Man-made vitreous fibres) | |
| Rubber industry | 28 (1982) (corr. 42, 261); Suppl. 7, 332 (1987) |
| *Rubia tinctorum* (see also Madder root, Traditional herbal medicines) | 82, 129 (2002) |
| Rugulosin | 40, 99 (1986); Suppl. 7, 71 (1987) |

**S**

| | |
|---|---|
| Saccharated iron oxide | 2, 161 (1973); Suppl. 7, 71 (1987) |
| Saccharin and its salts | 22, 111 (1980) (corr. 42, 259); Suppl. 7, 334 (1987); 73, 517 (1999) |
| Safrole | 1, 169 (1972); 10, 231 (1976); Suppl. 7, 71 (1987) |
| Salted fish | 56, 41 (1993) |
| Sawmill industry (including logging) (see Lumber and sawmill industry (including logging)) | |
| Scarlet Red | 8, 217 (1975); Suppl. 7, 71 (1987) |
| *Schistosoma haematobium* (infection with) | 61, 45 (1994) |
| *Schistosoma japonicum* (infection with) | 61, 45 (1994) |
| *Schistosoma mansoni* (infection with) | 61, 45 (1994) |
| Selenium and selenium compounds | 9, 245 (1975) (corr. 42, 255); Suppl. 7, 71 (1987) |
| Selenium dioxide (see Selenium and selenium compounds) | |
| Selenium oxide (see Selenium and selenium compounds) | |
| Semicarbazide hydrochloride | 12, 209 (1976) (corr. 42, 256); Suppl. 7, 71 (1987) |
| *Senecio jacobaea L.* (see also Pyrrolizidine alkaloids) | 10, 333 (1976) |
| *Senecio longilobus* (see also Pyrrolizidine alkaloids, Traditional herbal medicines) | 10, 334 (1976); 82, 153 (2002) |
| *Senecio riddellii* (see also Traditional herbal medicines) | 82, 153 (1982) |
| Seneciphylline | 10, 319, 335 (1976); Suppl. 7, 71 (1987) |
| Senkirkine | 10, 327 (1976); 31, 231 (1983); Suppl. 7, 71 (1987) |

| | |
|---|---|
| Sepiolite | *42*, 175 (1987); *Suppl. 7*, 71 (1987); *68*, 267 (1997) |
| Sequential oral contraceptives (*see also* Oestrogens, progestins and combinations) | *Suppl. 7*, 296 (1987) |
| Shale-oils | *35*, 161 (1985); *Suppl. 7*, 339 (1987) |
| Shikimic acid (*see also* Bracken fern) | *40*, 55 (1986); *Suppl. 7*, 71 (1987) |
| Shoe manufacture and repair (*see* Boot and shoe manufacture and repair) | |
| Silica (*see also* Amorphous silica; Crystalline silica) | *42*, 39 (1987) |
| Silicone (*see* Implants, surgical) | |
| Simazine | *53*, 495 (1991); *73*, 625 (1999) |
| Slag wool (*see* Man-made vitreous fibres) | |
| Sodium arsenate (*see* Arsenic and arsenic compounds) | |
| Sodium arsenite (*see* Arsenic and arsenic compounds) | |
| Sodium cacodylate (*see* Arsenic and arsenic compounds) | |
| Sodium chlorite | *52*, 145 (1991) |
| Sodium chromate (*see* Chromium and chromium compounds) | |
| Sodium cyclamate (*see* Cyclamates) | |
| Sodium dichromate (*see* Chromium and chromium compounds) | |
| Sodium diethyldithiocarbamate | *12*, 217 (1976); *Suppl. 7*, 71 (1987) |
| Sodium equilin sulfate (*see* Conjugated oestrogens) | |
| Sodium fluoride (*see* Fluorides) | |
| Sodium monofluorophosphate (*see* Fluorides) | |
| Sodium oestrone sulfate (*see* Conjugated oestrogens) | |
| Sodium *ortho*-phenylphenate (*see also ortho*-Phenylphenol) | *30*, 329 (1983); *Suppl. 7*, 71, 392 (1987); *73*, 451 (1999) |
| Sodium saccharin (*see* Saccharin) | |
| Sodium selenate (*see* Selenium and selenium compounds) | |
| Sodium selenite (*see* Selenium and selenium compounds) | |
| Sodium silicofluoride (*see* Fluorides) | |
| Solar radiation | *55* (1992) |
| Soots | *3*, 22 (1973); *35*, 219 (1985); *Suppl. 7*, 343 (1987) |
| Special-purpose glass fibres such as E-glass and '475' glass fibres (*see* Man-made vitreous fibres) | |
| Spironolactone | *24*, 259 (1980); *Suppl. 7*, 344 (1987); *79*, 317 (2001) |
| Stannous fluoride (*see* Fluorides) | |
| Static electric fields | *80* (2002) |
| Static magnetic fields | *80* (2002) |
| Steel founding (*see* Iron and steel founding) | |
| Steel, stainless (*see* Implants, surgical) | |
| Sterigmatocystin | *1*, 175 (1972); *10*, 245 (1976); *Suppl. 7*, 72 (1987) |
| Steroidal oestrogens | *Suppl. 7*, 280 (1987) |
| Streptozotocin | *4*, 221 (1974); *17*, 337 (1978); *Suppl. 7*, 72 (1987) |
| Strobane® (*see* Terpene polychlorinates) | |
| Strong-inorganic-acid mists containing sulfuric acid (*see* Mists and vapours from sulfuric acid and other strong inorganic acids) | |
| Strontium chromate (*see* Chromium and chromium compounds) | |

| | |
|---|---|
| Styrene | *19*, 231 (1979) (*corr. 42*, 258); *Suppl. 7*, 345 (1987); *60*, 233 (1994) (*corr. 65*, 549); *82*, 437 (2002) |
| Styrene–acrylonitrile copolymers | *19*, 97 (1979); *Suppl. 7*, 72 (1987) |
| Styrene–butadiene copolymers | *19*, 252 (1979); *Suppl. 7*, 72 (1987) |
| Styrene-7,8-oxide | *11*, 201 (1976); *19*, 275 (1979); *36*, 245 (1985); *Suppl. 7*, 72 (1987); *60*, 321 (1994) |
| Succinic anhydride | *15*, 265 (1977); *Suppl. 7*, 72 (1987) |
| Sudan I | *8*, 225 (1975); *Suppl. 7*, 72 (1987) |
| Sudan II | *8*, 233 (1975); *Suppl. 7*, 72 (1987) |
| Sudan III | *8*, 241 (1975); *Suppl. 7*, 72 (1987) |
| Sudan Brown RR | *8*, 249 (1975); *Suppl. 7*, 72 (1987) |
| Sudan Red 7B | *8*, 253 (1975); *Suppl. 7*, 72 (1987) |
| Sulfadimidine (*see* Sulfamethazine) | |
| Sulfafurazole | *24*, 275 (1980); *Suppl. 7*, 347 (1987) |
| Sulfallate | *30*, 283 (1983); *Suppl. 7*, 72 (1987) |
| Sulfamethazine and its sodium salt | *79*, 341 (2001) |
| Sulfamethoxazole | *24*, 285 (1980); *Suppl. 7*, 348 (1987); *79*, 361 (2001) |
| Sulfites (*see* Sulfur dioxide and some sulfites, bisulfites and metabisulfites) | |
| Sulfur dioxide and some sulfites, bisulfites and metabisulfites | *54*, 131 (1992) |
| Sulfur mustard (*see* Mustard gas) | |
| Sulfuric acid and other strong inorganic acids, occupational exposures to mists and vapours from | *54*, 41 (1992) |
| Sulfur trioxide | *54*, 121 (1992) |
| Sulphisoxazole (*see* Sulfafurazole) | |
| Sunset Yellow FCF | *8*, 257 (1975); *Suppl. 7*, 72 (1987) |
| Symphytine | *31*, 239 (1983); *Suppl. 7*, 72 (1987) |

## T

| | |
|---|---|
| 2,4,5-T (*see also* Chlorophenoxy herbicides; Chlorophenoxy herbicides, occupational exposures to) | *15*, 273 (1977) |
| Talc | *42*, 185 (1987); *Suppl. 7*, 349 (1987) |
| Tamoxifen | *66*, 253 (1996) |
| Tannic acid | *10*, 253 (1976) (*corr. 42*, 255); *Suppl. 7*, 72 (1987) |
| Tannins (*see* also Tannic acid) | *10*, 254 (1976); *Suppl. 7*, 72 (1987) |
| TCDD (*see* 2,3,7,8-Tetrachlorodibenzo-*para*-dioxin) | |
| TDE (*see* DDT) | |
| Tea | *51*, 207 (1991) |
| Temazepam | *66*, 161 (1996) |
| Teniposide | *76*, 259 (2000) |
| Terpene polychlorinates | *5*, 219 (1974); *Suppl. 7*, 72 (1987) |
| Testosterone (*see also* Androgenic (anabolic) steroids) | *6*, 209 (1974); *21*, 519 (1979) |
| Testosterone oenanthate (*see* Testosterone) | |
| Testosterone propionate (*see* Testosterone) | |
| 2,2′,5,5′-Tetrachlorobenzidine | *27*, 141 (1982); *Suppl. 7*, 72 (1987) |

| | |
|---|---|
| 2,3,7,8-Tetrachlorodibenzo-*para*-dioxin | *15*, 41 (1977); *Suppl. 7*, 350 (1987); *69*, 33 (1997) |
| 1,1,1,2-Tetrachloroethane | *41*, 87 (1986); *Suppl. 7*, 72 (1987); *71*, 1133 (1999) |
| 1,1,2,2-Tetrachloroethane | *20*, 477 (1979); *Suppl. 7*, 354 (1987); *71*, 817 (1999) |
| Tetrachloroethylene | *20*, 491 (1979); *Suppl. 7*, 355 (1987); *63*, 159 (1995) (*corr. 65*, 549) |
| 2,3,4,6-Tetrachlorophenol (*see* Chlorophenols; Chlorophenols, occupational exposures to; Polychlorophenols and their sodium salts) | |
| Tetrachlorvinphos | *30*, 197 (1983); *Suppl. 7*, 72 (1987) |
| Tetraethyllead (*see* Lead and lead compounds) | |
| Tetrafluoroethylene | *19*, 285 (1979); *Suppl. 7*, 72 (1987); *71*, 1143 (1999) |
| Tetrakis(hydroxymethyl)phosphonium salts | *48*, 95 (1990); *71*, 1529 (1999) |
| Tetramethyllead (*see* Lead and lead compounds) | |
| Tetranitromethane | *65*, 437 (1996) |
| Textile manufacturing industry, exposures in | *48*, 215 (1990) (*corr. 51*, 483) |
| Theobromine | *51*, 421 (1991) |
| Theophylline | *51*, 391 (1991) |
| Thioacetamide | *7*, 77 (1974); *Suppl. 7*, 72 (1987) |
| 4,4'-Thiodianiline | *16*, 343 (1978); *27*, 147 (1982); *Suppl. 7*, 72 (1987) |
| Thiotepa | *9*, 85 (1975); *Suppl. 7*, 368 (1987); *50*, 123 (1990) |
| Thiouracil | *7*, 85 (1974); *Suppl. 7*, 72 (1987); *79*, 127 (2001) |
| Thiourea | *7*, 95 (1974); *Suppl. 7*, 72 (1987); *79*, 703 (2001) |
| Thiram | *12*, 225 (1976); *Suppl. 7*, 72 (1987); *53*, 403 (1991) |
| Titanium (*see* Implants, surgical) | |
| Titanium dioxide | *47*, 307 (1989) |
| Tobacco habits other than smoking (*see* Tobacco products, smokeless) | |
| Tobacco products, smokeless | *37* (1985) (*corr. 42*, 263; *52*, 513); *Suppl. 7*, 357 (1987) |
| Tobacco smoke | *38* (1986) (*corr. 42*, 263); *Suppl. 7*, 359 (1987); *83*, 51 (2004) |
| Tobacco smoking (*see* Tobacco smoke) | |
| *ortho*-Tolidine (*see* 3,3'-Dimethylbenzidine) | |
| 2,4-Toluene diisocyanate (*see also* Toluene diisocyanates) | *19*, 303 (1979); *39*, 287 (1986) |
| 2,6-Toluene diisocyanate (*see also* Toluene diisocyanates) | *19*, 303 (1979); *39*, 289 (1986) |
| Toluene | *47*, 79 (1989); *71*, 829 (1999) |
| Toluene diisocyanates | *39*, 287 (1986) (*corr. 42*, 264); *Suppl. 7*, 72 (1987); *71*, 865 (1999) |
| Toluenes, α-chlorinated (*see* α-Chlorinated toluenes and benzoyl chloride) | |
| *ortho*-Toluenesulfonamide (*see* Saccharin) | |
| *ortho*-Toluidine | *16*, 349 (1978); *27*, 155 (1982) (*corr. 68*, 477); *Suppl. 7*, 362 (1987); *77*, 267 (2000) |
| Toremifene | *66*, 367 (1996) |
| Toxaphene | *20*, 327 (1979); *Suppl. 7*, 72 (1987); *79*, 569 (2001) |

T-2 Toxin (*see* Toxins derived from *Fusarium sporotrichioides*)
Toxins derived from *Fusarium graminearum*, *F. culmorum* and *F. crookwellense* — *11*, 169 (1976); *31*, 153, 279 (1983); *Suppl. 7*, 64, 74 (1987); *56*, 397 (1993)
Toxins derived from *Fusarium moniliforme* — *56*, 445 (1993)
Toxins derived from *Fusarium sporotrichioides* — *31*, 265 (1983); *Suppl. 7*, 73 (1987); *56*, 467 (1993)
Traditional herbal medicines — *82*, 41 (2002)
Tremolite (*see* Asbestos)
Treosulfan — *26*, 341 (1981); *Suppl. 7*, 363 (1987)

Triaziquone (*see* Tris(aziridinyl)-*para*-benzoquinone)
Trichlorfon — *30*, 207 (1983); *Suppl. 7*, 73 (1987)
Trichlormethine — *9*, 229 (1975); *Suppl. 7*, 73 (1987); *50*, 143 (1990)
Trichloroacetic acid — *63*, 291 (1995) (*corr. 65*, 549); *84* (2004)
Trichloroacetonitrile (*see also* Halogenated acetonitriles) — *71*, 1533 (1999)
1,1,1-Trichloroethane — *20*, 515 (1979); *Suppl. 7*, 73 (1987); *71*, 881 (1999)
1,1,2-Trichloroethane — *20*, 533 (1979); *Suppl. 7*, 73 (1987); *52*, 337 (1991); *71*, 1153 (1999)
Trichloroethylene — *11*, 263 (1976); *20*, 545 (1979); *Suppl. 7*, 364 (1987); *63*, 75 (1995) (*corr. 65*, 549)
2,4,5-Trichlorophenol (*see also* Chlorophenols; Chlorophenols, occupational exposures to; Polychlorophenols and their sodium salts) — *20*, 349 (1979)
2,4,6-Trichlorophenol (*see also* Chlorophenols; Chlorophenols, occupational exposures to; Polychlorophenols and their sodium salts) — *20*, 349 (1979)
(2,4,5-Trichlorophenoxy)acetic acid (*see* 2,4,5-T)
1,2,3-Trichloropropane — *63*, 223 (1995)
Trichlorotriethylamine-hydrochloride (*see* Trichlormethine)
$T_2$-Trichothecene (*see* Toxins derived from *Fusarium sporotrichioides*)
Tridymite (*see* Crystalline silica)
Triethanolamine — *77*, 381 (2000)
Triethylene glycol diglycidyl ether — *11*, 209 (1976); *Suppl. 7*, 73 (1987); *71*, 1539 (1999)
Trifluralin — *53*, 515 (1991)
4,4′,6-Trimethylangelicin plus ultraviolet radiation (*see also* Angelicin and some synthetic derivatives) — *Suppl. 7*, 57 (1987)
2,4,5-Trimethylaniline — *27*, 177 (1982); *Suppl. 7*, 73 (1987)
2,4,6-Trimethylaniline — *27*, 178 (1982); *Suppl. 7*, 73 (1987)
4,5′,8-Trimethylpsoralen — *40*, 357 (1986); *Suppl. 7*, 366 (1987)
Trimustine hydrochloride (*see* Trichlormethine)
2,4,6-Trinitrotoluene — *65*, 449 (1996)
Triphenylene — *32*, 447 (1983); *Suppl. 7*, 73 (1987)
Tris(aziridinyl)-*para*-benzoquinone — *9*, 67 (1975); *Suppl. 7*, 367 (1987)
Tris(1-aziridinyl)phosphine-oxide — *9*, 75 (1975); *Suppl. 7*, 73 (1987)
Tris(1-aziridinyl)phosphine-sulphide (*see* Thiotepa)
2,4,6-Tris(1-aziridinyl)-*s*-triazine — *9*, 95 (1975); *Suppl. 7*, 73 (1987)
Tris(2-chloroethyl) phosphate — *48*, 109 (1990); *71*, 1543 (1999)

| | |
|---|---|
| 1,2,3-Tris(chloromethoxy)propane | *15*, 301 (1977); *Suppl. 7*, 73 (1987); *71*, 1549 (1999) |
| Tris(2,3-dibromopropyl) phosphate | *20*, 575 (1979); *Suppl. 7*, 369 (1987); *71*, 905 (1999) |
| Tris(2-methyl-1-aziridinyl)phosphine-oxide | *9*, 107 (1975); *Suppl. 7*, 73 (1987) |
| Trp-P-1 | *31*, 247 (1983); *Suppl. 7*, 73 (1987) |
| Trp-P-2 | *31*, 255 (1983); *Suppl. 7*, 73 (1987) |
| Trypan blue | *8*, 267 (1975); *Suppl. 7*, 73 (1987) |
| *Tussilago farfara* L. (*see also* Pyrrolizidine alkaloids) | *10*, 334 (1976) |

## U

| | |
|---|---|
| Ultraviolet radiation | *40*, 379 (1986); *55* (1992) |
| Underground haematite mining with exposure to radon | *1*, 29 (1972); *Suppl. 7*, 216 (1987) |
| Uracil mustard | *9*, 235 (1975); *Suppl. 7*, 370 (1987) |
| Uranium, depleted (*see* Implants, surgical) | |
| Urethane | *7*, 111 (1974); *Suppl. 7*, 73 (1987) |

## V

| | |
|---|---|
| Vat Yellow 4 | *48*, 161 (1990) |
| Vinblastine sulfate | *26*, 349 (1981) (*corr. 42*, 261); *Suppl. 7*, 371 (1987) |
| Vincristine sulfate | *26*, 365 (1981); *Suppl. 7*, 372 (1987) |
| Vinyl acetate | *19*, 341 (1979); *39*, 113 (1986); *Suppl. 7*, 73 (1987); *63*, 443 (1995) |
| Vinyl bromide | *19*, 367 (1979); *39*, 133 (1986); *Suppl. 7*, 73 (1987); *71*, 923 (1999) |
| Vinyl chloride | *7*, 291 (1974); *19*, 377 (1979) (*corr. 42*, 258); *Suppl. 7*, 373 (1987) |
| Vinyl chloride-vinyl acetate copolymers | *7*, 311 (1976); *19*, 412 (1979) (*corr. 42*, 258); *Suppl. 7*, 73 (1987) |
| 4-Vinylcyclohexene | *11*, 277 (1976); *39*, 181 (1986) *Suppl. 7*, 73 (1987); *60*, 347 (1994) |
| 4-Vinylcyclohexene diepoxide | *11*, 141 (1976); *Suppl. 7*, 63 (1987); *60*, 361 (1994) |
| Vinyl fluoride | *39*, 147 (1986); *Suppl. 7*, 73 (1987); *63*, 467 (1995) |
| Vinylidene chloride | *19*, 439 (1979); *39*, 195 (1986); *Suppl. 7*, 376 (1987); *71*, 1163 (1999) |
| Vinylidene chloride-vinyl chloride copolymers | *19*, 448 (1979) (*corr. 42*, 258); *Suppl. 7*, 73 (1987) |
| Vinylidene fluoride | *39*, 227 (1986); *Suppl. 7*, 73 (1987); *71*, 1551 (1999) |
| *N*-Vinyl-2-pyrrolidone | *19*, 461 (1979); *Suppl. 7*, 73 (1987); *71*, 1181 (1999) |
| Vinyl toluene | *60*, 373 (1994) |
| Vitamin K substances | *76*, 417 (2000) |

## W

| | |
|---|---|
| Welding | 49, 447 (1990) (corr. 52, 513) |
| Wollastonite | 42, 145 (1987); Suppl. 7, 377 (1987); 68, 283 (1997) |
| Wood dust | 62, 35 (1995) |
| Wood industries | 25 (1981); Suppl. 7, 378 (1987) |

## X

| | |
|---|---|
| X-radiation | 75, 121 (2000) |
| Xylenes | 47, 125 (1989); 71, 1189 (1999) |
| 2,4-Xylidine | 16, 367 (1978); Suppl. 7, 74 (1987) |
| 2,5-Xylidine | 16, 377 (1978); Suppl. 7, 74 (1987) |
| 2,6-Xylidine (see 2,6-Dimethylaniline) | |

## Y

| | |
|---|---|
| Yellow AB | 8, 279 (1975); Suppl. 7, 74 (1987) |
| Yellow OB | 8, 287 (1975); Suppl. 7, 74 (1987) |

## Z

| | |
|---|---|
| Zalcitabine | 76, 129 (2000) |
| Zearalenone (see Toxins derived from *Fusarium graminearum, F. culmorum* and *F. crookwellense*) | |
| Zectran | 12, 237 (1976); Suppl. 7, 74 (1987) |
| Zeolites other than erionite | 68, 307 (1997) |
| Zidovudine | 76, 73 (2000) |
| Zinc beryllium silicate (see Beryllium and beryllium compounds) | |
| Zinc chromate (see Chromium and chromium compounds) | |
| Zinc chromate hydroxide (see Chromium and chromium compounds) | |
| Zinc potassium chromate (see Chromium and chromium compounds) | |
| Zinc yellow (see Chromium and chromium compounds) | |
| Zineb | 12, 245 (1976); Suppl. 7, 74 (1987) |
| Ziram | 12, 259 (1976); Suppl. 7, 74 (1987); 53, 423 (1991) |

# List of IARC Monographs on the Evaluation of Carcinogenic Risks to Humans*

**Volume 1**
**Some Inorganic Substances, Chlorinated Hydrocarbons, Aromatic Amines, *N*-Nitroso Compounds, and Natural Products**
*1972; 184 pages (out-of-print)*

**Volume 2**
**Some Inorganic and Organometallic Compounds**
*1973; 181 pages (out-of-print)*

**Volume 3**
**Certain Polycyclic Aromatic Hydrocarbons and Heterocyclic Compounds**
*1973; 271 pages (out-of-print)*

**Volume 4**
**Some Aromatic Amines, Hydrazine and Related Substances, *N*-Nitroso Compounds and Miscellaneous Alkylating Agents**
*1974; 286 pages (out-of-print)*

**Volume 5**
**Some Organochlorine Pesticides**
*1974; 241 pages (out-of-print)*

**Volume 6**
**Sex Hormones**
*1974; 243 pages (out-of-print)*

**Volume 7**
**Some Anti-Thyroid and Related Substances, Nitrofurans and Industrial Chemicals**
*1974; 326 pages (out-of-print)*

**Volume 8**
**Some Aromatic Azo Compounds**
*1975; 357 pages (out-of-print)*

**Volume 9**
**Some Aziridines, *N*-, *S*- and *O*-Mustards and Selenium**
*1975; 268 pages (out-of-print)*

**Volume 10**
**Some Naturally Occurring Substances**
*1976; 353 pages (out-of-print)*

**Volume 11**
**Cadmium, Nickel, Some Epoxides, Miscellaneous Industrial Chemicals and General Considerations on Volatile Anaesthetics**
*1976; 306 pages (out-of-print)*

**Volume 12**
**Some Carbamates, Thiocarbamates and Carbazides**
*1976; 282 pages (out-of-print)*

**Volume 13**
**Some Miscellaneous Pharmaceutical Substances**
*1977; 255 pages*

**Volume 14**
**Asbestos**
*1977; 106 pages (out-of-print)*

**Volume 15**
**Some Fumigants, the Herbicides 2,4-D and 2,4,5-T, Chlorinated Dibenzodioxins and Miscellaneous Industrial Chemicals**
*1977; 354 pages (out-of-print)*

**Volume 16**
**Some Aromatic Amines and Related Nitro Compounds—Hair Dyes, Colouring Agents and Miscellaneous Industrial Chemicals**
*1978; 400 pages*

**Volume 17**
**Some *N*-Nitroso Compounds**
*1978; 365 pages*

**Volume 18**
**Polychlorinated Biphenyls and Polybrominated Biphenyls**
*1978; 140 pages (out-of-print)*

**Volume 19**
**Some Monomers, Plastics and Synthetic Elastomers, and Acrolein**
*1979; 513 pages (out-of-print)*

**Volume 20**
**Some Halogenated Hydrocarbons**
*1979; 609 pages (out-of-print)*

**Volume 21**
**Sex Hormones (II)**
*1979; 583 pages*

**Volume 22**
**Some Non-Nutritive Sweetening Agents**
*1980; 208 pages*

**Volume 23**
**Some Metals and Metallic Compounds**
*1980; 438 pages (out-of-print)*

**Volume 24**
**Some Pharmaceutical Drugs**
*1980; 337 pages*

**Volume 25**
**Wood, Leather and Some Associated Industries**
*1981; 412 pages*

**Volume 26**
**Some Antineoplastic and Immunosuppressive Agents**
*1981; 411 pages (out-of-print)*

**Volume 27**
**Some Aromatic Amines, Anthraquinones and Nitroso Compounds, and Inorganic Fluorides Used in Drinking-water and Dental Preparations**
*1982; 341 pages (out-of-print)*

**Volume 28**
**The Rubber Industry**
*1982; 486 pages (out-of-print)*

**Volume 29**
**Some Industrial Chemicals and Dyestuffs**
*1982; 416 pages (out-of-print)*

**Volume 30**
**Miscellaneous Pesticides**
*1983; 424 pages (out-of-print)*

---

*Certain older volumes, marked out-of-print, are still available directly from IARCPress. Further, high-quality photocopies of all out-of-print volumes may be purchased from University Microfilms International, 300 North Zeeb Road, Ann Arbor, MI 48106-1346, USA (Tel.: +1 313-761-4700, +1 800-521-0600).

**Volume 31**
**Some Food Additives, Feed Additives and Naturally Occurring Substances**
*1983; 314 pages (out-of-print)*

**Volume 32**
**Polynuclear Aromatic Compounds, Part 1: Chemical, Environmental and Experimental Data**
*1983; 477 pages (out-of-print)*

**Volume 33**
**Polynuclear Aromatic Compounds, Part 2: Carbon Blacks, Mineral Oils and Some Nitroarenes**
*1984; 245 pages (out-of-print)*

**Volume 34**
**Polynuclear Aromatic Compounds, Part 3: Industrial Exposures in Aluminium Production, Coal Gasification, Coke Production, and Iron and Steel Founding**
*1984; 219 pages (out-of-print)*

**Volume 35**
**Polynuclear Aromatic Compounds, Part 4: Bitumens, Coal-tars and Derived Products, Shale-oils and Soots**
*1985; 271 pages*

**Volume 36**
**Allyl Compounds, Aldehydes, Epoxides and Peroxides**
*1985; 369 pages*

**Volume 37**
**Tobacco Habits Other than Smoking; Betel-Quid and Areca-Nut Chewing; and Some Related Nitrosamines**
*1985; 291 pages (out-of-print)*

**Volume 38**
**Tobacco Smoking**
*1986; 421 pages*

**Volume 39**
**Some Chemicals Used in Plastics and Elastomers**
*1986; 403 pages (out-of-print)*

**Volume 40**
**Some Naturally Occurring and Synthetic Food Components, Furocoumarins and Ultraviolet Radiation**
*1986; 444 pages (out-of-print)*

**Volume 41**
**Some Halogenated Hydrocarbons and Pesticide Exposures**
*1986; 434 pages (out-of-print)*

**Volume 42**
**Silica and Some Silicates**
*1987; 289 pages*

**Volume 43**
**Man-Made Mineral Fibres and Radon**
*1988; 300 pages (out-of-print)*

**Volume 44**
**Alcohol Drinking**
*1988; 416 pages*

**Volume 45**
**Occupational Exposures in Petroleum Refining; Crude Oil and Major Petroleum Fuels**
*1989; 322 pages*

**Volume 46**
**Diesel and Gasoline Engine Exhausts and Some Nitroarenes**
*1989; 458 pages*

**Volume 47**
**Some Organic Solvents, Resin Monomers and Related Compounds, Pigments and Occupational Exposures in Paint Manufacture and Painting**
*1989; 535 pages (out-of-print)*

**Volume 48**
**Some Flame Retardants and Textile Chemicals, and Exposures in the Textile Manufacturing Industry**
*1990; 345 pages*

**Volume 49**
**Chromium, Nickel and Welding**
*1990; 677 pages*

**Volume 50**
**Pharmaceutical Drugs**
*1990; 415 pages*

**Volume 51**
**Coffee, Tea, Mate, Methylxanthines and Methylglyoxal**
*1991; 513 pages*

**Volume 52**
**Chlorinated Drinking-water; Chlorination By-products; Some Other Halogenated Compounds; Cobalt and Cobalt Compounds**
*1991; 544 pages*

**Volume 53**
**Occupational Exposures in Insecticide Application, and Some Pesticides**
*1991; 612 pages*

**Volume 54**
**Occupational Exposures to Mists and Vapours from Strong Inorganic Acids; and Other Industrial Chemicals**
*1992; 336 pages*

**Volume 55**
**Solar and Ultraviolet Radiation**
*1992; 316 pages*

**Volume 56**
**Some Naturally Occurring Substances: Food Items and Constituents, Heterocyclic Aromatic Amines and Mycotoxins**
*1993; 599 pages*

**Volume 57**
**Occupational Exposures of Hairdressers and Barbers and Personal Use of Hair Colourants; Some Hair Dyes, Cosmetic Colourants, Industrial Dyestuffs and Aromatic Amines**
*1993; 428 pages*

**Volume 58**
**Beryllium, Cadmium, Mercury, and Exposures in the Glass Manufacturing Industry**
*1993; 444 pages*

**Volume 59**
**Hepatitis Viruses**
*1994; 286 pages*

**Volume 60**
**Some Industrial Chemicals**
*1994; 560 pages*

Volume 61
Schistosomes, Liver Flukes and *Helicobacter pylori*
1994; 270 pages

Volume 62
Wood Dust and Formaldehyde
1995; 405 pages

Volume 63
Dry Cleaning, Some Chlorinated Solvents and Other Industrial Chemicals
1995; 551 pages

Volume 64
Human Papillomaviruses
1995; 409 pages

Volume 65
Printing Processes and Printing Inks, Carbon Black and Some Nitro Compounds
1996; 578 pages

Volume 66
Some Pharmaceutical Drugs
1996; 514 pages

Volume 67
Human Immunodeficiency Viruses and Human T-Cell Lymphotropic Viruses
1996; 424 pages

Volume 68
Silica, Some Silicates, Coal Dust and *para*-Aramid Fibrils
1997; 506 pages

Volume 69
Polychlorinated Dibenzo-*para*-Dioxins and Polychlorinated Dibenzofurans
1997; 666 pages

Volume 70
Epstein-Barr Virus and Kaposi's Sarcoma Herpesvirus/Human Herpesvirus 8
1997; 524 pages

Volume 71
Re-evaluation of Some Organic Chemicals, Hydrazine and Hydrogen Peroxide
1999; 1586 pages

Volume 72
Hormonal Contraception and Post-menopausal Hormonal Therapy
1999; 660 pages

Volume 73
Some Chemicals that Cause Tumours of the Kidney or Urinary Bladder in Rodents and Some Other Substances
1999; 674 pages

Volume 74
Surgical Implants and Other Foreign Bodies
1999; 409 pages

Volume 75
Ionizing Radiation, Part 1, X-Radiation and γ-Radiation, and Neutrons
2000; 492 pages

Volume 76
Some Antiviral and Antineoplastic Drugs, and Other Pharmaceutical Agents
2000; 522 pages

Volume 77
Some Industrial Chemicals
2000; 563 pages

Volume 78
Ionizing Radiation, Part 2, Some Internally Deposited Radionuclides
2001; 595 pages

Volume 79
Some Thyrotropic Agents
2001; 763 pages

Volume 80
Non-Ionizing Radiation, Part 1: Static and Extremely Low-Frequency (ELF) Electric and Magnetic Fields
2002; 429 pages

Volume 81
Man-made Vitreous Fibres
2002; 418 pages

Volume 82
Some Traditional Herbal Medicines, Some Mycotoxins, Naphthalene and Styrene
2002; 590 pages

Volume 83
Tobacco Smoke and Involuntary Smoking
2004; 1452 pages

Volume 84
Some Drinking-Water Disinfectants and Contaminants, including Arsenic
2004

Volume 85
Betel-quid and Areca-nut Chewing and Some Areca-nut-derived Nitrosamines
2004; 334 pages

Supplement No. 1
Chemicals and Industrial Processes Associated with Cancer in Humans (*IARC Monographs*, Volumes 1 to 20)
1979; 71 pages (out-of-print)

Supplement No. 2
Long-term and Short-term Screening Assays for Carcinogens: A Critical Appraisal
1980; 426 pages (out-of-print)
(updated as IARC Scientific Publications No. 83, 1986)

Supplement No. 3
Cross Index of Synonyms and Trade Names in Volumes 1 to 26 of the *IARC Monographs*
1982; 199 pages (out-of-print)

Supplement No. 4
Chemicals, Industrial Processes and Industries Associated with Cancer in Humans (*IARC Monographs*, Volumes 1 to 29)
1982; 292 pages (out-of-print)

Supplement No. 5
Cross Index of Synonyms and Trade Names in Volumes 1 to 36 of the *IARC Monographs*
1985; 259 pages (out-of-print)

Supplement No. 6
Genetic and Related Effects: An Updating of Selected *IARC Monographs* from Volumes 1 to 42
1987; 729 pages (out-of-print)

Supplement No. 7
**Overall Evaluations of Carcinogenicity: An Updating of** *IARC Monographs* **Volumes 1–42**
*1987; 440 pages (out-of-print)*

Supplement No. 8
**Cross Index of Synonyms and Trade Names in Volumes 1 to 46 of the** *IARC Monographs*
*1990; 346 pages (out-of-print)*

All IARC publications are available directly from
IARCPress, 150 Cours Albert Thomas, 69372 Lyon cedex 08, France
(Fax: +33 4 72 73 83 02; E-mail: press@iarc.fr).

IARC Monographs and Technical Reports are also available from the
World Health Organization Marketing and Dissemination, 1211 Geneva 27, Switzerland
(Fax: +41 22 791 4857; E-mail: publications@who.int)
and from WHO Sales Agents worldwide.

IARC Scientific Publications, IARC Handbooks and IARC CancerBases are also available from
Oxford University Press, Walton Street, Oxford, UK OX2 6DP (Fax: +44 1865 267782).

IARC Monographs are also available in an electronic edition,
both on-line by internet and on CD-ROM, from GMA Industries, Inc.,
20 Ridgely Avenue, Suite 301, Annapolis, Maryland, USA
(Fax: +01 410 267 6602; internet: https//www.gmai.com/Order_Form.htm)

Achevé d'imprimer par l'Imprimerie Darantiere à Dijon-Quetigny en octobre 2004
Dépôt légal : octobre 2004 - N° d'impression : 24-1009

*Imprimé en France*

www.ingramcontent.com/pod-product-compliance
Lightning Source LLC
Chambersburg PA
CBHW081154020426
42333CB00020B/2496